EX LIBRIS

READER'S DIGEST

OUR
HUMAN
BODY

Its Wonders and Its Care

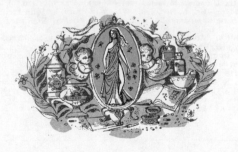

A LIBRARY OF FACT AND GUIDANCE

THE READER'S DIGEST ASSOCIATION

Pleasantville, N. Y.

Acknowledgments

The condensations reprinted in this book are used by permission of, and special arrangement with, the publishers holding the respective copyrights.

For excerpts: page 96, G. P. Putnam's Sons; pages 162, 425, Better Homes and Gardens, Aug. 1960; Meridith Pub. Co., pages 224, 389, Lifetime Living, May 1954; page 328, Doubleday & Co. Inc.; page 376, Oxford University Press; page 388, Simon and Schuster, Inc.; page 425, Dodd, Mead and Co.

THE LONG SEARCH, from the book, *The Human Body*, by Logan Clendening. © 1927, Alfred A. Knopf, Inc., N.Y., N.Y. MAN, THE UNKNOWN, from *Man, the Unknown*, by Alexis Carrel, Reader's Digest, Sept. '36. © 1935, Harper & Bros., N.Y., N.Y. SECRETS OF THE HUMAN CELL, by J. D. Ratcliff, Reader's Digest, June '58, from *Family Doctor*, June '58. Pub. by Brit. Med. Ass'n, London, England. © 1957, The Reader's Digest Ass'n, Inc. . . . and "The Exquisite Basic Molecule of Life," by Rutherford Platt. CONCEPTION, by J. D. Ratcliff, from "How Life Begins," Reader's Digest, Mar. '57. © 1957, The Reader's Digest Ass'n, Inc. BOY OR GIRL? THE MYSTERY OF SEX, by Amram Scheinfeld, Reader's Digest, Mar. '51, cond. from the book, *The New You and Heredity*. © 1950, the J. B. Lippincott Co., Phila., Pa. BIOGRAPHY OF THE UNBORN, from "Life Before Birth," by Herbert Thoms, M.D., and Bruce Bliven, Jr., Reader's Digest, Mar. '58, cond. from *McCall's*, Feb. '58. © 1958, McCall Corp., N.Y., N.Y. . . . and "Biography of the Unborn," by Margaret Shea Gilbert, Reader's Digest, Aug. '39, cond. from the book, *Biography of the Unknown*. © 1938 and pub. by the Williams & Wilkins Co., Balt., Md. NATURE'S WAY IN BIRTH, from "Birth, the Universal Miracle," by J. D. Ratcliff, Reader's Digest, Dec. '50, cond. from *Woman's Home Companion*, May, '50. © 1950, the Crowell-Collier Pub. Co., N.Y., N.Y. . . . and "Birth: Most Dangerous Experience in Life," by J. D. Ratcliff, Reader's Digest, Sept. '52, cond. from *Today's Health*, Sept. '52. © 1952, Amer. Med. Ass'n, Chi., Ill. WHAT IS A BABY? by Herbert Thoms, M.D., and Bruce Bliven, Jr., Reader's Digest, Feb. '57, cond. from *McCall's*, Jan. '57. © 1956, McCall Corp., N.Y., N.Y. OUR MIRACULOUS SYSTEM OF DEFENSES, from "The Wisdom of the Body," by Dr. Richard C. Cabot and Rev. Russell Dicks, Reader's Digest, Feb. '47, cond. from *The Art of Ministering to the Sick.* © 1936, the Macmillan Co., N.Y., N.Y. CLIMATE CONTROL — FROM WITHIN, from "Why Many are Cold but Few are Frozen," by Ruth and Edward Brecher, Reader's Digest, Dec. '56, cond. from *Today's Health*, Dec. '56. © 1956, Amer. Med. Ass'n, Chi., Ill. PAIN: FIRST SIGNAL OF DANGER, from "The Why of Aches and Pains," by Ruth and Edward Brecher, Reader's Digest, Apr. '55, cond. from *Farm Journal*, Apr. '55. © 1955, Farm Journal, Inc., Phila., Pa. WHEN YOU HAVE A FEVER, from "What It Means When You Have a Fever," by J. D. Ratcliff, Reader's Digest, Dec. '59, cond. from *The Atlantic Advocate*, Nov. '59. Pub. by University Press of New Brunswick, Ltd., Fredericton, N.B., Canada. © 1959, The Reader's Digest Ass'n, Inc. REPELLING THE UNSEEN INVADERS, from "Why Your Body Stays Well," by Ruth and Edward Brecher, Reader's Digest, Nov. '57, cond. from *Today's Health*, Nov. '57. © 1957, Amer. Med. Ass'n, Chi., Ill. . . . and "The Wonders of a Healing Wound," by J. D. Ratcliff, Reader's Digest, Sept. '59. © 1959, The Reader's Digest Ass'n, Inc. INTRODUCING THE BRAIN, abridgment of Chap. I of *The Human Brain*, by John Pfeiffer. © 1955, John Edward Pfeiffer. Reprinted by permission of Harper & Bros., N.Y., N.Y. THE MEMORY— REMARKABLE STORAGE BATTERY, from "Wondrous Storage Battery—the Brain," by Bruce Bliven, Reader's Digest, July '54, cond. from *Popular Science Monthly*, Apr. '53. © 1953, Popular Science Pub. Co., Inc., N.Y., N.Y. YOUR BRAIN'S UNREALIZED POWERS, by Bruce Bliven, Reader's Digest, Oct. '56. © 1956, The Reader's Digest Ass'n, Inc. WHY STROKES OCCUR, by Irvine H. Page, Reader's

Digest, Mar. '58, cond. from *Life*, Dec. 9, '57. © 1957, Time, Inc., N.Y., N.Y. . . . and "What You Should Know about Strokes," by Tom Mahoney, Reader's Digest, Mar. '54. © 1954, The Reader's Digest Ass'n, Inc. THE HEART — WONDROUS, COURAGEOUS ORGAN, from "The Heart, Wondrous & Courageous Organ," by Henry Morton Robinson, Reader's Digest, Feb. '48 and Feb. '60. © 1948, The Reader's Digest Ass'n, Inc. STEADY PACE OR HEARTBREAK? from "The World's Most Efficient Pump," by G. A. Skinner, Reader's Digest, Feb. '34, cond. from *Scientific American*, June '33. © 1933, Scientific American, Inc. . . . and "Stop Breaking Your Heart," by Howard Whitman, Reader's Digest, Aug. '59. © 1959, The Reader's Digest Ass'n, Inc. THE WHY AND HOW OF HEART ATTACKS, from "Stop Breaking Your Heart," by Howard Whitman, Reader's Digest, Aug. '59. © 1959, The Reader's Digest Ass'n, Inc. . . . and "Candidates for Heart Attack," by George Dock, Jr., Reader's Digest, Nov. '46, cond. from *Harper's Magazine*, Aug. '46. © 1946, Harper & Bros., N.Y., N.Y. HOW TO LIVE AFTER AN ATTACK, from "Your Heart's In Your Hands," by Peter F. Steincrohn, Reader's Digest, May '44, cond. from *Today's Health*, May '44. © 1944, Amer. Med. Ass'n, Chi., Ill. MAGIC IN BREATHING, from "Do You Really Know How to Breathe?" by W. P. Knowles, Reader's Digest, Mar. '59, cond. from *Today's Living*, Feb. 15, '59. © 1959, New York Herald Tribune, Inc., N.Y., N.Y. . . . and "Breathe Easier" by W. P. Knowles, Reader's Digest, Aug. '54, cond. from *The American Mercury*, Aug. '54. © 1954, American Mercury, Inc., N.Y., N.Y. OUR LUNGS — THOSE WONDERFUL WINDBAGS, by J. D. Ratcliff, Reader's Digest, Jan. '60, cond. from *Liberty*, Jan. '60, pub. by Liberty of Canada, Ltd., Toronto, Ont. © 1959, The Reader's Digest Ass'n, Inc. HOW HARMFUL IS SMOKING? from "How Harmful are Cigarettes?" by Roger William Riis, Reader's Digest, Jan. '50. © 1949, The Reader's Digest Ass'n, Inc. . . . and "Lung Cancer and Cigarettes—the Latest Findings," by Lois Mattox Miller, Reader's Digest, June, '62. © 1962, The Reader's Digest Ass'n, Inc. WHAT YOUR SKIN DOES FOR YOU, by Ruth and Edward Brecher, Reader's Digest, Aug. '56, cond. from *Journal of Lifetime Living*, Aug. '56. © 1956, Lifetime Living, Inc., Miami Beach, Fla. THE EVOLUTION OF EYES, by Thomas Hall Shastid, Reader's Digest, Dec. '33, reprinted from *The American Scholar*, Autumn, '33. © 1933, the United Chapters of Phi Beta Kappa. THE MYSTERIOUS POWER OF HUMAN SIGHT, by Sir Charles Sherrington, Reader's Digest, Sept. '52, cond. from *Man On His Nature*. © 1940, Cambridge University Press, N.Y., N.Y. . . . and "You Can Learn to See More," by Wolfgang Langewiesche, Reader's Digest, June '57. © 1957, The Reader's Digest Ass'n, Inc. THE EAR—A WONDERFUL MACHINE, from "They Can Hear Again," by Robert O'Brien, Reader's Digest, Feb. '62, cond. from *Today's*

Health, Dec. '61. © 1961, the Amer. Med. Ass'n, Chi., Ill. YOUR EDUCATED NOSE, from "Have You an Educated Nose?" by Roy Bedichek, Reader's Digest, Mar. '60, cond. from *The Sense of Smell*. © 1960, Doubleday & Co., N.Y., N.Y. . . . and "How Your Nose Knows," by Ruth and Edward Brecher, Reader's Digest, Mar. '56, cond. from *Science News Letter*, Feb. 18, '56. © 1956, Science Service, Inc., Wash., D.C. ALL ABOUT YOUR THROAT, by Evan Wylie, Reader's Digest, Nov. '58, cond. from *McCall's*, Mar. '58. © 1958, McCall Corp., N.Y., N.Y. THE MYTH OF THE "TERRIBLE TONSILS," by Lois Mattox Miller, Reader's Digest, May '51, cond. from *Today's Health*, May '51. © 1951, Amer. Med. Ass'n, Chi., Ill. HOW YOUR NERVOUS SYSTEM WORKS, by J. D. Ratcliff, Reader's Digest, May '56, cond. from *Today's Health*, May '56. © 1956, Amer. Med. Ass'n, Chi., Ill. THE MIRACLE OF MUSCLE, by J. D. Ratcliff, Reader's Digest, Jan. '56, cond. from *Today's Health*, Jan. '56. © 1955, Amer. Med. Ass'n, Chi., Ill. MUSCULAR ACHES AND PAINS, from "Why We Have Aches and Pains," Janet Travell, M.D., Reader's Digest, May 61, cond. from *U.S. News and World Report*, Feb. 20, '61. © 1961, U.S. News Pub. Corp., Wash., D.C. OUR BUSY BONES, by J. D. Ratcliff, Reader's Digest, Nov. '55, cond. from *Today's Health*, Nov. '55. © 1955, Amer. Med. Ass'n, Chi., Ill. . . . and "Our Living Bones," by Elsie McCormick, Reader's Digest, June '48, cond. from *Today's Health*, May '48. © 1948, Amer. Med. Ass'n, Chi., Ill. . . . and "The Skeleton Speaks," by Wilton Krogman, Reader's Digest, Aug. '38, *Scientific American*, Aug. '38. © 1938, Scientific American, Inc., N.Y., N.Y. THE HUMAN HAND: OUR GREATEST TOOL, from "The Marvels of the Human Hand," by Evan Wylie, Reader's Digest, July '62, cond. from *Today's Health*, July '62. © 1962, Amer. Med. Ass'n, Chi., Ill. WHAT YOU SHOULD KNOW ABOUT YOUR BACK, by C. Lester Walker, Reader's Digest, July '51. © 1951, The Reader's Digest Ass'n, Inc. LADIES AND GENTLEMEN, BE SEATED—PROPERLY, by Janet Travell, M.D., Reader's Digest, Aug. '61, cond. from *House Beautiful*, Oct. '55. © 1955, Hearst Corp., N.Y., N.Y. TREAT YOUR STOMACH WITH RESPECT, by Richard Carter, Reader's Digest, Feb. '59, cond. from *Life*, Nov. 17, '58. © 1958, Time, Inc., N.Y., N.Y. THE WINDOW IN ST. MARTIN'S STOMACH, by Richard Match, Reader's Digest, Oct. '51, cond. from *New Liberty*, Oct. '51. © 1951, Liberty of Canada, Ltd., Montreal, P.Q. YOUR LIVER IS YOUR LIFE, by Paul de Kruif, Reader's Digest, Jan. '58. © 1957, The Reader's Digest Ass'n, Inc. YOUR GALLBLADDER: TROUBLE HOT SPOT, by J. D. Ratcliff, Reader's Digest, Apr. '60, cond. from *Family Doctor*, Apr. '60, pub. by the Brit. Med. Ass'n, London, England. © The Reader's Digest Ass'n, Inc. THE KIDNEYS, from "Your Body's Master Chemists," by J. D. Ratcliff, Reader's Digest, Nov. '60, cond. from *Today's Health*, Dec. '60. © 1960, Amer. Med. Ass'n, Chi., Ill.

WHAT URINALYSIS TELLS THE DOCTOR, by J. D. Ratcliff, Reader's Digest, July '55, cond. from *Today's Health*, July '55. © 1955, Amer. Med. Ass'n, Chi., Ill. THE PANCREAS AND DIABETES, from "A Million Unknown Diabetics," by C. Lester Walker, Reader's Digest, Nov. '58, cond. from *Today's Health*, Nov. '58. © 1958, Amer. Med. Ass'n, Chi., Ill. . . . and "A New Day for Diabetics," by Paul de Kruif, Reader's Digest, Apr. '58. © 1958, The Reader's Digest Ass'n, Inc. YOUR LONG-SUFFERING COLON, from "Treat Your Colon Kindly," by William Glafke, M.D., Reader's Digest, Oct. '49. © 1949, The Reader's Digest Ass'n, Inc. THE BLOODSTREAM: CHEMISTRY IN ACTION, from "Your Amazing Circulatory System," by J. D. Ratcliff, Reader's Digest, Jan. '57, cond. from *Today's Health*, Jan. '57. © 1956, the Amer. Med. Ass'n, Chi., Ill....and "What Your Blood Tells the Doctor," by J. D. Ratcliff, Reader's Digest, June '62, cond. from *Family Doctor*, June '62, pub. by the Brit. Med. Ass'n, London, England. © 1962, The Reader's Digest Ass'n, Inc. LYMPH, THE MYSTERIOUS FLUID, from "Pay Your Respects to Lymph," by Henry Morton Robinson, Reader's Digest, Sept. '47, cond. from *Today's Health*, Sept. '47. © 1947, Amer. Med. Ass'n, Chi., Ill. INTRODUCTION TO THE BODY'S MASTER CHEMICALS, from "The Body's Mysterious Chemicals," by Bruce Bliven, Reader's Digest, Sept. '41, cond. from *The New Republic*, Aug. 18, '41. © 1941, Editorial Publications, Inc., N.Y., N.Y. THE ENDOCRINE GLANDS: CENTERS OF CONTROL, from "Your Amazing Glands," by J. D. Ratcliff, Reader's Digest, Nov. '58, cond. from *Family Doctor*, Nov. '58, pub. by the Brit. Med. Ass'n, London, England. © 1958, The Reader's Digest Ass'n, Inc. ENZYMES: NATURE'S "CONVERTERS," from "Enzymes, Medicine's Bright Hope," by J. D. Ratcliff, Reader's Digest, June '61, cond. from *Today's Health*, Sept. '60. © 1960, Amer. Med. Ass'n, Chi., Ill. VITAMINS – KEYS TO WELL-BEING, from "How to Prolong the Prime of Life," by Paul de Kruif, Reader's Digest, June '57. © 1957, The Reader's Digest Ass'n, Inc. . . . and "Vitamins, the Food – and Dr. Spies," Paul de Kruif, Reader's Digest, Sept. '58. © 1958, The Reader's Digest Ass'n, Inc. CHILDHOOD—WONDERFUL AND ALARMING, from "What Is a Child?" by Herbert S. Benjamin, M.D., *Coronet*, Feb. '58. © 1958, Esquire, Inc., N.Y., N.Y. WHY ADOLESCENTS ACT THAT WAY, by J. D. Ratcliff, Reader's Digest, Mar. '62, cond. from *Family Doctor*, Mar. '62, pub. by the Brit. Med. Ass'n, London, England. © 1962, The Reader's Digest Ass'n, Inc. ACNE—YOUTH'S MYSTERIOUS ENEMY, by Paul de Kruif, Reader's Digest, Mar. '57, cond. from *Today's Health*, Mar. '57. © 1957, Amer. Med. Ass'n, Chi., Ill. MENSTRUATION: NEW HELP FOR NEEDLESS MISERY, from "Pre-Menstrual Tension: the Needless Misery," by Dr. Robert B. Greenblatt with Richard L. Frey, Reader's Digest, May '55, cond. from *Woman's Life*, Summer '55. ©

1955, Woman's Life Publications, Inc., N.Y., N.Y. . . . and "The Truth About Menstruation," by Maxine Davis, Reader's Digest, June '43, cond. from *Good Housekeeping*, Jan. '43. © 1943, Hearst Magazines, Inc., N.Y., N.Y. WHAT TO DO ABOUT CHANGE OF LIFE, from "The Facts about Menopause," by Ruth and Edward Brecher, Reader's Digest, July '58, cond. from *Family Circle*, Mar. '58. © 1958, Family Circle, Inc., N.Y., N.Y. . . . and "New Help for Women's Change of Life," Paul de Kruif, Reader's Digest, Jan. '48. © 1948, The Reader's Digest Ass'n, Inc. . . . and "Changing Life Sensibly," by Lois Mattox Miller, Reader's Digest, Oct. '39, cond. from *Independent Woman*, Sept. '39. © 1939, Nat'l Federation of Business and Professional Women's Clubs, Inc., Wash., D.C. PROSTATE TROUBLE, by Paul de Kruif, Reader's Digest, Nov. '42. © 1942, The Reader's Digest Ass'n, Inc. SEX LIFE AFTER MIDDLE AGE, by Margaret Culkin Banning, Reader's Digest, Sept. '52. © 1952, The Reader's Digest Ass'n, Inc. CAN SCIENCE PROLONG OUR USEFUL YEARS? by Albert Q. Maisel, Reader's Digest, Jan. '62. © 1961, The Reader's Digest Ass'n, Inc. HOW TO KEEP YOUNG MENTALLY, by Mary B. Mullett, Reader's Digest, Feb. '62, reprinted from Feb. '22. © 1922, The Reader's Digest Ass'n, Inc. THE SECRET STRENGTH OF WOMEN, by Caroline Bird, Reader's Digest, Nov. '60, cond. from *Good Housekeeping*, Oct. '59. © 1959, the Hearst Corp., N.Y., N.Y. WHAT DOCTORS CAN DO TO PROMOTE FERTILITY, by Grace Naismith, Reader's Digest, May '62, cond. from *Today's Health*, Jan. '62. © 1961, Amer. Med. Ass'n, Chi., Ill. NUTRITION AND PREGNANCY, by Bruce Bliven, Reader's Digest, Jan. '48, cond. from the *Ladies' Home Journal*, Nov. '47. © 1947, the Curtis Pub. Co., Phila., Pa. THE RH FACTOR IN PREGNANCY, from "The Rh Factor in Blood," by J. D. Ratcliff, Reader's Digest, Oct. '45, cond. from *Woman's Home Companion*, Sept. '45. © 1945, Crowell-Collier Pub. Co., N.Y., N.Y. THE BREAST—ITS MYSTERIES, by J. D. Ratcliff, Reader's Digest, Oct. '61, from *Family Doctor*, Oct. '61, pub. by the Brit. Med. Ass'n, London, England. © 1961, The Reader's Digest Ass'n, Inc. BOSOM WORSHIP, from "This Bosom Business," by Goodrich C. Schauffler, M.D., Reader's Digest, Aug. '55. © 1955, The Reader's Digest Ass'n, Inc. BREAST-FED IS BEST FED, by Eleanor Lake, Reader's Digest, June '50. © 1950, The Reader's Digest Ass'n, Inc. CHILDBIRTH WITHOUT FEAR, by Grantly Dick Read, Reader's Digest, May '47, cond. from *Childbirth Without Fear*. © 1944, Grantly Dick Read, pub. by Harper & Bros., N.Y., N.Y. TRUTHS AND UNTRUTHS ABOUT MISCARRIAGE, by Edith L. Potter, M.D., Reader's Digest, Aug. '59. © 1959, The Reader's Digest Ass'n, Inc. BIRTH CONTROL, from "Where Do We Stand on the Birth-Control Pill?" by Albert Q. Maisel, Reader's Digest, Feb. '61. © 1961, The Reader's Digest Ass'n, Inc. STRESS – THE CAUSE OF ALL DISEASE? by J. D. Ratcliff, Reader's Digest, Jan. '55. © 1954, The Reader's Digest Ass'n, Inc. HOW TO DEAL WITH YOUR TENSIONS, by Dr. George S. Stevenson, Reader's Digest, Nov. '57, cond. from a booklet pub. and © by Nat'l Ass'n for Mental Health, Inc. N.Y., N.Y. HOW TO LIVE WITH YOUR NERVES, by Dr. Walter C. Alvarez, Reader's Digest, Apr. '51, cond. from booklet, *How to Live With Your Nerves*. © 1950, Wilcox & Follett Co., Chi., Ill. HOW TO STAND UP UNDER STRESS, Dr. Maxwell Maltz, Reader's Digest, June '61, cond. from *Psycho-Cybernetics*. © 1960, Prentice-Hall, Inc., Englewood Cliffs, N.J. YOUR MIND CAN KEEP YOU WELL, by Dr. John A. Schindler, Reader's Digest, Dec. '49, cond. from a talk over the University of Wisconsin Radio Station WHA. © 1949, The Reader's Digest Ass'n, Inc. THE CASE FOR CRYING, by Karl Huber, Reader's Digest, Feb. '61, cond. from *McCall's*, Nov. '60. © 1960, McCall Corp., N.Y., N.Y. IF YOU NEED A DRINK—DON'T TAKE IT! by Charles Stevenson, Reader's Digest, Oct. '47, cond. from *Nation's Business*, Aug. '47. © 1947, Chamber of Commerce of the United States, Wash., D.C. HOW TO LIVE WITHOUT FATIGUE, by Marguerite Clark, Reader's Digest, Mar. '62, cond. from *Why So Tired? The Why's of Fatigue and the Ways of Energy*. © 1962, Marguerite Clark, pub. by Duell, Sloan and Pearce, Inc., N.Y., N.Y. DESIGN FOR FATIGUE, Reader's Digest, Nov. '42, cond. from *Newsweek*, Aug. 17, '42. © 1942, Weekly Publications, Inc., N.Y., N.Y. SLEEP AND HOW TO GET MORE OF IT, by Robert Coughlan, Reader's Digest, Aug. '50, cond. from *Life*, Apr. 3, '50. © 1950, Time, Inc., N.Y., N.Y. WHAT DO YOU KNOW ABOUT SLEEP? by Gretta Palmer, Reader's Digest, June '45, cond. from *Woman's Home Companion*, Apr. '45. © 1945, Crowell-Collier Pub. Co., N.Y., N.Y. HEADACHES: WHY YOU HAVE THEM—WHAT YOU CAN DO ABOUT THEM, by Lin Root, Reader's Digest, Jan. '61, cond. from *Today's Living*, Dec. 4, '60. © 1960, The New York Herald Tribune, Inc., N.Y., N.Y. THE PESKY ALLERGIES, from "They Call It Allergy," by Lois Mattox Miller, Reader's Digest, Aug. '40. © 1940, Amer. Med. Ass'n, Chi., Ill. . . . and "Antidotes for Allergies," by Paul de Kruif, Reader's Digest, Sept. '47. © 1947, The Reader's Digest Ass'n, Inc. "ONE-SHOT" TREATMENT FOR HAY FEVER, from "What's the Truth About the 'One-Shot' Treatment for Hay Fever?" by Albert Q. Maisel, Reader's Digest, July '60, cond. from *Today's Health*, July '60. © 1960, Amer. Med. Ass'n, Chi., Ill. THE COMMON COLD, from "We Can't Cure a Cold," by Herbert A. Reimann, M.D., Reader's Digest, Nov. '47, cond. from the *Journal of the Amer. Med. Ass'n*, Nov. 2, '46. © 1946, Amer. Med. Ass'n, Chi., Ill. . . . and "Closing In On the Common Cold," by J. D. Ratcliff, Reader's Digest, Nov. '61, cond. from *Today's Health*, Oct. '61. © 1961, Amer. Med. Ass'n, Chi., Ill. THE FACTS ABOUT FOOD AND WEIGHT, from "The Facts About Your Weight," an interview with Dr. Frederick J. Stare, Reader's Digest, Apr. '55, cond. from *U.S. News & World Report*, Jan. 7, '55. © 1955, U.S. News Pub. Corp., Wash., D.C. . . . and "What Do You Know About Eating?" by Judith Chase Churchill, Reader's Digest, June '52, cond. from the *Woman's Home Companion*, Mar. '52. © 1952, Crowell-Collier Pub. Co., N.Y., N.Y. WHAT YOU SHOULD REALLY WEIGH, Reader's Digest, Feb. '60, from *U.S. News & World Report*, Nov. 2, '59. © 1959, U.S. News Pub. Corp., Wash., D.C. HOW TO REDUCE—THE QUESTION OF EATING, from "How to Reduce & Stay There," by Robert P. Goldman, Reader's Digest, Sept. '61, cond. from *Lose Weight and Live*. © 1961, Robert P. Goldman, pub. by Doubleday & Co., N.Y., N.Y. DOES EXERCISE HELP OR HINDER? from "One Sure Way to Reduce," by Blake Clark, Reader's Digest, Apr. '56. © 1956, The Reader's Digest Ass'n, Inc. WHAT DO YOU EAT FOR BREAKFAST? by Frederic Sondern, Jr., Reader's Digest, May '50, cond. from *The Christian Herald*, May '50. © 1950, Christian Herald Ass'n, Inc., N.Y., N.Y. STARVING TEEN-AGERS, by Myril Axelrod, Reader's Digest, Dec. '55. © 1955, The Reader's Digest Ass'n, Inc. THE CARE OF YOUR SKIN, from "Know Your Skin," by Elsie McCormick, Reader's Digest, Sept. '44, cond. from *Collier's*, July 1, '44. © 1944, Crowell-Collier Pub. Co. FACTS ABOUT EYE CARE, from "Facts and Non-Facts About Eye Care," by John K. Lagemann, Reader's Digest, Apr. '62, cond. from *Redbook*, May '60. © 1960, McCall Corp., N.Y., N.Y. . . . and "What You Should Know about Your Eyes," by Carle Hodge, Reader's Digest, Dec. '52, cond. from *Collier's*, Sept. 6, '52. © 1952, Crowell-Collier Pub. Co., N.Y., N.Y. WHAT YOU SHOULD KNOW ABOUT YOUR HAIR, by J. D. Ratcliff, Reader's Digest, Oct. '59, cond. from *Liberty*, Oct., '59, pub. by Liberty of Canada, Ltd., Toronto, Ont. © 1959, The Reader's Digest Ass'n, Inc. IF YOU REALLY WANT HEALTHY TEETH, by J. D. Ratcliff, Reader's Digest, Jan. '52, cond. from *The American Magazine*, Nov. '51. © 1951, Crowell-Collier Pub. Co., N.Y., N.Y. FLUORIDES: YOUR FAMILY'S PROTECTION AGAINST TOOTH DECAY, from "Your Family Can Have Healthy Teeth," by Merle E. Dowd, Reader's Digest, Jan. '62. © 1961, The Reader's Digest Ass'n, Inc. MIND YOUR OWN TWO FEET, by Lin Root, Reader's Digest, Mar. '61, cond. from *Today's Health*, Mar. '61. © 1961, Amer. Med. Ass'n, Chi., Ill. ARE AMERICANS PHYSICALLY FIT? from "Let's Close the Muscle Gap," by Max Eastman, Reader's Digest, Nov. '61. © 1961, The Reader's Digest Ass'n, Inc. DON'T JUST SIT THERE—EXERCISE! by Curtis Mitchell, Reader's Digest, July '61, cond. from *The N.Y. Times Magazine*, Apr. 23, '61. © 1961, New York Times Co., N.Y., N.Y. EVEN SIX SECONDS WILL HELP, from "Six Seconds for Exercise," by Keith Monroe, Reader's Digest, July '59. © 1959, The Reader's Digest Ass'n, Inc.

Illustrations

Contents

CHAPTER 1

Man Discovers His Body

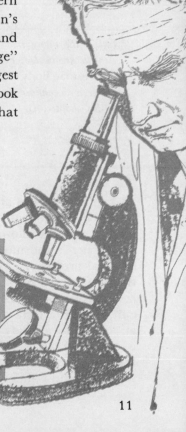

IT IS STRANGE that until the modern era, man studied the universe, yet never dared to investigate his own body. Here are condensations from two modern classics. The first tells the story of man's scientific exploration of himself, and what is known about the "average" man. The second is a Reader's Digest condensation from the most noted book in print that reveals for the layman what we know of the human body today.

11

The Long Search

A CONDENSATION FROM THE HUMAN BODY

by Logan Clendening, M.D.

Among the many innovations of the 1920s was the popularization of scientific knowledge. Perhaps the first outstanding book in physiology was The Human Body *by Dr. Logan Clendening. Highly personal, opinionated, written with confidence and vivacity, this book is as accurate as it is lively. In this chapter, Dr. Clendening reviews man's long search for knowledge of his own body.*

Man's world has always been grounded upon his body as its center; from it and its necessities he has circled out and learned what he knows about the universe. It is a true saying that "medicine is the mother of the sciences"—simply because the medical profession's primary interest was the human body, and the profession was for most of the world's history the only organized group of men using the scientific method—which is the accumulation of data without religious or political prejudice—in any field of the study of natural phenomena. There is a passage in Sinclair Lewis's *Main Street* in which Carol has been bewailing the lack of interest in literature and science in her little town, to which her husband, Will Kennicut, the country doctor, replies gravely and patiently: "Yes, I'm about all the science there is around here." That has been the position of medicine through many and long dark periods of the world's history and in many lonely and unlighted places. It was all the science that there was. But because it kept the lamp burning and because man's primary interest is his own body the other sciences were born.

Mathematics, for instance, derives its patterns from the human body. There is no reason why the numeral ten or the decimal system should be such a favorite except that we have ten fingers. When a primitive hunter saw a number of deer in the forest and conceived a perfectly natural desire to go home and tell how many there were, he counted them up on his fingers.

The stars and comets and the sun, the moon varying in its phases in the same time cycle with the issue of blood from his females—these became associated in the barbarian's thoughts with his destiny and his discomforts; he began to study them, and astronomy was born.

Plants, because they were found to be necessary as foods for his body, because he liked their taste, drew his interest. Somewhere, sometime, one of the greatest discoveries in the history of the race was made—that the plants he needed could be grown from their seeds—and botany was born.

The list of things man has learned about nature because of the necessities of his own body might be indefinitely extended.

The name of Hippocrates is familiar enough as a name. The average educated man would probably react to it by the words "the father of medicine." The average physician would be able to go little if any further.

Yet Hippocrates was one of the great human liberators. He was the first and greatest physician not because he was the only one of his day—the fifth century B.C.—not because he founded an ethical code with the Hippocratic oath, but because he first threw aside all the demonology of the priests and looked upon disease as part of the order of nature, having a natural cause and a certain course—a course which could be studied and recorded and, within certain limitations, be predicted and even altered.

Aristotle, too, was a great liberator, partly because he was interested in the human body. Not, strictly speaking, a physician, he first examined animal bodies in the scientific spirit, deducing from what he found in them speculation as to what went on in man's body (in *De Partibus Animalium*). No one, I think, has put Aristotelianism into a sentence, yet it can be done. He believed that man could master his world. Man unendowed save with his five senses, unaided by priestly advice or by divine inspiration, could find out the composition of the earth, what it contained that was useful, how human and other animal bodies worked, what were the wellsprings of joy (in the *Poetics*), how he could enter into the vastnesses of the sea (in a submarine) or launch himself into the airy firmament (in an airplane), what his enemy Disease was and how it could be combated. Such was the secret of that incredible activity of Aristotle's—studying now fishes and now politics, now ethics and now minerals. And man has justified Aristotle's conviction: man has conquered his world.

Galen, who with Aristotle shared the throne of scholastic authority in the Middle Ages, belonged to a later century and a different era. Galen lived in Rome and he wrote in Greek. His writings are so voluminous as to make the Holy Bible look like a pamphlet. He treated emperors, courtesans, wine merchants, generals, senators, vestal virgins, oriental rug dealers, philosophers and gladiators. He tells of all his patients, and of the little tricks he used to arrive at his diagnoses. Yet his knowledge of anatomy was learned entirely from dissections on animals. And for twelve hundred years the brilliance of his rhetoric prevented men from learning at first hand anything about the human body.

Finally the legions of light were drawn up and one other battle was fought in the name of the human body for human freedom. Its hero has been even more ignored than Hippocrates—the Flemish anatomist Vesalius, who first recorded completely and accurately the structure of the body. But not until 1543—when his *De Humani Corporis Fabrica* was printed. It is one of the great epoch-making books of the world.

In that long sleep of the intellect known as the Middle Ages there was no space for the study of nature, and there was determined opposition to human dissection both from the Church and the universities, from men ironically called Humanists. The influential scholars in the period of the revival of learning based their anatomy largely on the dictates of Galen, partly on Aristotle. The anatomy of Galen and Aristotle was based upon the dissection of animals. And the scholastic squabbles of the late fifteenth and early sixteenth centuries were due, incredible as it may seem, to debating whether or not the human body corresponded to Galen's description of it.

Against this massed tradition of ignorance and bigotry Vesalius launched himself with blunt vigor. The body was his bible, as he often said, and he cared not how he obtained copies. In Paris he found that he could steal bodies from Montfaucon, that spot which chatters in the pages of François Villon, where the bodies of criminals were hung upon the gibbets. In Louvain he sneaked by night to remove bodies from the gallows.

Under such difficult circumstances a knowledge of human anatomy was born into the world. Vesalius paid the penalty of his rashness. He was excommunicated; to lift the ban he went upon a penitential journey and we hear of him no more. But his work remains, *De Humani Corporis Fabrica*—"On the Fabric of the Human Body." Across the title page of a copy of that book which he presented to a medical library, the great modern Canadian physician, Sir William Osler, once wrote: "Modern medicine begins here." It was a long time to wait for a knowledge of the structure of the one object which is the most important and familiar to all of us. That knowledge is enshrined today in the minds and hearts of many men.

I DO NOT believe that God ever intended to disclose to man what man could find out for himself. —Abbé Georges Lemaître

Man, the Unknown

by Alexis Carrel

Excerpts from his notable best seller, of which Will Durant
wrote—"It is the profoundest, wisest and most valuable book
in the American literature of our century."

*The author, a surgeon world-famous for pioneer work in biological re-
search, was for twenty-seven years a distinguished member of the Rockefeller
Institute. He won the Nobel Prize in 1912 for his success in the suturing of
blood vessels and transplanting of organs.*

*Perhaps the most famous of his experiments was that in which for thirty-
four years he kept a section of chicken heart alive and growing by artificial
feeding and elimination of waste. Thus, instead of limiting his research to
the specific problems of disease, Dr. Carrel attacked the enigma at the very
core of our existence—the secret of life itself.*

Each man is characterized by his figure, his carriage, his face.
The outward form expresses the qualities, the powers, of the
body and mind. The man of the Renaissance, who was exposed
continuously to dangers and inclemencies, who was capable of as
great enthusiasm for the discoveries of Galileo as for the master-
pieces of Leonardo da Vinci, did not resemble modern man, who
lives in a steam-heated apartment, an air-conditioned office, who
contemplates absurd films and plays golf and bridge.

Each epoch puts its seal on human beings. We begin to observe the new types created by motor cars and athletics. Our form is molded by our physiological habits, and even by our usual thoughts. The shape and lines of the face and mouth are determined by the habitual condition of the muscles. And the state of these muscles depends on that of the mind. Unwittingly, the visage becomes more and more pregnant with the feelings, the appetites and the aspirations of the whole being; in this open book one can read not only the vices, the virtues, the intelligence, the stupidity, the most carefully concealed habits of an individual, but also the constitution of his body, and his tendencies to organic and mental diseases. The beauty of youth comes from the natural harmony of the lineaments of the human face. That, so rare, of an old man, from his soul.

The aspect of bones, muscles, skin and hair depends on the nutrition of tissues. And the nutrition of tissues is regulated by the composition of blood plasma; that is, by the activity of the glandular and digestive systems. The surface of the skin reflects the conditions of the endocrine glands, the stomach, the intestines and the nervous system. There are great functional disparities between tall and spare men and broad and short ones. The tall type is predisposed to tuberculosis and dementia praecox. The short, to cyclic mania, diabetes and rheumatism. In the diagnosis of diseases, ancient physicians quite rightly attributed great importance to temperament and idiosyncrasies. Each man bears on his face the description of his body and his soul.

The skin is the almost perfectly fortified frontier of a closed world. It is capable of destroying microbes living on its surface with the aid of substances secreted by its glands, and it is impermeable to water and gases. Its external face is exposed to light, wind, humidity, dryness, heat and cold. Its internal face is in contact with an aquatic world, warm and deprived of light, where cells live like marine animals. Its durability is due to its several layers of cells, which slowly and endlessly multiply. These cells die while remaining united to one another like the slates of a roof—like slates ceaselessly blown away by the wind and continually replaced by new slates.

Tactile corpuscles scattered all over the skin are sensitive to pressure, to pain, to heat or to cold. Those situated in the tongue are affected by certain qualities of food and also by temperature. Air vibrations act on the complex apparatus of the ear. The network of olfactory nerves is sensitive to odors. Thus the quality of an individual partly depends on that of his surface. For the brain is molded by the continual messages it receives from the outer world. Therefore the state of our envelope should not be modified thoughtlessly by new habits of life. For instance, we are far from knowing completely what effect exposure to sun rays has upon the development of the entire body. Exaggerated tanning of the skin, therefore, should not be blindly accepted.

One cannot understand the living being by studying the dead. For the tissues of a corpse have been deprived of their circulating blood and of their functions. In reality, an organ separated from its nutritive medium no longer exists. In the living body, blood is present everywhere, bathing all tissues in lymph. In order to apprehend this inner world as it is, we must study organs of living animals and of men as they are seen in surgical operations, and not simply those of cadavers. We must not separate cells from media, as anatomy has done. All living cells depend absolutely on the medium in which they are immersed. They modify this medium unceasingly, and are modified by it. In fact, they are inseparable from it.

The blood is composed of about twenty-five or thirty thousand billions of red cells, and of fifty billions of white cells. These cells are suspended in a liquid, the plasma. Blood carries to each tissue the proper nourishment, but acts, at the same time, as a sewer that takes away the waste products set free by living tissues. It also contains chemical substances and cells capable of repairing organs wherever necessary. These properties are indeed strange. When carrying out such astonishing duties, the bloodstream behaves like a torrent which, with the help of the mud and the trees drifting in its stream, would set about repairing the houses on its banks.

Blood plasma, incomparably richer than generally believed, contains proteins, acids, sugars, fats and the secretions of all glands and tissues. The nature of the majority of these substances and the immense complexity of their functions are very imper-. fectly known. The blood also contains antibodies, which appear when the tissues have to defend themselves against invading microbes. In addition there is in blood plasma a protein, fibrinogen, whose shreds adhere to wounds and stop hemorrhages.

The entire body is traversed by this stream of nutritive substances. The digestive membranes, with extraordinarily vast surfaces, are not only a filter, but also a chemical factory. The mucosas covering our inner surfaces secrete and absorb large quantities of fluids. Their cells allow the foodstuffs, when digested, to enter the body. But they resist the penetration of the bacteria that swarm in the digestive tract. These dangerous enemies are always a menace. Viruses thrive in the pharynx and the nose, streptococci and microbes of diphtheria in the tonsils. The bacilli of typhoid fever and of dysentery multiply with ease in the intestines. The soundness of the respiratory and digestive membranes governs, in a large measure, the resistance of the organism to infectious diseases, its equilibrium, its effectivity, its intellectual attitude.

The sexual glands intensify all physiological, mental and spiritual activities. No eunuch has ever become a great philosopher, a great scientist or even a great criminal. Testicles and ovaries secrete into the blood certain substances which give to all our functions their character. The testicle engenders audacity, violence and brutality, the qualities distinguishing the fighting bull from the ox drawing the plow along the furrow. The ovary affects the organism of the woman in an analogous manner.

A fragment of living tissue, in a flask, must be given a volume of liquid equal to 2000 times its own volume, in order not to be poisoned within a few days by its waste products. Consequently, a human body reduced to pulp and artificially cultivated would demand about 200,000 quarts of nutritive fluid. It is on account of the marvelous perfection of the apparatuses responsible for the circulation of the blood, its wealth of nutritive substances and the constant elimination of the waste products that our tissues can live in 6 or 7 quarts of fluid, instead of 200,000.

The speed of circulation is sufficiently great to prevent the composition of blood from being modified by waste products. Each organ regulates the volume and the rapidity of its blood flow by means of vasomotor nerves. Brain and other organs demand a certain tension of the blood. Our conduct depends, in large measure, on the state of our circulatory apparatus. All human activities are regulated by the condition of the nutritive medium.

When blood returns from the muscles and the organs, the pulsations of the heart drive it into the immense network of the lung capillaries, where each red corpuscle takes up atmospheric oxygen. Carbon dioxide simultaneously is expelled into the outside atmosphere by the respiratory movements. The purification of the blood is completed in the kidneys, which separate from the blood certain substances that are eliminated in the urine. They also regulate the quantity of salts indispensable to plasma. The functioning of the kidneys and of the lungs is of a prodigious efficiency. It is their intense activity that permits the fluid medium required by living tissues to be so limited, and the human body to possess such compactness and agility.

Another kind of nutritive substance contained in blood, in addition to atmospheric oxygen and to products of intestinal digestion, consists of the secretions of the endocrine glands, which have the peculiar quality of manufacturing new compounds from the chemical substances of the blood. These compounds serve to feed certain tissues and to stimulate certain functions. This sort of creation of itself by itself is analogous to the training of the will by an effort of the will. Glands, such as the thyroid, the suprarenal (or adrenal), the pancreas, synthetize new compounds—thyroxin, adrenalin, insulin and corticoids (or hormones of the cortisone family). They are true chemical transformers. In this way, substances indispensable for the nutrition of cells and organs, and for physiological and mental activities, are produced. Such a phenomenon is as strange as if certain parts of a motor should create the oil used by other parts of the machine, the substances accelerating the combustion of the fuel, and even the thoughts of the engineer. To these glands is due the existence of the body with its manifold activities.

Man is, first of all, a nutritive process. He consists of a ceaseless motion of chemical substances. Matter perpetually flows through all the cells of the body, yielding to tissues the energy they need, and also the chemicals which build the temporary and fragile structure of our organs and humors.

Functions of the body are much less precisely located than organs. The skeleton, for example, is not merely the framework of the body. It also constitutes a part of the circulatory, respiratory and nutritive systems, since, with the aid of the bone marrow, it manufactures leucocytes (white cells) and red cells. The liver secretes bile, destroys poisons and microbes, stores glycogen and regulates sugar metabolism in the entire organism. In a like manner, the pancreas, the suprarenals and the spleen do not confine themselves to one function. Each possesses multiple activities and takes part in almost all the events of the body.

An organ is not limited by its surface. It reaches as far as the substance it secretes. Each gland extends, by means of its secretions, over the whole organism. Suppose the substances set free in the blood by testicles to be blue. The entire body of the male would be blue. The testicles themselves would be more intensely colored. But their specific hue would be diffused in all tissues and organs, even in the cartilages of the bones.

An organ builds itself by techniques very foreign to the human mind. It is not made of extraneous material, like a house. Neither is it a cellular construction, a mere assemblage of cells. It is, of course, composed of cells, as a house is of bricks. But it is born from a cell, as if the house originated from one brick, a magic brick that would set about manufacturing other bricks. Those bricks, without waiting for the architect's drawings or the coming of the bricklayers, would assemble themselves and form the walls. They would also metamorphose into windowpanes, roofing slates, coal for heating and water for the kitchen and bathroom. An organ develops by means such as those attributed to fairies in the tales told to children. It is engendered by cells which, to all appearances, have a knowledge of the future edifice, and synthetize from substances contained in blood plasma the building material and even the workers.

The body is extremely robust. It adapts itself to all climates—Arctic cold as well as tropical heat. It also resists starvation, weather inclemencies, fatigue, hardships. Man is the hardiest of all animals. We always unconsciously compare the body with a machine. The strength of a machine depends on the metal used in it. But the endurance of man comes from the elasticity of the tissues, their tenacity, their property of growing instead of wearing out; from their strange power of adaptive change. Resistance to disease, work and worries, capacity for effort, and nervous equilibrium are the signs of the superiority of a man.

Many people, although not ill, are not in good health. Perhaps the quality of some of their tissues is defective. The secretions of such gland, or such mucosa, may be insufficient or too abundant. The excitability of their nervous system, exaggerated. Or their tissues, not as capable of resisting infections as they should be. These deficiencies bring these individuals much misery. The future discoverer of a method for inducing tissues and organs to develop harmoniously will be a greater benefactor of humanity than Pasteur himself.

In illness the body preserves the same unity as in health. It is sick as a whole. No disturbance remains strictly confined to a single organ. Physicians have been led to consider each disease as a specialty by the old anatomical conception of the human being. Only those physicians who know man both in his parts and in his entirety, physically and mentally, are capable of understanding him when he is sick.

The cerebral centers consist partly of fluids containing the gland and tissue secretions that diffuse through the entire body. Thus every organ is present in the cerebral cortex. When blood and lymph are deprived of the secretions of the suprarenal glands, the patient falls into a depression. Everyone knows how human personality is modified by diseases of the liver, the stomach and the intestines. Obviously, the cells of the organs discharge into the bodily fluids certain substances that react upon our mental and spiritual functions.

The testicle exerts a profound influence upon the strength and quality of the mind. In general, great poets, artists and saints, as well as conquerors, are strongly sexed. The removal of the genital glands produces some modifications of the mental state. Inspiration seems to depend on a certain condition of the sexual glands. Love stimulates the mind when it does not attain its object. If Beatrice had been the mistress of Dante, there would perhaps be no *Divine Comedy*. It is well known that sexual excesses impede intellectual activity. In order to reach its full power, intelligence seems to require both the presence of well-developed sexual glands and the temporary repression of the sexual appetite.

Envy, hate, fear, when these sentiments are habitual, are capable of starting organic changes and genuine diseases. Moral suffering profoundly disturbs health. Businessmen die young who do not know how to fight worry. Emotions affect the dilation or the contraction of the small arteries, through the vasomotor nerves. They are, therefore, accompanied by changes in blood circulation. Pleasure causes the skin of the face to flush. Fear turns it white. The affective states stimulate or stop the gland secretions, or modify their chemical constitution. It has been proved that a moral shock may cause marked changes in the blood. Thought can generate organic lesions. The instability of modern life, the ceaseless agitation, create states of consciousness which bring about nervous and organic disorders of the stomach and of the intestines, defective nutrition and passage of intestinal microbes into the circulatory apparatus. Such diseases are almost unknown in social groups where life is simpler, where anxiety is less constant. Likewise, those who keep the peace of their inner self in the midst of tumult are immune from nervous and organic disorders. Man thinks, invents, loves, suffers, admires and prays with his brain and all his organs.

Mental activities improve with exercise. Intelligence has to be molded by the habit of logical thinking. Every human being is born with different intellectual capacities. But, great or small, these potentialities require constant exercise. Intellectual power is augmented by the habit of precise reasoning, the study of logic, mental discipline and deep observation of things. On the contrary, superficial observations, a rapid succession of impressions and lack of intellectual discipline hinder the development of the mind.

In order to reach its highest development the mind probably demands an ensemble of conditions, which has occurred only at certain epochs. What were the mode of existence, the diet and the education of the men of the great periods of the history of civilization? We are almost totally ignorant of the genesis of intelligence. And we believe that the minds of children can be developed by the mere training of their memory and by exercises practiced in modern schools!

There is a striking contrast between the durability of our body and the transitory character of its elements. Man is composed of a soft, alterable matter, susceptible of disintegrating in a few hours. However, he lasts longer than if made of steel. He accommodates himself, much better than animals do, to changing conditions, to physical, economic and social upheavals. Instead of wearing out, the body changes. Our organs improvise means of meeting every new situation.

When one half of the thyroid gland is removed, the remaining half increases in volume, generally increasing more than is necessary. The extirpation of a kidney is followed by the enlargement of the other one, although the secretion of urine is amply assured by a single normal kidney. If the secretion of a gland is insufficient, other glands augment their activity to supplement its work.

Each element of the body adjusts itself to the others, and the others to it through a correlation of the organic fluids and the nervous system. Each part seems to know the present and future needs of the whole, and acts accordingly. The body perceives the remote as well as the present. When pregnancy is nearly completed, the tissues of the vulva and vagina are invaded by fluids. They become soft and extensible, rendering the passage of the fetus possible a few days later. At the same time, the mammary glands multiply their cells. Before confinement, they begin to function. They are ready and waiting to feed the child. All these processes are obviously a preparation for a future event.

During the entire history of the embryo the tissues prepare for the future. The component parts of the eye, for example, associate for a definite, although future, purpose. The brain causes a part of itself, the optic nerve and the retina, to shoot out toward the surface. The skin overlying the young retina undergoes an astonishing modification. It becomes transparent, forms the cornea and the crystalline lens, building up the prodigious optical system which we call the eye. By what means does the future retina induce the skin to manufacture a lens capable of projecting upon its nerve endings the image of the outer world? In front of the lens the iris shapes itself into a diaphragm. This diaphragm dilates or contracts according to the intensity of the light. In addition, the form of the lens automatically adjusts itself to near or distant vision. These correlations cannot be explained.

The correlation of organic processes is evident after a hemorrhage. First, all the vessels contract. The relative volume of the remaining blood automatically increases. The heart beats faster. Thus arterial pressure is sufficiently restored for blood circulation to continue. The fluids of the tissues pass through the wall of the capillary vessels and invade the circulatory system. The patient feels intense thirst. The blood immediately absorbs the fluids that enter the stomach and re-establishes its normal volume. The reserves of red cells escape from the organs where they were stored. Finally, the bone marrow begins manufacturing red corpuscles, which will complete the regeneration of the blood. In sum, all parts of the body contribute to the phenomena.

When skin, muscles, blood vessels or bones are injured, the organism immediately adapts itself. Everything happens as if a series of measures were taken by the body in order to repair the damage. As in blood regeneration, converging mechanisms come into play. An artery is cut. Blood gushes in abundance. Arterial pressure is lowered. The patient feels a sudden faintness. The hemorrhage decreases. A clot of fibrin forms in the wound. Then the hemorrhage stops. During the following days, leucocytes and tissue cells invade the clot and progressively regenerate the wall of the artery.

When a limb is broken, the sharp ends of the fractured bones tear muscles and blood vessels. They are soon surrounded by a bloody clot. Then, circulation becomes more active. The limb swells. The nutritive substances necessary for the regeneration of the tissues are brought into the wounded area. All processes are directed toward repair. Tissues become what they have to be in order to accomplish the common task. For example, a shred of muscle close to the fracture metamorphoses into cartilage. This cartilage later transforms into bony tissue. During the period of repair, an immense number of chemical, nervous, circulatory and structural phenomena take place. They are all linked together. The blood flowing from the vessels at the time of the accident sets in motion the physiological processes of regeneration. Each phenomenon results from the preceding one.

Knowledge of these healing processes has brought about modern surgery. Surgeons would not be able to treat wounds if adaptation did not exist. They have no influence on the healing mechanisms. They content themselves with guiding the spontaneous activity of those mechanisms.

It seems that the work of the adaptive mechanisms stimulates all organic functions. Man attains his highest development when he is exposed to the rigors of the seasons, when his meals are sometimes abundant and sometimes scanty, when he conquers food and shelter by strenuous effort. He has also to train his muscles, to tire himself and rest, to fight, to suffer and to be happy, to love and to hate. His will needs alternately to strain and to relax. He must strive against his fellow men or against himself. He is made for such an existence, just as the stomach is made for digesting food. When his adaptive processes work most intensely, he develops his virility to the fullest extent. We know how strong physically and morally are those who, since childhood, have been submitted to intelligent discipline, who have endured some privations and adapted themselves to adverse conditions. When an individual, insufficiently clothed, has to maintain his inner temperature by violent exercise, all his organic systems work with great intensity. On the contrary, these systems remain in a condition of repose if cold weather is fought by furs and warm clothing, by the heating apparatus of a closed car or by the walls of a steam-heated room. The skin of modern man is never whipped by the wind. It never has to defend itself for hours against snow, rain or sun. In former times the mechanisms responsible for regulating the temperature of blood and humors were maintained in constant activity by the struggle against the rigors of the weather. Today they are in a state of perpetual rest.

Rougher conditions of existence and more responsibility would restore man's moral energy and audacity. More virile habits should be substituted for the uniformity and softness of life in schools. The adaptation of the individual to discipline determines definite changes in the nervous system, the endocrine glands and the mind. The organism thus acquires a better integration, and greater vigor to overcome the difficulties of existence.

Man naturally tends toward the satisfaction of his appetites, such as the cravings for alcohol, speed and ceaseless change. But he degenerates when he satisfies these appetites completely. He must accustom himself to dominating his hunger, his sexual impulses, his laziness, his fondness for alcohol, his need of sleep.

Modern man sleeps too much or not enough. He does not easily adapt himself in this respect. It is useful to accustom oneself to remain awake when one wants to sleep. The struggle against sleep sets in motion organic apparatuses whose strength develops by exercise. It also calls for an effort of the will. This effort, together with many others, has been suppressed by modern habits.

The individual and the race are weakened by extreme poverty. Wealth is just as dangerous. In the poor, as well as in the rich, leisure engenders degeneration. Cinemas, concerts, automobiles and athletics are no substitute for intelligent work. Two essential conditions for the progress of the individual are relative isolation and discipline. Every individual can submit himself to these conditions. One has the power of refusing to go to certain cinemas, to listen to music and entertainment programs, to read certain newspapers or books. But it is chiefly through intellectual and moral discipline, and the rejection of the habits of the herd, that we can reconstruct ourselves. Such discipline is particularly essential in middle and old age. Senescence seems to be delayed when body and mind are kept working. Work is more effective than alcohol and morphine in helping to bear adverse conditions.

Inaction augments all sufferings. Man is indelibly marked by prolonged and intense mental effort.

All physiological and mental functions are improved by work. The more the muscle works, the more it develops. Activity strengthens it, instead of wearing it out. An organ atrophies when not used. Like muscles and organs, intelligence and moral sense atrophy for want of exercise. Effort is indispensable to the optimum development of the individual.

Sunset on McBurney's Point

YOU'LL NEVER SAIL among the Islands of Langerhans or drift lazily down the Aqueduct of Sylvius. And don't expect to stroll along the banks of Hunter's Canal, or watch the sun go down behind McBurney's Point, explore the Fissure of Rolando or ride through the Tunnel of Corti. You'll never trundle the Bundle of Vicq d'Azyr, or pillow your head on Passavant's Cushion, or vacation in Wernicke's Center. Nor will you walk under the Palmar Arch, or loop the Loop of Henle. And you may travel the whole world over and never gaze down upon the Pacchionian Depression or stand in the shadow of the Pyramids of Malpighi.

Because—they are all parts of the human body!

The Islands of Langerhans are small masses of tissue in the pancreas (named after the German anatomist who first described them) whose disordered functioning causes diabetes. The Aqueduct of Sylvius, the Bundle of Vicq d'Azyr, the Fissure of Rolando and Wernicke's Center are all parts of the brain. Hunter's Canal is an area in the thigh.

McBurney's Point is a spot on the right side of the body that's tender to the touch in acute appendicitis. The Palmar Arch is in the hand. Passavant's Cushion is to be found in the throat; the Tunnel of Corti in the inner ear; and the Pacchionian Depression on the inner surface of the skull.

The Pyramids of Malpighi? You'll find them in the kidney—quite near the Loop of Henle!   —Ruth M. Clark

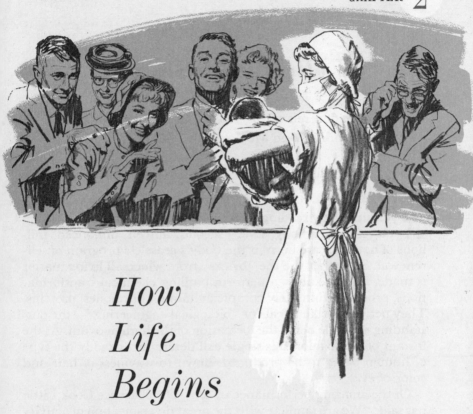

CHAPTER 2

How Life Begins

FROM CONCEPTION UNTIL BIRTH there is a miraculous process in which a speck of protoplasm grows into a new human being. In these selections are set forth the latest remarkable scientific discoveries about the creation of life.

Secrets
of the Human Cell

*Adapted from "Secrets of the Human Cell" by J. D. Ratcliff and
"The Exquisite Basic Molecule of Life" by Rutherford Platt*

As you sit quietly reading these lines, a whirl of activity is taking
place in your body. Every second, unseen, unnoticed, millions of new cells are born in the body's ceaseless program of self-
renewal. Since they are the "bricks" from which all living matter
is made, cells are able to perform baffling chemical transformations, producing infinitely complex vitamins, hormones, proteins.
They perform striking feats of "biological engineering"—the outstanding example being the formation of the human ovum. At the
instant of fertilization this single cell determines exactly the type
of human being to be produced, down to waviness of hair and
color of eyes.

Of the amazing performance of cells, Dr. Clarence Cook Little
has said: "We are familiar with the great diversification of activity
in a large city. It does not seem possible that our own bodies could
quietly and steadily be carrying on a more complicated and extraordinary process of manufacturing, storage, repair, communication, transportation, police, waste disposal, administration,
food production, temperature control." Yet that is the case.

If anything, Dr. Little's statement is conservative. The cells of
our bodies are more like the population of a planet. But though
they number in the trillions, they normally work in harmony,
each member of the complex society contributing to the welfare
of the others.

Today the exploration of this most minute fragment of life is underway in dozens of laboratories, and there is a growing conviction that cell studies will answer many biological mysteries, including the mystery of cancer.

Look more closely at this remarkable little bundle of life, the human cell. It has three principal parts: nucleus, cytoplasm and outer membrane. The nucleus, the "executive" part of the cell, governs structure, so that cells produce only exact copies of themselves—lung cells make only lung cells, kidney cells only kidney cells. Cytoplasm is the jellylike substance in which the all-important nucleus floats; it controls cellular respiration, growth, waste disposal. Enclosing the entire cell is the gossamer membrane, which acts as a molecular sieve. Through it, nourishment passes into the cell to be distributed by a minute system of canals; and through the same membrane wastes are passed outward for disposal.

Each human cell nucleus contains approximately forty-six chromosomes—with the exception of egg and sperm cells, which contain half as many. (When these combine in the fertilized egg, the normal cell complement of chromosomes is reached.) Each chromosome contains genes—the seeds of inheritance—of which there are believed to be thousands in the human body.

Since the mother and the father contribute an equal number of genes for a new life, the number of possible combinations is staggering. Genes are passed directly from parents to children, and have been so passed since man first appeared on earth. Thus in every cell in our bodies we have bits of matter that are directly descended from Dawn Man. "Our ancestors," says Dr. A. E. Mirsky of the Rockefeller Institute, "are present in our chromosomes and reach down to influence the chemistry of every cell in our bodies."

There are four general "types" of cell: the nerve cells, which form the body's communication system; epithelial cells, which line and cover—they line the digestive tract, for example, and make the skin which covers the body; connective-tissue cells, which bind the body together; and muscle cells, which move the body's members.

Cells come in a vast variety of shapes and sizes: globular, disc-shaped, elongated. Some are relatively large—a nerve cell, for example, may have a "tail" three feet long. Nerve cells cannot reproduce themselves; we have our lifetime complement at birth and once one is destroyed it is destroyed for good. Other cells usually reproduce by simple division: they narrow in the middle and finally split into two, the daughter cells being exact duplicates of the original.

The speed with which cell reproduction occurs varies from place to place in the body according to local need. It is estimated that half of all the body's protein—mainly muscle tissue—is replaced every eighty days. The life span of the skin cell is four to five days. New skin is steadily forming from underneath and pushing to the surface, where it dies and is washed away.

One of the most fascinating features of cells is their potential immortality. In 1912 the late Alexis Carrel of the Rockefeller Institute snipped out a piece of chicken heart. Periodically it was fed nourishing broth, and from time to time excess tissue was trimmed away. The cells remained alive for thirty-four years—

HUMAN CELL

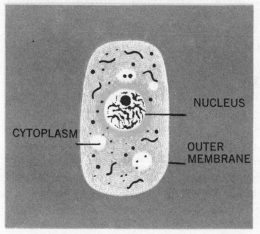

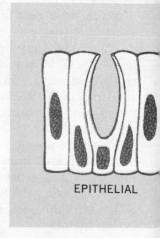

and were permitted to die only when the experiment had fulfilled its usefulness.

In general, cells have two main lines of responsibility: their own housekeeping activities and their community responsibilities. The first includes such functions as eating and waste disposal. The second includes the responsibility of each cell to all others. Tiny cells in the pancreas, for example, produce minute squirts of the insulin which controls sugar use by all other cells; fat cells store droplets of oil to be used as fuel to warm the rest of the body; stomach cells manufacture enzymes which aid in protein digestion.

Some cells demonstrate an uncanny ability to protect the body from harm. The white blood cells normally float idly in the bloodstream. Yet if a finger is cut and bacteria invade the wound, they swarm to the hurt spot and consume the bacteria. If the infection is great they reproduce in enormous numbers to meet the challenge.

Researchers probing the secrets of cells have bumped into a number of problems which have so far proved baffling. For example, since cells generally show a remarkable specificity—lung

TYPES OF HUMAN CELLS

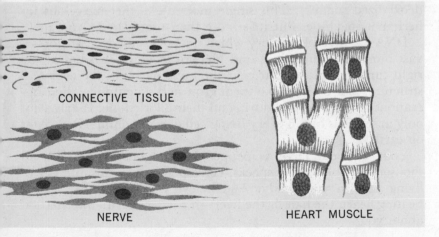

CONNECTIVE TISSUE

NERVE

HEART MUSCLE

cells, and so on—why doesn't the original fertilized ovum simply duplicate itself instead of going through an amazingly intricate series of divisions and differentiations to produce a mouse, a whale or a man? Cell students have found no satisfactory answers, although they have made many interesting observations. They have, for example, studied fertilized frog's eggs and watched the division take place which marks the first steps toward a new life: one cell into two, two into four, etc. They have taken the first 32 cells from this process—cells which would have ultimately made one new frog—divided them and produced 32 frogs! But after the 32-cell stage such interference brings only death to the entire cell mass. Why? No one knows.

There is another great, and pressing, mystery. Normally, cellular division is a perfectly orderly process. But at times cells go on a wild, uncontrolled, reproductive spree. This is cancer. Why do cells suddenly go berserk? Again, no one knows.

In some of the most portentous research of our day, scientists are seeking basic information about the chemical composition of cells—in effect, how we are put together.

The focus of many of these studies is an exquisite and astonishing structure called DNA, a handy nickname for deoxyribonucleic acid (translated: "an acid, in the nuclei of cells, made of deoxydized sugar"). This single molecule is the marvelous inheritance machine. But it is more than that. *DNA is life itself.*

DNA has a vivid memory which time does not dim. It stores a vast number of directions and blueprints which it issues at the right time and place to trigger the building of all the cells and structures of a body, make them grow and synchronize their operations at every second during all their allotted life. It exists not only in sex cells but in every living cell of every animal and plant on earth!

Your personal DNA is peppered throughout your body in thousands of billions of specks, corresponding to the number of living cells in your body. And in every cell—whether in the beating heart, the hair or the liver—it carries the full information about you.

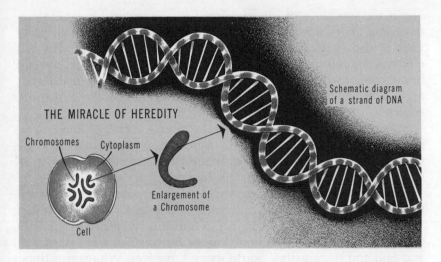

THE MIRACLE OF HEREDITY

Chromosomes

Cytoplasm

Enlargement of
a Chromosome

Cell

Schematic diagram
of a strand of DNA

Your DNA specks have the same chemical composition, are about the same size and look like the DNAs in your dog, or in a housefly, a bread mold, a blade of grass or a sequoia. Yet somehow DNA makes every living thing different from every other living thing. It makes dogs different from fish or birds, bread mold from apple trees, elephants from mosquitoes.

The coded directions in your DNA were compiled by chance selection from those of your mother and father at the conception of your egg cell. That first cell was a complete you, your first person singular. Its DNA was prepared to generate on a prearranged schedule your heart, lungs and kidneys, your seven quarts of blood, twenty-five feet of intestines—all of you. It held advance reservations for all the body functions of your life span, bestowed all the equipments and talents you will ever have. The number of jobs DNAs control vary according to the organism. A one-celled amoeba has little growing to do, it does not think about anything and it has no heart, liver, lungs or limbs to operate, so its DNAs have few responsibilities. On the other hand, the number of DNA jobs in a human being is estimated at 700,000.

In decades of remarkable research, much had been learned

about the workings of inheritance. But the astonishing physical nature of genes was not revealed to scientists until after the advent in the 1940s of such spectacular new laboratory tools as: electron microscopes that can magnify part of a quarter into an image which would make the quarter bigger than Central Park, and X-ray devices which can "see" the actual patterns of molecules.

Surprisingly, DNA has a basically simple form. It consists of two intertwined, tapelike coils, connected by crosspieces at regular intervals—like a spiral staircase. Thus it can shorten and elongate, compress and open up, by coiling and uncoiling.

Since ordinary molecules are apt to be chunky, scientists marveled at the extreme slenderness and length of the spiraling tapes. Dr. George W. Beadle, a DNA authority, estimates that if the tapes inside the nucleus of a *single* human cell were uncoiled and laid end to end they would extend five feet. What utter fineness of tapes and tightness of coils, where all this is neatly packed inside an ultramicroscopic speck! There is surprising logic in the long, slender form of DNA—this gives it a capacity, like magnetic recording tape, for storing all the vast number of informations needed in a lifetime.

Countless atoms make up the internal structure of the giant DNA molecule. The tapes themselves are sugar. Evenly embossed along the outside are spots of phosphoric acid; and on the inside, nubs of four kinds of nitrogen compounds—the steps of the spiral staircase.

The nitrogens together spell out a mysterious code. For it is the sequence of these four nitrogen nubs on the DNA tapes that spells out the events which make bodies grow and turns out wood or muscles, leaves or lungs, fins, wings or legs, as the case may be—much as the electronic specks on magnetic tapes produce, according to their order, the sounds of music.

Does that alphabet seem too simple for all the information and instructions it must carry? Dr. Beadle says that if we were to put the DNA code of a single human cell into English letters and a typist copied them, they would fill a 1000-volume encyclopedia!

What the final results will be from these exciting studies now underway in virtually every country in the world, no one will venture to say. Besides contributing new knowledge to the problem of cancer and other diseases, they will almost certainly shed more light on the mechanics of inheritance. In the words of E. B. Wilson in *The Cell in Development and Heredity:* "The key to every biological problem must finally be sought in the cell; for every living organism is, or at some time has been, a cell."

Conception

by J. D. Ratcliff

"The fertilization of an egg by a sperm cell is one of the greatest wonders of nature. If it were a rare event, or if it occurred only in some distant land, our museums and universities would organize expeditions to witness it, and newspapers would record its outcome with enthusiasm."

DR. GEORGE W. CORNER, *Embryologist at the Rockefeller Institute*

Of all the thousands of billions of cells in the human body, the female egg—though barely visible to the eye—is the largest, the male sperm the smallest. Apparently a woman is born with a lifetime supply of immature eggs already present in the ovaries. Normally the two ovaries produce one egg per month, with no known pattern as to which ovary is selected each time for the egg-producing job. From puberty until ovulation ends, about the

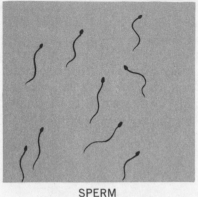

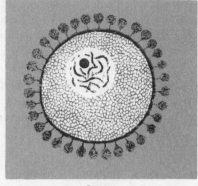

SPERM   OVUM

time of menopause, a woman will thus produce between four
hundred and five hundred eggs.

Before the egg is cast free from the ovary, a fluid-filled "follicle," or nest, forms around the immature egg cell. Gradually
the follicle enlarges until it makes a bubblelike protuberance the
size of a large marble. Eventually, its membranes stretch and
burst, liberating the egg.

The liberated ovum is a tiny glistening sphere about the con-
sistency of hard gelatin. The eggs of all mammals—whales, mice,
human beings—are approximately the same size: two million
would fit in a tablespoon.

Cast free from the ovary, the egg appears to face enormous
perils. Unless fertilized, it will expire in about twenty-four hours.
During this critical period "nurse" cells cluster protectively
around it. From the ovary it drifts into the funnel-like mouth of
the Fallopian tube. The tube—warm, moist, dark—provides an
ideal environment. Gently the egg is moved along the tube, by
muscular movements of the tube itself, by fluid currents and by
tiny fingerlike cilia. All this activity has but a single purpose: to
move the egg into position for its meeting with the sperm. It is in
the tube that fertilization takes place. Then, normally, the egg is
moved along to the womb.

The egg contains only microscopic amounts of food—a supply of starch, protein and sugar which will last until about the eighth day, when the egg will attach itself to the wall of the womb and draw on the resources of the mother.

In many respects the spermatozoön is even more remarkable than the egg. It has a minute, oval head and a whiplike tail about nine times as long. It is almost incomprehensibly small—probably about 1/500 of an inch in length. Yet, tiny as it is, the sperm is able to propel itself with its thrashing tail on a journey of staggering proportions for its size. The sperm's five-inch journey to the egg is the equivalent of a man's five-mile swim upstream.

Sperm cells are deposited by most men in overwhelming numbers—some five hundred million at a time. There are clearly apparent reasons for the need of so many. In general, the environ-

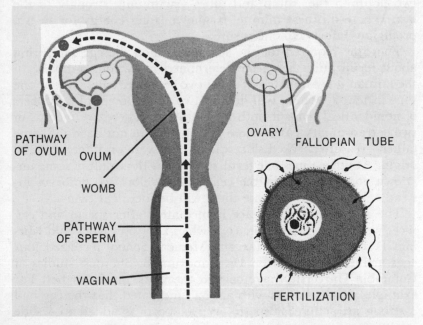

FERTILIZATION OF THE OVUM IN THE FEMALE REPRODUCTIVE TRACT

ment they face is hostile. The vagina, where they are deposited, is acid—and sperm must have an alkaline environment for survival. When deposited, sperm are almost motionless; within a minute there is an outburst of energy, and the great migration begins.

Of the five hundred million sperm deposited, millions perish in the vagina. For those that reach the cervix, the mouth of the womb, great rigors lie ahead. The pear-sized womb must be crossed, where each fold of tissue represents a challenge as great as Mount Everest to a man. Probably not more than a few thousand get as far as the next goal—the upper portion of the womb where the two Fallopian tubes splice in. Only a few thousand start the journey up the tubes—fighting fluid currents—and half of these survivors will be in the wrong tube, since only one contains an egg.

Although sperm can survive for only a few hours in the hostile environment of the vagina, some manage to live as long as seventy-two hours in the womb and tubes—swimming strongly to the last. Where do these minute, fragile cells get energy for such a prodigious effort? No one is sure.

The time required for the sperm to reach the egg and bring about fertilization has been determined in various animals. In the human it is estimated at some two or three hours. About one time in ten, a woman will deposit two eggs, potential producers of nonidentical twins if both are fertilized. There are records of two extraordinary cases where such twins did not have the same father—readily checked since the fathers were of different racial origin. At other times one fertilized egg, as the result of some unknown condition within the cell, will develop two embryos instead of one—in which case there will be identical twins.

The events that take place immediately after sperm and egg meet were first witnessed in 1944 when Dr. John Rock and Miriam F. Menkin of the Harvard Medical School fertilized four eggs artificially. Recently, Dr. Landrum B. Shettles' studies at Columbia University have carried the work much further. For example, earlier studies with animals indicated that the egg had a strong attraction for sperm. When sperm is added to a slide containing a sea urchin's egg, a pell-mell rush is observed under the microscope. It was guessed that this might also happen in humans. Dr. Shettles' findings indicate otherwise. While he watched, sperm swam indifferently past the egg. Fertilization in human beings, he concluded, is a chancy affair, depending on a random sperm hitting the egg by accident. But once a strike is made, the sperm holds on tenaciously.

Most researchers had assumed that once the all-important head of the sperm, which contains the nucleus, penetrated the egg, the propelling tail dropped off. Dr. Shettles found that the *entire* sperm entered the egg.

Research in recent decades on the egg and sperm has yielded information of immediate usefulness. Greater knowledge of conception is helping childless couples to produce the children they so badly want.

How We Started

To LEARN from chimpanzees why their distant human cousins have big brains and walk on their hind legs, Dr. Sydney W. Britton installed a female chimp named Bonga on a small island in a lake at Charlottesville, Virginia. Bonga could not swim and therefore had to make the best of it, even though the Virginia winter soon brought snow. When there was snow on the ground, Bonga walked upright, apparently to keep her hands and belly from getting cold and wet.

This, thinks Dr. Britton, may be how it all started. When glaciers crept down a million years ago, chilling the climate, the ape men began to walk upright. Their brains then got more blood and grew bigger. This started the long intellectual climb that turned ape men into men. — *Time*

EVERY child comes with the message that God is not yet discouraged of man. —Tagore

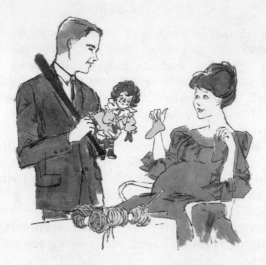

Boy or Girl?

THE MYSTERY OF SEX

by Amram Scheinfeld

Despite a fascinating variety of potions, midwives' formulas, "thought applications," diets, drugs and quasi-medical treatments still being employed by expectant mothers to influence the sex of a child, science says flatly: The sex of every child is fixed at the instant of conception—from the moment the father's sperm enters the mother's egg, nothing can change what is to be a girl into a boy, or vice versa.

The human egg and sperm each carry 23 minute chromosomes, which contain the hereditary material contributed by mother or father. (Until recently there were believed to be 24.)

With regard to the sex factor, the mother produces only one kind of egg, each containing an "X" chromosome. But the father produces two kinds of sperm in exactly equal numbers, one bearing an "X" chromosome and the other a "Y." If a sperm with an

X gets to the egg first, it pairs up with the X already there, and a girl is produced. But should a Y-bearing sperm win the race, the result will be a boy.

Records show that more boys are born than girls. In most Western countries the ratio for many years has been about 105.5 boys to 100 girls. It may vary slightly, but always with an excess of boys. Why?

The old theory was that boy embryos are "stronger, on the average, and thus better able to survive through to birth."

But evidence shows that the male baby is much more susceptible to defect or death on the road to birth. Far more boys than girls are miscarried, die before or immediately after birth or come into the world defective. Among stillborn babies the average has been about 125 boys to 100 girls. In short, males—not females—are biologically the weaker sex, not only before birth but in infancy and thereafter.

Thus, if despite their greater weakness, and the greater toll taken of them on the road to birth, there still are more boys born than girls, it can only be because more boys are conceived—perhaps 20 to 30 percent more.

How can this be, if the male-producing and female-producing sperm are equal in number? Apparently the small Y-bearing sperm have some advantage over the X sperm in speed, or in their chemical reaction to the uterine environment.

At every stage of life males seem destined to die off at a higher rate; it can well be that nature starts the sexes off with a surplus of males partly to provide for the greater drain upon their number later.

Where prenatal conditions are most favorable, the chances of a boy's achieving birth are greater. Young, healthy mothers on the average produce a considerably higher ratio of boys than do older mothers. In some groups the ratio among young mothers, 18 to 22, has been reported as high as 120 boys to 100 girls, while the ratio among mothers aged 38 to 42 has been reported as low as 90 boys to 100 girls.

Another belief of long standing is that the ratio of boys born goes up in wartime through some mysterious influence of nature, presumably an attempt to make up for the men killed. Statistically, there may seem to be some support for this.

Among births in the United States during the years from 1942 to 1946, the ratio was 106.1 boys to 100 girls, as compared with a ratio of 105.8 boys to 100 girls for the preceding five years. However, the reason might be chiefly that during or following wars there is a large increase in childbearing among the younger, healthier or more favored mothers, who normally produce a higher ratio of boys.

Does a tendency to bear sons run in certain families or individuals? Quite possibly, yes. Ordinarily, a "run" of either sons or daughters in a given family may be just a matter of chance. Yet the strikingly high disproportion of sons or daughters in some large families for successive generations suggests that hereditary factors may influence the sex ratios—perhaps directly through the genes, or indirectly through making the uterine environments of mothers either more or less favorable for sons, or else through making the male-producing sperms of fathers either more or less active and potent than in average cases.

Can where you happen to live influence the chances of bearing a son or daughter? Studies in the United States over a ten-year period show that the sex ratios average about the same in one part of the country as in another, despite marked differences in climate.

Can the "acid-alkali" treatment before conception (acid for a girl, alkali for a boy) influence sex determination? Apparently not. Despite the wide publicity given to this in recent years, careful follow-up studies have produced no corroborative results. Nor has any kind of drug or diet been found effective. (It has been reported that the time of conception—earlier or later in the woman's fertile period—might have an influence on whether a boy or girl was conceived, with the earlier conception presumably favoring a female birth. But this, at best, remains to be proved.)

Some method may eventually be found which will give parents power to have a child of the sex they desire. The strongest possibility may lie in finding a way to separate the Y-bearing from the X-bearing sperm, and then, through artificial insemination, using either kind of sperm. Or, if chemical differences can be found in the two types of sperm, a way may be devised to give one or the other a marked advantage in the race for conception. No doubt if parents could have a boy or girl baby as they wish, it would bring happiness in many individual cases. But for society at large, it might open up a Pandora's box of new, unpredictable headaches.

So the natural process of sex determination, whatever its shortcomings, may still be the best.

Biography of the Unborn

Adapted from "Life Before Birth" *by Herbert Thoms, M.D., and Bruce Bliven, Jr., and* "Biography of the Unborn" *by Margaret Shea Gilbert*

From conception to birth, the growth of a baby proceeds with astonishing speed. In the first month alone the tiny organism increases to nearly ten thousand times its initial weight. In the first three months it progresses from a speck of watery material to an infinitely complicated human form—unfinished, to be sure, but recognizably a baby-to-be.

The whole process is a marvel of refinement that staggers the imagination. One change prepares the way for the next, and the plan, for all its subtlety, is marked by incredible accuracy. This transformation, taking about 267 days, is the unbelievable manner in which one's own, and everybody's, biography begins.

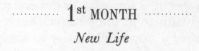

1ˢᵗ MONTH

New Life

At conception the female egg is joined by the male sperm, and immediately the forty-six chromosomes in the nucleus of this completed cell begin to churn about, a prelude to the first cell division. In the first month we change from a small round egg cell into a creature with a head, a body and, it must be admitted, a tail; with a heart that beats and blood that circulates; with the beginnings of arms and legs, eyes and ears, stomach and brain. In fact, within the first thirty days of our life almost every organ that serves us during our allotted time (as well as some organs that disappear before birth) has started to form.

In addition to this astounding growth and development we must also make our first struggle for food. For this purpose a special "feeding layer"—the trophoblast—forms on the outer edge of the little ball of cells, and "eats its way" into the tissues of the uterus. As these tissues are digested, the uterus forms a protective wall—the placenta—which coöperates in feeding the growing embryo. The maternal blood carries food, oxygen (the essential component of the air we breathe) and water to the placenta, where they are absorbed by the trophoblast and passed on to the embryo through the blood vessels in the umbilical cord. In return, the waste products of the embryo are brought to the placenta and transferred to the mother's blood, which carries them to her kidneys and lungs to be thrown out. In no case does the mother's blood actually circulate through the embryo—a prevalent but quite unfounded belief.

Meanwhile the new individual has been moving slowly along the path of changes which it is hoped will make a man of him. While the trophoblast has been creating a nest for the egg in the uterine wall, the inner cell mass has changed from a solid ball of cells into a small hollow organ resembling a figure eight—that is, it contains two cavities separated in the middle by a double-layered plate called the embryonic disc which, *alone*, develops into a human being. The lower half of our hypothetical figure eight becomes a small empty vesicle, called the yolk sac, which eventually (in the second month) is severed from the embryo. The upper half forms a water sac (called the amnion) completely surrounding the embryo except at the thick umbilical cord. The embryo then floats in a water jacket which acts as a shock absorber, deadening any jolts or severe blows which may strike the mother's body. Pregnant women have had hair-raising accidents without losing their babies.

Having now made sure of its safety, the truly embryonic part of the egg—the double-layered plate—can enter wholeheartedly into the business of becoming a human being. Oddly enough, it is his heart and his brain, in their simplest forms, which first develop.

Almost at once (by the age of seventeen days at most) the first special cells whose exact future we can predict appear. They are young blood cells, occurring in groups called "blood islands" which soon fuse to form a single tube, the heart tube, in the region that is to be the head end of the embryonic disc. This simple tube must undergo many changes before it becomes the typical human heart, but rather than wait for that distant day before starting work, it begins pulsating at once. First a slight twitch runs through the tube, then another, and soon the heart is rhythmically contracting and expanding, forcing the blood to circulate through the blood vessels in the embryonic disc. It must continue to beat until the end of life.

About the same time the nervous system also arises. In the embryonic disc a thickened oval plate forms, called the neural plate, the edges of which rise as ridges from the flat surface and roll together into a round tube exactly in the middle of what will be the embryo's back. The front end of this tube will later develop into the brain; the back part will become the spinal cord. Thus, in this fourth week of life, this simple tube represents the beginning of the nervous system—the dawn of the brain, man's most precious possession.

The embryo now turns his attention to the food canal. The hungry man calls this structure his stomach, but the embryologist briefly and indelicately speaks of the "gut." The flat embryonic disc becomes humped up in the middle into a long ridgelike pocket which has a blind recess at either end. Very shortly an opening breaks through from the foregut upon the under surface of the future head to form the primitive mouth, though a similar outlet at the hind end remains closed for some time.

Within twenty-five days after the simple egg was fertilized by the sperm, the embryo is a small creature about one tenth of an inch long with head and tail ends, a back and a belly. He has no arms or legs, and he lacks a face or neck, so his heart lies close against his brain. Within this unhuman exterior, however, he has started to form also his lungs, which first appear as a shallow groove in the floor of the foregut; his liver is arising as a thickening in the wall of the foregut just behind the heart; and he has entered on a long and devious path which will ultimately lead to the formation of his kidneys.

The development of the human kidneys presents a striking example of a phenomenon which might be called an "evolutionary hangover." Instead of forming at once the type of organ which

DEVELOPMENT OF THE FETUS

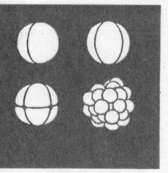

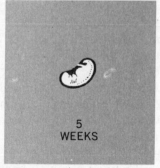

5
WEEKS

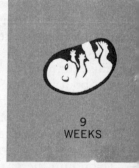

9
WEEKS

Following fertilization, the ovum enters a period of rapid cell division, increasing its initial weight nearly 10,000 times in the first month alone.

The embryo is now about one fourth of an inch long. Already it has the basic structures of the brain, heart, liver and other vital organs.

The internal sex organs have now begun to develop and the fetus, as it is now called, is capable of movement and is taking on more human characteristics.

he as a human will use, the embryo forms a type which a much simpler animal (say the fish) possesses. Then he scraps this "fish organ" and forms another which a higher animal such as the frog uses. Again the embryo scraps the organ and then, perhaps out of the fragments of these preceding structures, forms his own human organ. It is as if, every time a modern locomotive was built, the builder first made the oldest, simplest locomotive ever made, took this engine apart, and out of the old and some new parts built a later locomotive; and after several such trials finally built a modern locomotive, perhaps using some metal which had gone into the first. Scientists interpret this strange process common to the development of all higher animals as a hasty, sketchy repetition of the long process of evolution.

By the end of the month the embryo is about one fourth of an inch long, curled almost in a circle, with a short pointed tail below his belly, and small nubbins on the sides of his body—incipient arms and legs. On the sides of his short neck appear four clefts, comparable to the gill slits of a fish—another "evolutionary hangover." Almost all the organs of the human body have begun to form. In the head the eyes have arisen as two small pouches thrust out from the young brain tube. The skin over the

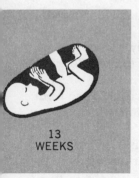

13 WEEKS

The respiratory and digestive systems are beginning to show their first signs of activity and the fetal liver and kidneys have begun to function.

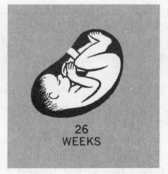

26 WEEKS

The six-month fetus has developed hair and nails and his eyes have begun to open. If born, he has a slight chance of survival.

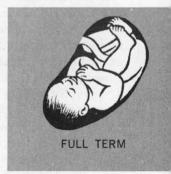

FULL TERM

The mature fetus usually weighs 6 to 7 pounds and is about 19 inches long. It should now assume a head-down position in the womb, waiting to be born.

front of the head shows two sunken patches of thickened tissue which are the beginning of a nose. At a short distance behind each eye an ear has started to develop—not the external ear, but the sensitive tissue which will later enable the individual to hear. In thirty days the new human being has traveled the path from the mysteriously simple egg and sperm to the threshold of humanity.

············ 2ⁿᵈ MONTH ············

The Face of Man

From tadpole to man: so one might characterize the changes that occur during the second month of life. True, the embryo is not a tadpole, but it looks not unlike one. The tailed bulbous creature with its enormous drooping head, fishlike gill slits, and formless stubs for arms and legs bears little resemblance to a human form. By the end of the second month, however, the embryo has a recognizable human character, although it is during this period that the human tail reaches its greatest development. In this month the embryo increases sixfold in length (to almost an inch and a half) and approximately five hundred times in weight. Bones and muscles, developing between the skin and the internal organs, round out the contours of the body.

But the developing face and neck are the main features that give a human appearance, however grotesque. The mouth, now bounded by upper and lower jaws, is gradually reduced in size as the fused material forms cheeks. The nasal sacs gradually move closer together until they form a broad nose. The eyes, which at first lie on the sides of the head, are shifted around to the front. During the last week of the month eyelids develop, which shortly afterwards close down.

The forehead is prominent and bulging, giving the embryo a very brainy appearance. In fact, the embryo is truly brainy in the sense that the brain forms by far the largest part of the head. It will take the face many years to overcome this early dominance of the brain and to reach the relative size the face has in the adult.

The limbs similarly pass through a surprising series of changes. The limb "buds" elongate, and the free end of the limb becomes flattened into a paddlelike ridge which forms the finger plate or toe plate. Soon five parallel ridges separated by shallow grooves appear within each plate; the grooves are gradually cut through, thus setting off five distinct fingers and toes. Transverse constrictions within each limb mark off elbow and wrist, knee and ankle.

The human tail reaches its greatest development during the fifth week, and the muscles which move the tail in lower animals are present. But from this time it regresses, and only in abnormal cases is it present in the newborn infant. Along with the muscles develop the bones. In most instances of bone development a pattern of the bone is first formed in cartilage, a softer translucent material, and later a hard bony substance is laid down in and around the cartilage model. As a sculptor first fashions his work in clay and then, when he knows that his design is adequate, casts the statue in bronze, so the developing embryo seems to plan out its skeleton in cartilage and then cast it in bone. This process continues through every month of life before birth, and throughout childhood and adolescence. Not until maturity is the skeleton finally cast.

Perhaps the most interesting feature of the second month of life is the development of the sexual organs. At the beginning of the month there is no way of telling the sex of the embryo except by identifying the sex chromosomes. By the end of the month the sex is clearly evident in the internal sex organs and is usually indicated externally. The most surprising aspect of sexual development is that the first-formed organs are identical in the two sexes. Even milk glands start to develop in both sexes near the end of the second month. Nature seems to lay down in each individual all the sexual organs of the race, then by emphasizing certain of these organs and allowing the remainder to degenerate, transforms the indifferent embryo into male or female.

So the second month of life closes with the stamp of human likeness clearly imprinted on the embryo. During the remaining seven months the young human being is called a fetus, and the chief changes will be growth and detailed development.

············ 3rd MONTH ············

Emergence of Sex

Now the future "lords of all they survey" assert their ascendency over the timid female, for the male child during the third month plunges into the business of sexual development, while the female dallies nearer the neutral ground of sexual indifference. Or if sexual differences are overlooked, the third month could be marked the "tooth month," for early in this period buds for all twenty of the temporary teeth of childhood are laid down, and the sockets for these teeth arise in the hardening jawbones.

Although six months must pass before the first cry of the infant will be heard, the vocal cords whose vibrations produce such cries now appear, at present as ineffective as a broken violin string. Only during the first six months after birth do they take on the form of effective human vocal cords. It must be remembered that during the period of life within the uterus no air passes through the larynx into the lungs. The fetus lives in a watery world where breathing would merely flood the lungs with amniotic fluid, and the vocal cords remain thick, soft and lax.

The fetus has also begun to swallow small amounts of the amniotic fluid, an exercise not only in swallowing but in something like breathing. The liquid enters its lungs, then the fetus expels it, using the breathing muscles. It is now just practice; until birth the fetus gets all its oxygen and food from the mother's blood.

The digestive system of the three-month-old fetus begins to show signs of activity. The cells lining the stomach have started to secrete mucus—the fluid which acts as a lubricant in the passage of food through the digestive organs. The liver starts pouring bile into the intestine. The kidneys likewise start functioning, secreting urine, which gradually seeps out of the fetal bladder into the amniotic fluid, although most of the waste products of the fetus are still passed through the placenta into the mother's blood.

Overlying the internal organs are the bones and muscles which, with their steady development, determine the form, contours and strength of the fetal body. In the face, the developing jawbones, the cheekbones and even the nasal bones that form the bridge of the nose begin to give human contours and modeling to the small, wizened fetal face. Centers of bone formation have appeared in the cartilages of the hands and feet, but the wrists and ankles are still supported only by cartilage.

No longer is there any question about whether or not the fetus is a living, individual member of mankind. Not only have several of the internal organs taken on their permanent functions, but the well-developed muscles now produce spontaneous movements of the arms, legs and shoulders, and even of the fingers.

············ 4th MONTH ············

The Quickening

Death throws its shadow over man before he is born, for the stream of life flows most swiftly through the embryo and young fetus and then inexorably slows down, even within the uterus. The period of greatest growth occurs during the third and fourth fetal months, when the fetus grows approximately six to eight inches in length, reaching almost one half its height at birth. Thereafter the rate of growth decreases steadily.

However, the young fetus is not a miniature man, but a gnome-like creature whose head is too large, trunk too broad and legs too short. At two months the head forms almost one half of the body; from the third to fifth months it is one third, at birth one fourth, and in the adult about one tenth the body height.

Nevertheless, the four-month fetus is not an unhandsome creature. With his head held more or less erect, and his back reasonably straight, he bears a real resemblance to a normal infant. The face is wide but well modeled, with widely spaced eyes. The hands and feet are well formed. The fingers and toes are rather broad, and are usually flexed. At the tip of each finger and toe patterned whorls of skin ridges appear—the basis of future fingerprints and toeprints. As might be expected, the pattern of these skin ridges is characteristically different for each fetus; at four months each human being is marked for life with an individual, unchangeable stamp of identity.

The skin of the body is in general dark red and quite wrinkled at this time; the redness indicates that the skin is so thin that the blood coursing through the underlying vessels determines its color. Very little fat is stored in the fetus's body before the sixth month, and the skin remains loose and wrinkled until underlain by fat.

Now the still, silent march of the fetus along the road from conception to birth becomes enlivened and quickened. The fetus stirs, stretches, and vigorously thrusts out arms and legs. The first movements to be perceived by the mother may seem to her like the fluttering of wings, but before long his blows against the uterine wall inform her in unmistakable terms that life is beating at the door of the womb. For this is the time of the "quickening in the womb" of folklore.

5th MONTH

Hair, Nails and Skin

Now that the internal organs are well laid down, the skin and the structures derived from it hasten to attain their final form. The surface of the skin becomes covered with tough dried and dead cells which form a protective barrier between the environment and the soft tissues of the body. Even as in life after birth, the outer dead cells are being constantly sloughed off and replaced from below by the continually growing skin. Sweat glands are formed, and sebaceous glands, which secrete oil at the base of each hair. During the fifth month these glands pour out a fatty secretion which, becoming mixed with the dead cells sloughed off from the skin, forms a cheesy paste covering the entire body. This material, called the vernix caseosa, is thought to serve the fetus as a protective cloak from the surrounding amniotic fluid, which by this time contains waste products which might erode the still tender skin.

Derivatives of the skin likewise undergo marked development. Fine hair is generally present all over the scalp at this time. Nails appear on the fingers and toes. In the developing tooth germs of the "milk teeth," the pearly enamel cap and the underlying bonelike dentine are formed.

But the most striking feature of the month's development is the straightening of the body axis. Early in the second month the embryo forms almost a closed circle, with its tail not far from its head. At three months the head has been raised considerably and the back forms a shallow curve. At five months the head is erectly balanced on the newly formed neck, and the back is still less curved. At birth the head is perfectly erect and the back is almost unbelievably straight. In fact, it is more nearly straight than it will ever be again, for as soon as the child learns to sit and walk, secondary curvatures appear in the spinal column as aids in body balance.

The five-month fetus is a lean creature with wrinkled skin, about a foot long and weighing about one pound. If born (or, strictly speaking, aborted) it may live for a few minutes, take a few breaths and perhaps cry. But it soon gives up the struggle and dies. Although able to move its arms and legs actively, it seems to be unable to maintain the complex movements necessary for continued breathing.

6th MONTH

Eyes That Open on Darkness

Now the expectant parents of the six-month-old human fetus may become overwhelmingly curious about the sex of their offspring, especially when they realize that the sex is readily perceived in the fetus. Yet to the external world no sign is given. During the sixth month the eyelids, fused shut since the third month, reopen. Completely formed eyes are disclosed, which during the seventh month become responsive to light. Eyelashes and eyebrows usually develop in the sixth or seventh month.

Within the mouth, taste buds are present all over the surface of the tongue, and on the roof and walls of the mouth and throat, being relatively more numerous than in the infant or adult. It seems odd that the fetus, with no occasion for tasting, should be the more plentifully equipped, and some biologists believe that this phenomenon is but another evidence of the recurrence of evolutionary stages in development, since in many lower animals taste organs are more widely and generously distributed than they are in man.

The six-month fetus, if born, will breathe, cry, squirm and perhaps live for several hours, but the chances of such a premature child surviving are extremely slight unless it is protected in an incubator. The vitality, the strength to live, is a very weak flame, easily snuffed out by the first adverse contact with the external world.

··········· 7th MONTH ···········

The Dormant Brain

Now the waiting fetus crosses the unknown ground lying between dependence and independence. For although he normally spends two more months within the sure haven of the uterus, he is nonetheless capable of independent life. If circumstances require it and the conditions of birth are favorable, the seven-month fetus is frequently able to survive premature birth.

One of the prime causes of the failure of younger fetuses to survive birth is believed to be the inadequate development of the nervous system, especially of those parts concerned in maintaining constant rhythmic breathing movements, in carrying out the sequence of muscular contractions involved in swallowing, and in controlling the intricate mechanism for maintaining body temperature.

The human nervous system consists of a complex network of nerves connecting all the organs of the body with the brain and spinal cord, the centralized "clearinghouse" for all the nervous impulses brought in from the sense organs and sent out to the muscles. By the third month of life special regions and structures have developed within the brain: the cerebellum, an expanded part of the brain that receives fibers coming mostly from the ear; and two large saclike outpocketings, the cerebral hemispheres, which are the most distinctive feature of man's brain. They are destined to become the most complex and elaborately developed structures known in the nervous system of any animal. They are alleged by some to be the prime factor in man's dominance over other animals.

At seven months these hemispheres cover almost all the brain, and some vague, undefined change in the minute nerve cells and fibers accomplishes their maturation. Henceforth the nervous system of the fetus is capable of successful functioning.

The seven-month fetus is a red-skinned, wrinkled, old-looking child about sixteen inches long and weighing approximately three pounds. If born he will cry, breathe and swallow. He is, however, very susceptible to infection and needs extra protection from the shocks which this new life in the external world administers to his delicate body. He is sensitive to a light touch on the palm. He probably perceives the difference between light and dark. Best of all—he has a chance to survive.

8th and 9th MONTHS

Beauty That Is Skin-Deep

Now the young human being, ready for birth, with all his essential organs well formed and able to function, spends two more months putting the finishing touches on his anatomy, and improving his rather questionable beauty. Fat is formed rapidly all over his body, smoothing out the wrinkled, flabby skin and rounding out his contours. The dull red color of the skin fades gradually to a flesh-pink shade. The fetus loses the wizened, old-man look and attains the more acceptable lineaments of a human infant.

Pigmentation of the skin is usually very slight, so that even the offspring of colored races are relatively light-skinned at birth. Even the iris of the eye is affected; at birth the eyes of most infants are a blue-gray shade (which means that very little pigment is present) and it is usually impossible to foretell their future color.

The fetus is by no means a quiet, passive creature saving all his activity until after birth. He thrashes out with arms and legs, and may even change his position within the somewhat crowded quarters of the uterus. He seems to show alternate periods of activity and quiescence, as if perhaps he slept a bit and then took a little exercise.

There is nothing sacrosanct about the proverbial "nine months and ten days" as the duration of pregnancy; but 10 percent of the fetuses are born on the 280th day after the onset of the last true menstrual period and approximately 75 percent are born within two weeks of that day.

The mature fetus usually weighs something between 6 and 7 pounds; it is close to 19 inches tall. Its arms are folded across its chest and its thighs drawn up against its stomach, a position that takes up the least possible space. Most of the time it is quiet (and presumably in a state very much like sleep), but now when it thrusts its arms or legs the movements are really powerful. If the doctor places the palm of his hand over the womb, the fetus is likely to answer with blows of protest.

This is a small but complete human being. Any day now he will face his first great ordeal, the process of being born. Everything for him is in a sense still to come. And yet no one would deny that his experience already has been a truly marvelous one.

এ৹

Two seven-year-olds were passing the time of day. "What's your Dad do?" one asked the other.

"He's a doctor."

"Well, what kind? A dog doctor, or a dentist, or a specialist, or what?"

"No, none of those," was the reply. "He's a woman's organist."

—Sally A. Daugherty

Nature's Way in Birth

by J. D. Ratcliff

At each tick of the second hand of your watch a baby is born somewhere in the world—an event so frequent that much of its wonder is lost. The woman who has borne several children considers herself an authority on the subject. But the studious medical-research man lacks this assurance. *He* wonders. He admits there are great gaps in his knowledge. Indeed, he doesn't even know why a baby is born when it is.

Why does the mother-body suddenly decide to rid itself of an infant it has sheltered for nine months? What causes the dramatic changes that take place in the bodies of mother and child at the moment of birth? What forces act to make the infant take its first gasping breath on which its life depends? The thoughtful obstetrician wishes he knew.

But while many of the basic facts about birth are still mysterious, a great fund of practical knowledge has accumulated. Impending birth is announced by an unmistakable sign: a slight pain, caused by contractions of the uterus. These contractions are quite beyond the mother's control, yet any woman intuitively recognizes their significance. The first primitive woman needed no tutoring to assist her at childbirth, the process being as automatic as breathing.

The woman's body has prepared for this moment in a number of remarkable ways. Her heart has enlarged slightly and her blood volume is up perhaps 25 percent in order to care for the requirements of her baby. Under pressure of increased sex hormones, breasts have enlarged, developing an intricate network of milk ducts and an even more elaborate system of blood vessels to feed those ducts.

The mouth of the womb, instead of being hard and fibrous, is now soft and pliable. There is a good reason for this change. The cervix, or opening of the womb, is normally no larger than a soda straw. It will have to enlarge by five or six inches to permit passage of the baby.

The birth canal itself has undergone remarkable alteration. Muscle fibers have elongated to become more elastic. The shorter fibers normally present would never meet the stresses imposed at birth. There is a new system of blood vessels; and the tissues of the birth canal have begun to secrete a starchy stuff called glycogen, which changes into glucose and thence into lactic acid. Bacteria have a difficult time surviving in this highly acid environment. Apparently this is nature's way of warding off infection.

The ovaries and placenta have begun manufacture of a remarkable hormone, discovered not long ago. Dr. Frederick L. Hisaw of Harvard noted that the pocket gopher had pelvic bones which acted as a barrier in the birth canal. At the time of birth some of these bones disappeared, others opened more widely. He sought the reason and found a hormone responsible—a hormone christened relaxin. In the human being it appears shortly before delivery. Its function, apparently, is to relax ligaments and other tissues in the pelvic area.

At the time of birth the uterus also undergoes change. At the first birth pain the stretched muscle fibers in the upper portion of the uterus begin to contract. The effect is to pull the lower uterus, which remains passive, over the baby's head.

At the time of birth most infants—about 96 percent—have assumed a head-down position. Gravity may have played a part in placing them in this position, or the shape of the uterus. Only about 3½ percent are buttocks-down. Since nature obviously intended a head-down position, an obstetrician will attempt, by external pressures, to maneuver an abnormally placed baby into this position. This is usually done about the eighth month of pregnancy.

The kinds of contraction associated with delivery are varied. The first, usually mild, come at intervals of ten to thirty minutes and usually last about one minute. Gradually the tempo quickens. Toward the end they come at two- to three-minute intervals and the abdominal muscles come into play, exerting even greater force than the uterus itself.

In the first stage of labor, contractions of the uterus push the head of the baby against the cervix. Each pressure dilates this tiny opening a little more. Dilating it to its greatest diameter is a trying and time-consuming process—one which cannot be hurried. With first babies an average of sixteen hours is required. Later children require less time—eight to twelve hours is a good average. But "average" figures are often meaningless. One woman may remain in labor for three days; with another the baby arrives in the taxicab which is rushing the patient to the hospital.

As a rule the amniotic sac, the "bag of waters" which encloses the baby, breaks when the cervix is fully dilated. The breaking of this sac often acts as a stimulant to labor. It is even possible to induce labor by puncturing this membrane.

Once the cervix permits passage of the baby's head, the second stage of labor begins. The baby passes through the cervix and finally the perineum, the muscle bed at the bottom of the pelvis. Nature has seen to it that the baby's head bones are not knit firmly together; if its head is too large for passage the bones can slide to adapt to the narrow opening. Thus, many babies are born with distressingly misshapen heads. But they return to normal within the first week or so. The time required for the second stage of labor varies from forty-five minutes with women who have borne several babies to two hours for the firstborn.

The most critical point in human life is the moment of birth. Up to then lungs have been useless—tiny collapsed balloons, not needed, since the mother supplied the baby with oxygen. The first breath sets off an intricate series of events. Since the baby's lungs gathered no oxygen in the watery uterus, there was no point in circulating blood to them. Thus, in the unborn infant, blood is diverted from the right to the left side of the heart—instead of being sent to lungs to pick up oxygen. At the moment of birth the tiny opening in the heart closes and blood is sent through the lungs. Note in passing that when this opening fails to close properly the world has another "blue baby"—a condition that requires elaborate surgery later.

Formerly it was the custom to cut the cord almost as soon as the baby was born—clamping it to prevent loss of blood and taping it with linen. Then physicians noted that a few minutes after birth there is a final surge of blood from the placenta into the baby's body. So they now wait for this last ration of blood before cutting the link with the mother.

After delivery of the baby the mother enters the third stage of labor—a period lasting under half an hour. The placenta is still partially attached to the upper portion of the uterus. At its point of attachment there is a rich network of blood vessels. If suddenly exposed they might hemorrhage. To solve this problem, nature has acted ingeniously. Immediately after birth the uterus has a short period of rest. Then it starts its kneading motions again, to expel the placenta, and contracts sufficiently to close off exposed blood vessels.

This, then, is the process by which a new life comes into the world. For all its universality, it remains the supreme miracle.

The average human life span in the U.S. and Canada is nearly seventy years. It would be only three months if the death rate that prevails the first day of life were to continue. A generation ago, 15 out of every 1000 infants born alive died the first day. Even today, the rate is just under 11—a total of 38,000 per year.

Why does the newborn infant face such deadly danger his first day on earth? Many infants are born prematurely—unfinished products thrust into a hostile world too soon. Occasionally babies are poorly formed. Physicians cannot prevent some of these things. But they *can* reduce the toll taken by one of the top baby-killers: neonatal asphyxia, or oxygen starvation of the newborn.

In the womb a baby faces no oxygen problems; his mother supplies all requirements. At birth, something, no one knows what, prompts the baby to take his first vital breath. From then on, the respiratory center in the brain must trigger each succeeding breath. There is always the possibility of failure at any point in this intricate process, and nature has provided for it. Babies have a notable faculty: they can withstand periods of oxygen starvation that would mean death for adults. Usually everything goes without a hitch. In a distressing number of cases, however, babies do not breathe properly. They are victims of neonatal asphyxia.

In some cases the placenta becomes detached before the baby is born. In others, the umbilical cord is compressed. Either of these things can reduce or shut off the oxygen supply to the baby. In still others, a membrane covers the baby's lung surfaces, excluding air.

Mounting evidence indicates that a too free use of obstetrical analgesia (drugs) and anesthesia may be one of the causes of breathing difficulties in the newborn. Many physicians feel that this situation warrants serious and immediate study.

A barbiturate given to calm the mother finds its way into the baby's bloodstream within fifteen minutes. An anesthetic which puts the mother to sleep also puts the baby to sleep. The doctor can check the mother's responses from minute to minute. Beyond listening to the baby's heartbeat, however, he has little knowledge of how his other patient is doing.

Everything indicates that babies on the point of being born are more susceptible to anesthetics and pain-killing drugs than the mother. Frequently, women are given a sedative to allay fear and lessen pain in the earliest stages of labor. This sometimes reduces the supply of oxygen to the baby. Drugs given within four hours before birth depress the respiratory center in the baby's brain — dulling its urge to breathe.

Observe what happens to infants when anesthetics and pain-killing analgesics are *not* used: Babies are generally born awake and alert; about 98 percent of them take the first breath without help from the physician. In contrast, when pain-killing drugs are used, babies have breathing difficulties—26 to 55 percent of the time, depending on amounts used.

Damage to the baby doesn't end with breathing difficulties. Brain cells can survive the lack of oxygen for only the briefest periods. If oxygen is denied too long, permanent damage is done. Considerable evidence points to the fact that such ailments as epilepsy, cerebral palsy and other convulsive states may sometimes trace to oxygen hunger at birth.

Since experimentation with human beings along this line is out of the question, most evidence of damage caused by lack of oxygen comes from experiments with animals. Newborn rats and guinea pigs are denied oxygen; then, later in life, they are checked against their litter mates. Almost always, animals that get normal oxygen appear healthier, more intelligent. In maze tests the oxygen-starved animals are markedly slower than their brothers and sisters; many have paralysis and tremors suggestive of cerebral palsy in humans.

Observing a number of these experiments at Northwestern University, Dr. William F. Windle said: "We are prone to blame inferior human mentalities on poor environment or defects of the germ plasm. Can it be that asphyxia at birth is partly responsible?"

A number of studies indicate that this is the case. One study of the birth records of nine hundred children who were mentally retarded, or suffered from epilepsy, cerebral palsy or other convulsive states showed that 70 percent of them had suffered from asphyxia at birth.

These facts are not recited to frighten prospective parents, or to indicate that a few whiffs of ether will lead to death or convulsive illness. Many infants survive the most profound oxygen starvation without ill effect. One prominent obstetrician told me: "Years ago I witnessed a serious case of asphyxia which required over an hour's hard work to inaugurate regular breathing in an infant boy. Last year he graduated from a leading university in the top third of his class."

Still, everything indicates that greater wisdom and greater caution are needed in obstetrical anesthesia. Dr. Nicholson J. Eastman, emeritus professor of obstetrics at Johns Hopkins University, notes: "Reluctant though we may be to admit it, we still have no medicinal means of relieving the pain of labor which does not carry with it some slight hazard to both mother and child. As a matter of fact, the hazards imposed on both by obstetrical analgesia and anesthesia constitute one of the most important problems in all obstetrics."

Some doctors defend the use of large amounts of pain-erasing drugs on the ground that women demand that birth be as painless as possible. Many mothers, indeed, ask for a complete blackout. Physicians say that when they fail to meet these demands they find themselves without patients.

Increasingly, however, women are asking for the "natural" method of childbirth propounded by Dr. Grantly Dick Read, of England. This consists mainly of conditioning the mind of the mother to the fact that birth is a natural process and is not to be feared. Fear only tenses muscles and makes delivery more difficult. In addition, the natural method includes a series of elaborate exercises which strengthen the muscles that will assist in the birth process. Thus prepared, many women are able to have their babies without anesthesia; others get by with minimal amounts.

Miss Hazel Corbin, of the Maternity Center Association in New York, observes: "When they think of labor most women think of pain. They should be taught to think of it as work."

For a growing number of women, "natural" childbirth offers the allure of healthier babies given a better start in the world. Yet many women are not able, physically or emotionally, to face childbearing without some relief of pain. Many doctors are proposing a middle course. They believe in telling women frankly that there is no such thing as a completely safe method of obliterating childbirth pain, and that the too liberal use of analgesia and anesthesia may endanger the life or health of the baby. They encourage patients to face as many pains as possible without requesting sedation; once patients do ask for relief, however, they are given it. Under such guidance, many women will face the first stages of labor with a minimum of drugs.

Thus, part of the solution appears to lie in better patient-physician coöperation. Better care of the newborn would also lessen damage done by oxygen starvation. Many hospitals are still using antiquated methods of initiating the first breath. They slap and pound babies, and "tub" them—dip them alternately in tubs of hot and cold water. These things failing, the physician may cup his hands over the baby's mouth and attempt to inflate the baby's lungs with his own breath. All such efforts consume precious time and increase the hazard of permanent damage to the brain.

Infant resuscitators are far more effective. These range from tiny face masks, which administer oxygen, to elaborate heated bassinets equipped with intricate oxygen apparatus. Resuscitators have been on the market for years, but many hospitals still don't have them. If your hospital does not have a resuscitator, perhaps some civic group in which you are interested will provide one.

We can do much to reduce the hazards of the first day of life. Women can play a major part by facing with greater courage the pains of childbirth. Doctors can contribute by boasting less of painless deliveries and more about the health and vigor of infants they deliver. Hospitals can help by seeing that everything, including oxygen equipment, is instantly available for the newborn. When these steps are taken, a greater proportion of pregnancies will have a happy ending.

An EIGHT-YEAR-OLD taken to the hospital to see a new baby was asked what she thought of him. Disappointed but polite, she stammered, "He's—he's—just my favorite shade of red."   —Laura Rountree

What Is a Baby?

by Herbert Thoms, M.D., and Bruce Bliven, Jr.

This small, squirming object is a newborn baby. One of the 13,000 born daily in the United States and Canada, he resembles every other newborn. Yet he deserves attention, for there never has been and never will be another baby exactly like him. He is a brand-new person, different from either of his parents and something other than a blend of both. He is unique.

Biologically, however, newborn babies do have common characteristics. This baby weighs an average 7.13 pounds, and is about 19 inches long. (If the baby had been a girl, it probably would have been two tenths of a pound lighter.)

He looks top-heavy, and is. His head is remarkably large—almost one fourth as long as his entire body. His seven pounds are concentrated in this big head and in the other disproportionately large part of his body, his abdomen.

The baby's arms and legs are ridiculously short. His bones, composed mainly of cartilage, are soft and almost rubbery. His backbone is so elastic that, if he were put in traction, it could be stretched out another couple of inches. His wristbones are not even formed. There is an open spot in his skull called the fontanel, but it is covered by an extremely tough membrane which protects his brain. His muscles are poorly developed; they haven't been used much and are soft and flabby—a condition which he sets out to rectify almost immediately by doing an extraordinary amount of squirming.

His eyes are blue-gray, no matter what color they are going to be. They will not acquire their individual pigmentation for another ninety days or more.

His temperature at birth is slightly higher than normal, and since he's naked and wet, and since evaporation produces sudden chilling, he must be swathed in blankets almost immediately in order to survive. He is, in fact, the most helpless of all newborn creatures.

Yet this baby is considerably tougher than he appears. He has already lived through a good deal. The Chinese system of counting age gives a baby credit at birth for having lived a full year. It considers his nine months of prenatal life as equivalent to any subsequent twelve, and certainly they were as eventful. None of the changes in store for the newborn quite compares with the drama of his development from a single fertilized cell to a well-organized many-billion-cell individual.

That is the main thing to understand about the baby's birth: it is not an abrupt beginning. Except for crying, yawning and sneezing, which he can perform for the first time today, he has been practicing his entire repertoire for months—sometimes with marked vigor, as his mother is well aware.

The newborn baby *has* to cry within a minute or two after delivery in order to start breathing air. This cry is an emergency gasp, a bellowslike action of his diaphragm which sucks air into his lungs and drives the fluids out of his nose and throat. The noise he makes is entirely incidental; his vocal cords just happen to be there, and the air rushing past them sets them in motion.

Now, having established breathing with his first cry, the baby is prepared to cry for a host of other reasons—such as hunger, followed closely by wet diapers. Then, as he learns that crying brings help, he develops a vocabulary of shrieks, whines and grunts, which his mother soon understands, even if no one else does.

Besides crying, he can grimace, smile and scowl. But his expressions only *seem* meaningful. They are attributable to his rapidly adjusting nervous system; he is simply trying on various faces for size rather than portraying emotion.

He also has a number of reflex reactions to discomfort or pain.

He can shiver. If he is pinched he will draw away. Put him face down and he will turn his head to one side so that he can continue to breathe. He hates to have his head held still or his hands held against his sides; in either case he will struggle with surprising violence to work himself free.

His strength on such occasions is comparable to his extraordinary grasping ability. His grip is so strong that if a rod is put into his hand he will grasp it and hold on while he is lifted off his bed. He may hang from it with a one-hand grasp for as long as thirty seconds. This grasp is a pure reflex; it will disappear in a few months when he begins to coördinate his hand movements with what he sees.

He can blink his eyes, although he doesn't do so until his eyeball is actually touched. It will take time for this protective reflex to develop to the point of making him blink, as grown-ups do, when somebody makes a threatening motion. Perceiving light is about the best his eyes can do, although within sixty days he will be able to recognize a number of familiar objects.

Probably the first sensations he feels, however vaguely, have to do with his sense of touch. But it is his skin that is sensitive rather than his fingertips. When, after a few weeks, he begins to explore the world around him, he will start by feeling things with the palms of his hands, not his fingers. As a more reliable method, he will try to taste things, for of his five senses taste is the best developed. While he may not distinguish clearly among sweet, sour, salt and bitter, he reacts to them—he likes them or he doesn't—about as emphatically as an adult.

But this newborn baby amounts to much more than all these physical facts. He brings something unique into the world with him: his heredity, present physically in every cell of his small body in the form of genes. These genes are his inborn endowment, not only from his parents but from all his ancestors back through history. They have determined not only his sex, his size and how much his nose today looks like his father's, but they have directed his development from a single cell—a cell startlingly similar to the first cell of every other creature—into a human being rather than, say, a dog or a hamster.

Above all, they have established the potentialities for his unique personality. No matter what his future environmental influences may be, he is the only person in the whole world with exactly this set of genes.

But the most impressive and accurate way of looking at this newborn baby is to consider him as a being in the midst of an almost incomprehensibly rapid process of growth. His capacity for development is unparalleled. For most of the coming year his rate of learning will be slightly inferior to that of a baby chimpanzee. From then on, however, the contest is over. After age one he will race ahead into a realm where no other creature can follow. His power to perceive and to act will go on growing for decades, and his power to understand will increase until the day he dies. At the pinnacle of his capabilities his brain will be able not only to assimilate an infinite variety of ideas but to arrange them in patterns and draw conclusions and proceed, perhaps, toward answering the greatest of all questions: "What is Man?"

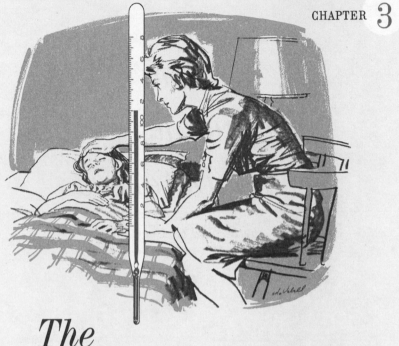

CHAPTER 3

The
Wisdom of the Body

SOME OF the most dramatic and wonderful things that happen in the human body are the result of its own natural system of defenses against injury and the disease germs that attack us by the billions. If you would have greater confidence in your body's innate ability to withstand such assaults, consider these marvels that occur daily.

Our
Miraculous System
of Defenses

by Richard C. Cabot, M.D.,
and the Reverend Russell L. Dicks

❧

In Boston an elderly man, with a ruddy, fresh complexion, stepped off the curb without looking and was struck by an automobile. Taken to the Massachusetts General Hospital, he died within an hour. When his wife was asked about her husband, she declared that he had never been sick in his life. He was a most active person both in mind and body.

Yet this is what was found upon examination: (1) healed tuberculosis of both lungs; (2) cirrhosis of the liver, with all the blood going around by a new set of roads above and below his liver; (3) chronic kidney trouble, but with enough reserve kidney tissue to function despite the destruction of portions of both kidneys; (4) hardening of the arteries and compensatory enlargement of his heart. No doubt he had had high blood pressure for a long time. All this he never knew. He was a well man despite four potentially fatal diseases inside of him.

When a vessel's rudder is damaged in a storm a "jury rudder" is often rigged. This man's body was full of "jury" arrangements. Four vital organs had these compensatory defenses, *but he was a going concern.*

"When you understand a great deal about the human body and its resources for health, you wonder why anyone is ever sick," the late Dr. Walter Cannon once said. Any physician knows that if given rest, proper food and ease of mind 90 percent or more of his patients get well. As a ship rights herself after a squall has keeled her over, so the body rights itself after the minor squalls that strike it daily in health and after the tempests of disease.

The organs of the body have a reserve that can be called upon in need. When a man suffers from tuberculosis of the lungs, part of the lung is destroyed; but he has a great deal more lung tissue than he needs. He can call upon his reserve and get along, as the great Dr. Trudeau did at Saranac for nearly forty years of hard work, though he had only a part of one lung still healthy.

Experiments have shown that one can remove more than two fifths of the liver, and still the remaining part will carry on. When we see a surgeon cut and tie thirty or forty blood vessels in the course of an operation, we may wonder what is to become of the blood that should circulate through them. The answer is that we have many more blood vessels than we need. Each of us has, too, about twenty-five feet of intestine. Three or four feet can be removed and hardly be missed.

When heart disease takes the form of valvular inflammation and deforms the valve, the situation is as if one of the doors of a room were stuck halfway open. A person could not live if it were not that, as the deformity gradually occurs in the valve, the heart gradually thickens and so strengthens its own muscle. A heart that is ordinarily the size of a fist will become as big as two or even four fists, because it must.

How does a surgeon dare to remove a diseased kidney? Because, as one kidney is removed, the other begins to grow to as much as double its size, and does the work of two. All the details are rebuilt, and the architecture of a kidney is far more complicated and differentiated than the architecture of any ordinary building. This ingenious ability has been called "the wisdom of the body."

Another natural defense of the body is rest. If you sprain your wrist, even before the doctor comes nature splints it by making it so sore and stiff that you hesitate to move it. If a person is strained emotionally or physically beyond a certain point of exertion or terror, nature says, "Take a rest," and he faints.

If you wound your finger with a dirty splinter, festering occurs. This is one of the most dramatic and wonderful things that happens in the human body. What is this stuff called "pus"? It is the dead bodies of the white corpuscles which have come to fight the bacteria and have died in the attack. They make a wall of defense between the attacking bacteria on one side and the free circulation on the other. Almost every case of appendicitis would be fatal if this wall were not built by nature around the diseased appendix. It shuts in the inflammation until the surgeon operates.

God's plan provides a great healing power in ourselves that makes for health, a never-slumbering intelligence which doctors try to imitate and supplement with medical and surgical work. In our fight against disease we always have this prodigiously ingenious and powerful force at work on our side.

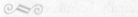

HEALTH is the thing that makes you feel that now is the best time of the year.   —Franklin P. Adams

NATURAL forces within us are the true healers of disease. —Hippocrates

Climate Control— from Within

by Ruth and Edward Brecher

We human beings are essentially semitropical animals. Our bodies at rest and unclothed are designed to maintain their internal temperature effortlessly with the thermometer at about 85° Fahrenheit. But built into us are various methods of coping with much lower temperatures—methods so effective that Indians living in the near-freezing temperatures of Tierra del Fuego, near the Antarctic tip of South America, have been able to survive for generations without any clothing whatever, and with very little shelter.

We achieve cold-weather comfort in part by generating more heat in our internal furnaces, in part by conserving that heat.

The most important sources of internal heat are our muscles, which use about 70 percent of the food energy they consume in the generation of heat. Under average conditions, body muscles produce enough heat to boil a quart of freezing-cold water every hour, and when you wave your arms or stomp your feet you stoke your muscle furnaces to a still higher level of heat production.

The extent to which muscular activity enables you to ward off cold has been strikingly illustrated by experiments of Canada's National Research Council. These experiments show that the same clothing needed to keep you comfortably warm when you're sitting quietly at 70° will keep you warm at 40° if you're walking briskly—or at 5° *below zero* if you're running.

If you don't ward off the cold by exercising voluntarily, your muscles take over willy-nilly and warm themselves by shivering. "It's shivering," one physiologist has said, "which largely explains why so many are cold but so few are frozen." Under extreme exposure, in fact, intensive shivering may even save you from freezing to death.

Because your muscles produce more heat in cold weather, they use up more food energy; but nature compensates for this by turning up your appetite a few notches. On the average you eat 15 more calories per day for every 1° drop in the thermometer. Soldiers allowed to eat as much as they please when stationed in the tropics at 92° have been found to select a diet totaling about 3000 calories daily. In the polar regions at 25° below zero their food intake rises to nearly 5000 calories a day.

Instead of increasing your heat production in cold weather, you can achieve much the same result by conserving what heat there is. One simple method is familiar to everyone: When you're cold you instinctively curl up into a ball, thus reducing the surface area through which your internal heat is dissipated. Less familiar are your automatic blood and skin changes. Ordinarily the blood and skin act as a cooling system like the water in a car radiator: hot blood emerging from your internal organs is cooled by flowing through your skin at the rate of 50 to 80 gallons per hour. When you're chilled, however, many small blood vessels in your skin close up, reducing the flow to one fifth of normal or less, with the result that your skin is converted from a radiator dissipating heat into a blanket that conserves it.

The efficiency of this skin blanket depends in part upon the thickness of the fat layer beneath it. In general, persons with well-distributed fat survive extreme cold better than their thinner fellows. But fat people aren't necessarily more comfortable in the cold. For the nerve endings which complain, "I'm cold," to the brain are located near the skin's surface, and if these endings are insulated by layers of fat from internal sources of heat, a fat man may actually end up feeling colder than a thin one.

Fur insulates the same way. Many animals are able to conserve their body heat by means of tiny muscles which erect the hairs and thus thicken the furry layer when the animal begins to chill. We humans still have hair-erecting muscles in our skin, which contract when we're suddenly chilled, producing "goose pimples."

Conserving body heat depends in part on what your body or clothing makes contact with. Thus the tile floor of your bathroom feels colder to your feet than the bathmat, even when both are the same temperature. Heat flows more rapidly from your skin to a good heat conductor like tile.

Quiet air, fortunately, is a poor conductor of heat—much poorer than water, for example. The human body, which maintains its heat balance without effort in still air at 85° Fahrenheit, requires water at more than 90° to achieve a similar balance. A man may die of exhaustion after sixty minutes in ice-cold water, but he can survive much longer in air at the same temperature. Wool socks and boots may keep your feet warm at sub-zero temperatures while they're dry; but if water seeps in, your toes will soon start to numb.

The mother who bundles five-year-old Stevie up in layers of wool before sending him out in the cold to play has forgotten that Stevie is going to run and jump, increasing his internal heat production many times over, and will soon be perspiring in his heavy togs. When he sits down to rest, his internal heat production falls while his heat loss increases due to the dampness of his clothing. Soon he comes home, chilled to the bone.

A wiser mother sends a child out for strenuous play in relatively light clothing, but with adequate protection for his hands and feet; and she'll remind him to come in for something warmer if he begins to feel cold.

Whereas quiet air is an excellent insulating material, moving air carries heat away with it quickly. Even a breeze blowing at five miles an hour carries away about eight times as much body heat as quiet air. A soldier's winter uniform loses about a quarter of its insulating efficiency when he's walking fast rather than standing, because breezes are generated within his clothing.

The loosely tailored sealskin and walrus-skin clothing of the

Eskimos is very nearly ideal for cold weather. When an Eskimo chases his quarry in a hunt, the chill air flows into and out of his flapping garments to prevent overheating. Later, when he rests, his clothing settles around him and achieves an insulating efficiency that is hard to surpass.

Most of us think of wool as the ideal textile for heat conservation, and scientific studies have confirmed its excellence. Experts point out, however, that the insulating effect is not achieved by the fabric itself but by the air trapped among its fibers. Thickness of trapped air is what counts. Wool's superiority to cotton, accordingly, is due largely to its springiness. Damp or dry, it tends to regain its thickness more readily after compression, and to trap more air.

Understanding the importance of thickness in clothing has enabled scientists to improve gloves for Arctic wear. Our fingers are held partially curved most of the time, yet manufacturers ordinarily tailor gloves to fit the fully extended hand. As a result, most gloves are compressed at the joints and knuckles where our fingers bend—and heat leaks out. Military gloves are now shaped to the natural curve of the relaxed fingers.

Keeping warm while asleep offers a particular challenge. No doubt you have had the experience of falling asleep in a comfortably heated room and awakening to find that you're cold and stiff. The room didn't chill while you slept; as was to be expected, your internal heat production dropped off. It's wise, therefore, to use a cover when you take a nap—even though you're sure you won't need it.

Electric blankets may seem an exception to the general rule that bedding and clothing are designed to conserve body heat: an electric blanket feels as if it were sending heat to your skin. But this is an illusion. Such a blanket rarely reaches the temperature of your skin; it slows down the loss of your internal heat like any ordinary blanket. Its chief advantages are three: it warms itself, so that you don't have to curl up and shiver in order to warm it initially from your own inner heat; it provides a maximum of heat conservation with a minimum of weight; a good electric blanket automatically adjusts so that you don't have to add or take off a blanket as the temperature of the air changes. How much cold can the human body survive? Scientists haven't answered that question definitely. But when Dorothy Mae Stevens was found unconscious and almost unclothed in a Chicago alley one winter morning in 1951, her internal temperature had fallen to 64.4°—more than 34° below normal. Yet the hospital where Miss Stevens was taken was able to save her life through the use of stimulants, blood plasma, oxygen, anti-blood-clotting drugs and other means. Even more astounding was the 1955 case of two-year-old Vickie Davis, who survived after being found unconscious in her nightclothes with an internal temperature of 60°.

Medical scientists began in the 1930s to experiment cautiously with a deliberate lowering of body temperature for treating certain illnesses. Because pain is numbed when body temperature drops, internal chilling is occasionally used to soothe some types of otherwise unsuppressible pain. Even more remarkable is the recent successful use of internal cold to control blood flow while delicate operations are performed inside the human heart. With the internal human temperature at 75° or 80° instead of 99°, all bodily processes slow down, and only about one fourth as much oxygen is needed per minute as normally. Thus the flow of blood through the heart can safely be stopped for eight minutes or even more—long enough to enable the surgeon to do his work.

If you're caught in sub-zero temperatures and reach shelter chilled to the bone, with nipped fingers, toes, cheeks, nose or ears, what should you do about it? Don't follow Grandma's suggestion to rub the frostbitten parts with snow or ice. Recent research has shown that the immediate application of warmth leaves you with less tissue damage and less likelihood of infection or gangrene.

A supplement to the authoritative American Red Cross *First Aid Textbook* now recommends that the victim be brought into a warm room as soon as possible, given a warm drink and either wrapped in warm blankets or else placed in a tub of warm—not hot—water. Just as you lose more heat from your body in cold water, so your body absorbs heat more rapidly from warm water. Too much heat should be avoided—don't use a heat lamp or hot-water bottle or expose frostbitten areas to a hot stove. And don't rub or massage a frozen finger, toe or ear. After the part is warmed, however, the victim should be encouraged to move his fingers and toes.

The best approach to frostbite is to prevent its occurrence. Dress warmly and dryly enough. Exercise to keep warm, especially your toes and fingers. And don't be one of those foolhardy heroes who hasn't sense enough to come in out of the cold.

Pain:
First Signal of Danger

by Ruth and Edward Brecher

A twenty-eight-year old stenographer named Lucy, who lives in western Canada, has never felt an ache or pain in her life. Just as some people are born deaf or blind, she was born without the sense of pain.

But you wouldn't envy Lucy if you knew her. Her body is a mass of scars and bruises. Because she lacks the warning of danger that pain provides, she has several times suffered serious burns; the smell of scorched flesh was her first inkling of injury. She has been repeatedly hospitalized for infections of a kind which the rest of us avoid because pain warns us that we are in need of medical care.

Lucy also lacks the internal responses to pain which protect the rest of us. When you suffer an injury your body responds to the "pain alarm" in a number of ways. Blood which ordinarily circulates through your skin and abdominal organs is rerouted to your brain, lungs and muscles; your heart beats faster and your blood pressure rises—all preparations for taking action against the source of the pain. Your liver secretes stored-up sugar into your bloodstream, and this energy-providing sugar is rapidly carried to your muscles. If the injury is in the vicinity of your head, tears probably flow and your nose runs—the body's method of washing away harmful substances. Chemical changes occur in your blood to make it clot more quickly, so that less blood will be lost.

If the pain is from an internal source, an entirely different set of protective responses may be ushered in. Your blood pressure may drop, and nausea and other unpleasant symptoms may make you want to lie down and curl up—an excellent posture for recovery.

Pain has yet another kind of usefulness. After a period of excessive exercise which leaves you with painful muscles, the initial soreness fades away; but the abused muscles immediately become painful again if they are exercised before recovery is complete. This increased sensitivity—known as "hyperalgesia"—is one of nature's most effective ways of protecting us following an injury.

Pain is a sense like vision, taste or smell. Pain-sensitive nerve endings are distributed through your skin and organs, and when these endings are stimulated you feel pain. Years of research by three scientists—Dr. James D. Hardy of the University of Pennsylvania Medical School and the U.S. Naval Air Development Center, and Dr. Harold G. Wolff and Miss Helen Goodell of the Cornell University Medical College—have shown that the intensity of pain does not depend upon the *amount* of tissue injury but upon the *rate* of injury. Thus if you immerse your body in hot water at 112° Fahrenheit for six hours you will feel only the slightest pain. Yet at the end of the period your skin will be thoroughly cooked. Conversely, a white-hot iron touched to your skin for a fraction of a second may not even produce a burn, yet you may suffer excruciating pain.

"Pain is a sort of speedometer which measures the speed with which tissue damage is occurring," Dr. Hardy says. "It tells you little about the seriousness of your injuries, but it warns you how rapidly injury will proceed if you don't take action."

The nerve endings which produce pain are distributed through your body in accordance with an intelligible plan. They are relatively less exposed on the palms of your hands and soles of your feet, where minor injuries are frequent and unimportant. In the region of the groin and neck, where injuries might threaten your life, pain-sensitive nerve endings are closer to the surface. The gray matter of your brain is protected by your skull and lacks pain nerves altogether. But the arteries which transport blood to the brain are richly supplied with them. Thus headaches are not really brain aches; most are aches in the blood vessels of the head.

Drs. Hardy and Wolff and Miss Goodell classified pain into three types. One they called "pricking" pain; this reaches your consciousness immediately after your skin is cut, bruised or burned. It is sharp, and tells you precisely where the injury occurred. A second or two later you feel the "burning" pain; this is duller, lasts longer and spreads vaguely over a larger area. The third type is "aching" pain; it arises from nerve endings in your internal structures rather than your skin. The pain suffered in real life, however, may be very different from pain produced in laboratory tests. It may be compounded with worry, fear, nausea and other feelings more important to the victim than the actual pain from the injury.

We often suspect that people whom we call "stoical" are less sensitive to pain than other people, but research says this isn't so. Most people experience pain in about the same degree. Some just make less fuss about it. Dr. Hardy, Dr. Wolff and Miss Goodell have demonstrated this by means of a pain thermometer called a "dolorimeter," from the Latin word for pain, *dolor*. They define each degree measured on the dolorimeter as one "dol."

A pinprick or other slight pain which you can barely feel is a ½-dol pain; an ordinary headache may measure 2 or 3 dols. The pain during passing of a kidney stone measures 10½ dols; this is the ceiling above which pain does not rise, even though the cause of the pain continues to increase in intensity. The stoical person may stand an 8-dol pain with less screaming or writhing than others who suffer a 2- or 3-dol pain. Some people—as your dentist will assure you—react to a 1-dol pain as if they were suffering the tortures of hell.

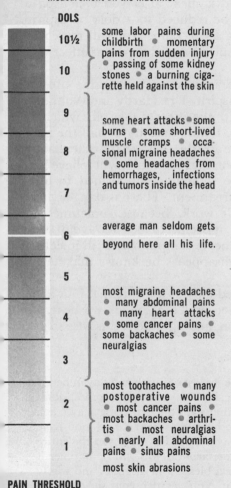

PAIN CHART

The chart shows severity of various types of pain. It is based on the results of tests with pain-measuring dolorimeter. A dol is unit of measurement on the machine.

DOLS

10½ } some labor pains during childbirth • momentary pains from sudden injury • passing of some kidney stones • a burning cigarette held against the skin

10

9 } some heart attacks • some burns • some short-lived muscle cramps • occasional migraine headaches • some headaches from hemorrhages, infections and tumors inside the head

8

7

6 average man seldom gets beyond here all his life.

5 } most migraine headaches • many abdominal pains • many heart attacks • some cancer pains • some backaches • some neuralgias

4

3

2 } most toothaches • many postoperative wounds • most cancer pains • most backaches • arthritis • most neuralgias • nearly all abdominal pains • sinus pains

1

most skin abrasions

PAIN THRESHOLD

Each of us may react differently, too, at different times. A prize fighter who ignores intense pain in the ring may squeal like a baby in the dentist's chair. A football player who hurts his ankle in a crucial play may not feel pain until two or three plays later.

In many illnesses pain lasts long after its warning function has been served—and long-lasting pain, even of minor intensity, can change the gentlest and happiest person into an irritable, angry beast or a depressed and cowering whimperer.

Distractions are sometimes effective in alleviating pain. (Primitive medicine men, wearing grotesque masks, use music, dancing and bitter medicines to distract the patient from his pains.) Work is also a distraction; a backache or headache which you ignore on the job all day may seem excruciating when you have nothing to do in the evening except think about your suffering.

You can find relief from pain by reading or watching television. For this reason volunteers who bring entertainment or other distractions into hospitals are helping to alleviate pain as well as to speed the idle hours.

The Hardy-Wolff-Goodell experiments show that simple pain relievers such as aspirin act primarily by increasing the amount of nerve stimulation needed to produce pain. A headache which is producing a 2-dol pain may disappear after you take aspirin. But a 4-dol headache will not be reduced to 2 dols by aspirin. In fact aspirin will not affect a 4-dol pain. Nor will increasing the dosage help. One or two aspirins at a time are as effective as five or six—and far safer.

Mental expectation of pain relief has much the same effect as chemical pain relievers such as aspirin. Drs. Hardy and Wolff have compared the effect of aspirin with the effect of fake pills which the patient thinks are aspirin. They report that about half the pain-relieving effect is produced by the aspirin itself and the other half by the patient's confident expectation that the tablet will relieve him.

Nerve-cutting operations are sometimes performed to quiet pains which yield to no other treatment. There is danger, however, that nerve cutting won't work, because sometimes the source of the pain isn't where it seems to be. To avoid being fooled, the surgeon paralyzes a nerve temporarily with injections before cutting it. If the pain disappears he knows that he has located the right nerve.

Such surgery, however, is used only as a last resort. Our aches and pains, like the sights we see and the sounds we hear, are useful possessions. For this reason, among others, it is wise to grin and bear them.

IF YOU HAVE NEVER BEEN SICK, never lost so much as a day in bed— then you have missed something! When your turn comes, don't be dismayed. Remind yourself that pain and suffering may teach you something valuable, something that you could not have learned otherwise. Possibly it may change for the better the entire course of your life. You and those around you will be happier if you can look upon any illness as a blessing in disguise, and wisely determine to make the most of it. You *can* turn your sickness into an asset.   —Louis Bisch

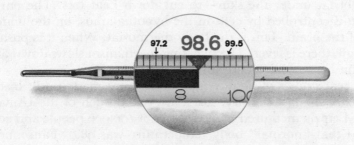

When You Have
a Fever

by J. D. Ratcliff

Millions of people each day slip thermometers under their tongues, wait a few minutes, then consult the little arrow. Most laymen believe that the higher the body temperature the graver the illness. Physicians aren't so sure. For upwards of two thousand years medical men have been debating the question: is fever friend or foe? Is it an indicator of how sick a person is—or of how vigorous an effort his body is making to get well?

What *is* fever? It is simply an indication that the body is generating heat faster than it is losing it. Your body's remarkable heating system is in many respects strikingly like a home heating system. The food you eat is burned, mainly in muscle tissue. The resultant heat is piped around the body by the blood in blood vessels. Like a well-built home, the body has its insulation—a layer of fat under the skin—to cut down heat loss. The entire system is controlled by cells in the hypothalamus, on the underside of the brain. This is the body thermostat. When it is pushed too high, there is fever. The sweating mechanism slows down and the skin becomes dry and hot.

No real studies of body temperature were made until, in the middle of the last century, Dr. Carl Wunderlich of the University of Leipzig measured temperatures of 100,000 people and concluded that "normal" body temperature was 98.6° Fahrenheit.

Today's research men note that body temperature varies widely during a day—being lowest in the early-morning hours, highest in the late afternoon. Therefore, physicians think it would be better to speak of a normal "zone"—from 97.2° to 99.5°.

Although the blood is highly efficient as a distributor of heat, it doesn't do a perfect job. If the mouth temperature is 98.6°, the rectal temperature is usually a degree higher. The liver, hottest organ in the body, is around 101°. The groin area is usually at least a degree lower than the interior of the body. Survival of the human race depends on its rising no higher. Above this level, male reproductive glands are unable to produce sperm.

What induces fever? A surprising variety of causes. Anxiety is one. Children frightened by going to the hospital often run fevers in the 101° to 103° range. One draft-board physician found that the temperatures of 324 draft examinees, anxious about their status, averaged nearly a degree above normal. Also, injury to the brain thermostat—caused by accidents or by tumors growing into the area—often produces raging fevers.

By far the largest producers of fever are bacterial and viral diseases. The exact means by which these microbes cause fever is not known. But Dr. Paul B. Beeson of Yale believes that under microbial attack white blood cells release fever-producing chemicals called pyrogens which prod the brain thermostat into action.

Are fevers harmful? There is no cut-and-dried answer. Some fevers are clearly dangerous—particularly those caused by brain injury, tumors, sunstroke. They soar to levels where temperature itself becomes a menace to life. A fever of 109°, for example, does irreparable damage to the brain if not brought under quick control by ice-water enemas or immersion in tubs of ice water.

Fevers following heart attacks are also grave affairs. The danger here is this: in fever the rate of cellular activity in the body (metabolism) may be greatly increased. At this faster clip the cells require more oxygen. Thus there is an added load on an already damaged heart.

These are the exceptional cases. About the more common fevers that accompany colds, sore throats and such, one point should be remembered: fever is not a *disease* but a *symptom*— often a valuable and revealing one. Many physicians are today questioning the wisdom of fighting common fevers with temperature-reducing drugs—such as aspirin. Speaking mainly of childhood diseases, Dr. Alan K. Done of Stanford University school of medicine observes: "Antifever therapy is often employed more for the benefit of parents, or the physician, than the child. It is doubtful whether body temperatures in the range of 104° are harmful, even if prolonged for several days."

Fever may be the best, or the only, available sign for following the course of an illness, as many diseases have readily recognized temperature patterns. In typhus, for example, fever is continuous. Malaria has a relapsing pattern—normal for a few days, followed by an upward swing. In typhoid there is a remittent pattern (marked fluctuations remaining above normal); in bone infections and abdominal abscesses there is an intermittent fever (where normal is approached at some time during the day).

What are safe limits for fever? There is no hard and fast rule. It has been observed that people rarely survive temperatures above 109°. However, temperatures almost never rise above 106°. Apparently, the body has some emergency mechanism that takes over at this point. A chain of lifesaving events gets under way. The patient usually goes into coma, blood flow to the blood vessels near the surface of the body is increased and sweating becomes profuse. These events produce a cooling effect, and the fever begins to fall to safer levels.

Fearsome as fever may be to laymen, it has many beneficial effects. It prods the body into greater production of bacteria-fighting white blood cells and bacteria-killing antibodies. Recent evidence indicates that it increases production of the hormone ACTH, which in turn combats the stress placed on the body by disease. It appears to enhance the action of such antibiotics as penicillin.

At certain reasonably safe temperature levels some bacteria are simply cooked to death. Last century, for example, physicians noted that after bouts with certain feverish diseases (malaria, typhus) many patients were cured of syphilis. This led Dr. Julius Wagner-Jauregg, Austrian physician, to infect patients with malaria as a treatment for syphilis, and led later on to production of artificial fevers with high-frequency electric current.

As wider knowledge of fever has accumulated, many old rules have been rewritten. A generation ago it was standard practice to "starve a fever"—which undoubtedly killed many badly debilitated patients. Since fever hoists the metabolic rate, the need for food and fluids is increased. Today's rule: a high-protein, high-vitamin diet, with all the liquid the patient can take.

Another old rule was to cover the feverish patient with blankets and heat up the sickroom—so he could "sweat it out." This was the worst possible treatment. In fever, the body is struggling to get rid of heat. Why make the job more difficult? Today's rule: a comfortably coolish room, light bed covering.

Until recently it has been customary to keep feverish patients in bed. Under certain circumstances this rule, too, may be ready for discard. Not long ago Dr. John P. Gibson, a Texas physician, collected records of 1082 feverish youngsters. Some were confined to bed, some were allowed up and about the home. Temperatures returned to normal at almost exactly the same rate with each group. Concluded Dr. Gibson: "This study seems to indicate that in 'ordinary' or 'self-limiting' illnesses . . . children may rest as they desire, and play quietly in the house."

To sum up: Fever is no longer the frightening thing it once was. According to present-day thinking, the great majority of fevers are more apt to be friends than foes.

Repelling
the
Unseen Invaders

by Ruth and Edward Brecher

❦

"Not sickness but *health*," a famous physician once remarked, "is the greatest of medical mysteries."

Your own good health is an example. Every day your body is assailed by billions of germs, many of which can produce illness or even death. *Yet you stay well.* Countless bacteria and viruses gain entry into your body with the food you eat or the air you breathe or through breaks in your skin. *Yet you stay well.* Some of them establish permanent residence in your mouth, your nose and throat or your intestines, where they may multiply fantastically. *Yet you stay well.*

What protects you from these ceaseless assaults by bacteria and viruses?

Through decades of study scientists have been slowly finding out. Your health is safeguarded, they report, by an ingenious series of defenses arranged in depth like the successive lines of an army entrenched to ward off invaders.

Suppose, for example, that a germ-laden fleck of dust floats into your eye. In all probability there is nothing to worry about.

Your eye surface is constantly bathed in tears, which contain a bacteria-destroying antiseptic called lysozyme. Lysozyme is so powerful that a single teardrop diluted with half a gallon of water will still destroy at least one species of germs.

Your saliva and the other fluids manufactured by your body also contain antiseptic chemicals. Even your bare skin has considerable germicidal power. For example, virulent-dysentery bacteria in a drop of fluid placed on a glass slide will survive for hours, while those in a drop placed on the clean palm of your hand will be dead within about twenty minutes.

Some kinds of germs can survive these external defenses and even multiply on your skin. Before they can harm you, however, they must gain entry into your body and then run an amazing gantlet of other defenses. Germs entering through your mouth, for instance, are attacked by the antiseptics in your saliva. For those that are swallowed and washed into your stomach, powerful digestive juices lie in wait. Few reach your intestines alive.

Germs which gain entry through your nose must thread the complicated maze of your air-filtering nasal passages. The surfaces of these passages are kept moist by a mucous fluid for catching germs. If the germs cause irritation, they are sneezed out; or your nose starts to run and they are flushed out. Germs which manage to reach the tubes to the lungs are also trapped in a mucous fluid, and are coughed out, or if swallowed, meet their fate in the well-guarded gastrointestinal tract.

When germs get into your body through breaks in your skin or mucous surfaces—breaks so small that they may be unnoticed—the peril is seemingly greater. Let's say that you step on a germ-laden nail. Each germ thus entering your tissues may divide into two after twenty minutes or so, and divide again in another twenty minutes. If this rate were to continue, you would be host to a million descendants within seven hours, and to several quadrillion the next day. By then your entire body would, of course, be overwhelmed. But before this can happen another type of defense will have come to your aid.

One of the most awe-inspiring marvels of life is the ability of the body to renew itself, to repair damage and go forward. Every time you so much as nick yourself with a razor or paring knife, a construction job far more complex than building a skyscraper gets underway. We take this healing power for granted, yet without it surgery couldn't exist; the slightest injury could lead to death.

Inflammation begins when various chemicals are released at the site of a germ invasion by the invaders or by the injured cells in your body. These chemicals seep outward in all directions until they reach the nearest blood vessels. There they cause a relaxing of the vessel walls that enables plasma, the watery part of the blood, to seep out. Accompanying the blood plasma are white blood cells called leucocytes, and various chemicals that curb bacterial growth.

Leucocytes are among the most curious and most effective of your body's defenses. In appearance they resemble the one-celled animal called amoeba, and like the amoeba they can propel themselves from place to place within your body. In some way not yet understood, leucocytes are attracted as if by a magnet to the site of a bacterial invasion. When they arrive they gobble up any invading particles they find.

It is fascinating to watch this gobbling-up process through a microscope. A leucocyte slithers up to an invading bacterium, crowds it against a solid surface, then flows its jellylike body around the bacterium to "corner" it. Next it opens a hole in its skinlike membrane, and the bacterium is completely engulfed. A moment later the leucocyte slithers off after its next quarry. Millions of leucocytes are often mobilized at the site of an infection.

Other factors involved in inflammation help the leucocytes in their work. In the blood plasma is a chemical called fibrinogen, which quickly solidifies into a network of strands and, with other plasma substances and the leucocytes, forms a wall around the battlefield, trapping the germs so that the infection is localized. Boils and abscesses are typical examples of how this walling-off process safeguards the rest of your body from germ invaders.

Even though bacteria are thus contained, the resources of your entire body are mobilized to defeat them. Some of the chemicals released during the battle enter your bloodstream and carry the alarm to storehouses throughout your body where leucocyte reserves are maintained. Within minutes millions of additional leucocytes are released into your blood, which carries them to all your tissues. While this is going on, your bone marrow is also alerted and it speeds up the manufacture of new leucocyte reserves.

Some germs are coated with a repellent which keeps leucocytes away, and some have the power to kill the leucocytes that engulf them. Even in death, however, the leucocytes continue to release chemicals injurious to germs.

If the leucocytes cannot complete the mopping-up operation, they are joined by larger (but still microscopic) cells called macrophages. These can gobble up not only bacteria but also leucocytes that are harboring bacteria.

Usually when a leucocyte or a macrophage engulfs a germ it means death to the germ, but not always. Some bacteria can survive for long periods within cells which have gobbled them up. Indeed, a cell may occasionally prolong the life of a bacterium by protecting it from antiseptic blood substances and from the drugs your physician prescribes to help combat the infection. Your body requires a way to dispose of these germs after they have been engulfed, and to get rid of other waste products.

To provide for this, your body tissues are drained by a network of channels called the lymphatic system. Leucocytes, macrophages and invading particles enter the vessels of this network and are carried by the lymph fluid to "regional lymph nodes," or glands, situated at strategic points throughout your body. Each node

LEUCOCYTE ABSORBING BACTERIUM

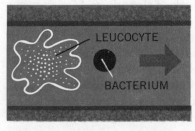
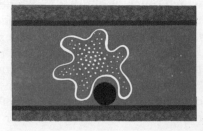

serves as a filter, holding back bacteria and other particles. The lymph fluid flows on from one node to another until it reaches the ones in the neck, where it is discharged into the bloodstream. By then, generally, all germs have been filtered out of the lymph fluid.

Following an illness, however, disease germs may survive for days or even weeks within the lymph nodes. The glands in your neck are the final barriers which prevent germs from reaching your bloodstream, and the survival of germs in them for long periods explains why these glands sometimes remain swollen and tender long after other symptoms have disappeared.

Even if a few germs reach the bloodstream, another line of defense stands ready. Your bone marrow, liver, spleen and a few smaller organs are equipped with multitudes of macrophages to filter invading particles out of your blood just as the lymph nodes filter your lymph fluid.

How are the leucocytes and macrophages able to distinguish between invading germs or other particles and the cells or molecules of your own body? Your body has a built-in identification system which *labels* invading particles. These labels, which attach themselves to invaders, are called antibodies. Leucocytes and macrophages will occasionally engulf almost any particle they happen upon, but the ones they search out and devour with the greatest voracity are those which have been labeled as invaders by antibodies.

Most cases of recovery from an infection are traceable in large part to antibody action. If you have never had scarlet fever, your

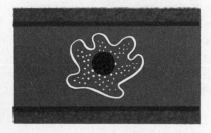 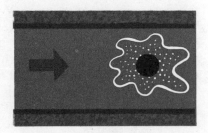

body lacks antibodies tailored to fit the streptococci which cause that disease. But if streptococci secure a sufficient toehold in your body to multiply, your antibody factories start tooling up. For several days, perhaps, the germs continue to multiply and you get sicker and sicker. By then, however, full-scale antibody production has begun and antibodies are turned out in large amounts. These latch onto the scarlet-fever streptococci, which, as soon as they are labeled, fall prey to the voracious leucocytes and macrophages, and your recovery begins. Other substances in your blood help out by destroying bacteria to which antibodies are attached.

It is chiefly your antibodies which make you immune to second attacks of many common illnesses. The first time you suffer from a disease such as scarlet fever or measles your antibody factories take several days to learn the right pattern. Once the lesson is learned, however, production can begin much more promptly, and large amounts of antibodies of the desired pattern may be turned out within a few hours after the entry of a few thousand germs. Thus the second invasion and subsequent entries of a particular type of germ are frequently wiped out before you even suspect that you've been infected.

Antibodies are also the agents which make it possible to control infectious diseases through vaccination. A vaccine is a substance which teaches your body in advance how to manufacture antibodies promptly against a disease you have not yet encountered.

A few kinds of germs have learned how to evade our antibody defenses. The influenza virus is the most striking example. Every few years a type of flu virus comes along which is unaffected by the common flu antibodies. When this happens, an influenza "pandemic" sweeps the world, as with the "Asian flu." Within a few years almost everybody gets the new kind of flu and develops antibodies against it—whereupon a different flu virus pops up. Each type of flu requires a separate antibody.

Most of the antibodies circulating in your blood are found in a part of the blood plasma called gamma globulin. This antibody-rich substance can be extracted from the blood of donors and stored for considerable periods. Small injections of gamma globulin will provide temporary immunity to measles and infectious hepatitis; the "borrowed antibodies" in the gamma globulin act in just the same way as the antibodies you manufacture yourself.

Newborn babies also stay well on borrowed antibodies. Their antibody factories operate poorly or not at all during the first few weeks of life, but antibodies received from their mothers before birth protect them for a time from most of the diseases to which the mothers themselves are immune. Babies also get protective antibodies in mother's milk, especially in the milk secreted during the first few days of nursing.

Some germs attack only cells in their immediate vicinity; others release poisonous molecules called toxins which may circulate to other parts of your body. Diphtheria and tetanus bacteria are examples of these toxin producers. When attacked by toxins your body manufactures antitoxins—that is, antibodies against toxin molecules. And just as you can be immunized against virus diseases by means of vaccines containing denatured viruses, so you can be immunized against diphtheria and tetanus toxins by injections of denatured toxins called toxoids.

In the economy of the body a wound always gets first priority. Even people starving in World War II concentration camps retained the ability to heal. Whatever materials are needed for the healing process are provided by tearing down tissues elsewhere in the body. Thus, muscle is broken down into amino acids, which build new tissue at the wound site. That is why badly injured people "waste away."

Gradually a wound fills with granulation tissue—a beefy, spongy patching material which will be replaced by firm, fibrous scar tissue.

The construction of new tissue is one of the true wonders of nature. In response to some mysterious directive force, fiber cells arrange themselves in neat geometric patterns, like chemical crystals. Since these more complex tissues need a reliable blood supply, an intricate plumbing system of capillaries must be installed. Researchers can watch this when the ear of a rabbit is injured: little blood vessels, so delicate that they bleed at the touch, start drilling their way through the new tissue. Their ends remain sealed; otherwise, blood would leak away. Progressing in random fashion, they finally strike another capillary. The ends magically dissolve and the two join, laying down the elements of a new circulatory system. By a process still more complex, nerve tails push their way into the new tissue.

All this has been taking place deep under the scab. Meanwhile directly beneath the scab, new skin is forming. Around the margins of the wound, skin cells start playing their all-important role. They start elongating—reaching their way toward the center of the denuded area, just as bark grows over a blaze on a tree. The first skin to cover the wound is thin, fragile, living. Eventually it will mature, with uppermost cells dying and hardening to form a permanent, inert covering.

A week or so after the injury the wound looks healed. Actually, some of the most remarkable steps in the healing process are to come. In the months following injury, tiny muscle fibers start growing outward from either side of the wound, finally meeting and splicing together. Fat joins to fat, connective tissue to connective tissue. In time, perhaps a year, the scar tissue is replaced by functioning tissue. The reconstruction job is completed.

Could mankind survive without the human body's miraculously coördinated "defense in depth"? It seems unlikely.

Pain makes man think. Thinking makes man wise. Wisdom makes life endurable.   —John Patrick, *Teahouse of the August Moon*

Never does nature say one thing and wisdom another.   —Juvenal, *Satires*

CHAPTER 4

Giants
of the Body

EVEN primitive man sensed that the brain, the heart and the lungs played the most dramatic roles within the human body, though the nature of their functions long remained cloaked in mystery and superstition.

The more medical knowledge advances, the more awe-inspiring does the magnitude of the tasks performed by these great organs become.

Introducing the Brain

by John Pfeiffer

This vivid account of the human brain in all its aspects is from the most out-standing work written for laymen in the English language on the subject of this organ of the human body. The condensation of the opening chapter of The Human Brain *by John Pfeiffer is an exciting invitation to self-understanding.*

The human brain is perched like a flower on the top of a slender stalk, which in a six-foot man is not quite a yard long. The top three inches of the stalk, a thick white cable of nerve fibers known as the brain stem, lies entirely within the skull and is partly buried by the bulging halves or hemispheres of the brain. The rest of the long stalk, the spinal cord, is a direct continuation of the cable outside the skull. It runs down through holes in the vertebrae of the spine and ends at the small of the back. Many branches extend from the central stalk, like the roads that feed traffic in and out of a superhighway. Through their finest fibers they reach into the remotest places, and into every nook and cranny from the roots of hairs and teeth to the tips of the toes.

The brain itself is three pounds of "messy substance shut in a dark warm place"—a pinkish-gray mass, moist and rubbery to the touch, about the size of a softball. Shock-absorbing fluid cushions it against bumps, sharp blows and other impacts. It is wrapped in three membranes, including an extra-tough outer envelope, and is set snugly into its crate of bone.

Under the microscope a single brain cell with its fibers may resemble the crown of a tree. Growing out from each branch are smaller branches, and from each of them comes a succession of smaller and smaller offshoots down to the most delicate twig. The brain contains some thirteen billion such cells, five times more than the total number of people in the world.

These units form masses of twisted fibers, a tangle which one investigator has called the "cerebral jungle." Until recently most investigators assumed that nerve fibers occupied fixed positions, or at least moved only as they grew, like the roots of plants. But new studies (at the University of Texas) indicate that brain tissue is far more active than this. As you read this sentence, fibers in your head are swaying like seaweed swept by tides. Tentacles of protoplasm are slowly moving forward, retreating, swelling and shrinking, waving from side to side.

What is the brain for? Judging by what we know today, it is the great organ of adjustment. It plays the basic biological role of keeping us adjusted to unpredictable events in the outside world, of preserving our identities in an environment of swift and ceaseless chemical change.

The brain keeps us alive by balancing the processes of birth and decay. These basic reactions have top priority. Everything else either helps in carrying them out, or else waits its turn. We pay a high price when the balance of any vital process is upset. For example, sugar is one of the body's energy-providing substances and we must have just the right amount, no more and no less. We walk a biological tightrope between coma and convulsion, the possible results of relatively slight changes in blood-sugar levels.

But the brain usually receives advance notice of impending trouble. It receives a steady flow of information about current sugar levels, and makes adjustments as effectively as a pilot guiding an airplane through a storm. If there is too much sugar, the excess is burned up and excreted. If there is too little, the liver is instructed to release the proper amount of reserve sugar. Notice what such control implies. The brain must "know" the desired sugar level, about a sixtieth of an ounce for every pint of blood, on the average. It must go by similar standards in regulating breathing (most of us inhale and exhale eighteen to twenty times a minute) and heartbeat rates (about seventy times a minute), and in holding body temperature at 98.6° Fahrenheit.

The brain must also be in constant communication with all parts of the body. Indeed, it turns out to be the headquarters of the most elaborate communications network ever devised. Its activities are the result of the combined and patterned activities of billions of nerve cells. A nerve cell is a living wire which produces and conducts rapid electrical impulses. It keeps itself "loaded" and ready for action with the aid of a built-in battery which runs on an oxygen-sugar mixture and recharges automatically. It fires—that is, emits up to several hundred impulses a second—when triggering impulses reach it from sense organs or from other nerve cells.

These outside signals enter the body of the cell through special receiving fibers which are usually short, fine and highly branched. The slenderest fibers, about 1/25,000 of an inch in diameter, have speed limits of a foot a second or two thirds of a mile an hour. But in large-gauge fibers, which measure about ten times thicker, nerve impulses flash along at speeds up to 150 yards a second, a respectable 300 miles an hour. Thick, fast fibers generally connect remote parts of the nervous system; thin, slow fibers connect neighboring regions. Thus, if a cell communicates with several other cells at varying distances, the messages all tend to arrive at about the same time. This means that widely scattered parts of the nervous system can be stimulated, inhibited or alerted at once—a distinct advantage in coördinating very complex behavior.

The brain uses this network to adjust us to the outside world. Generally speaking, its operation can be divided into three parts:

(1) it receives input in the form of messages from the sense organs; (2) it organizes the input on the basis of past experience, current events and future plans; and (3) it selects and produces an appropriate output, an action or series of actions.

The brain keeps in constant touch with the flow of events. It is stirred up by lights, sounds, odors and other disturbances in the environment. Each sensation produces electrical impulses in nerves leading to the brain, "shocks" which stream into higher nerve centers and cause cell after cell to fire in a series of chain reactions.

The sense organs most remote from your brain are those located in your toes. Fibers originating in these outlying stations carry messages concerning heat, cold, muscle tension, touch, pain. They are joined by more and more fibers from your foot, leg, knee and thigh.

By the time the collected fibers reach the lower part of the spinal cord they form a thick cable. The cable continues to thicken as it climbs and is joined by millions of fibers from other organs of the body on the way up to the brain. It subjects the brain to constant proddings. Although its lines are less busy during sleep, even then it is occupied with various duties—keeping your heart and lungs going, dreaming, and listening with a somewhat reduced vigilance. The brain relaxes, but as long as it is alive it finds no rest.

The brain's informers are sense organs, sentinels located at strategic points throughout the body. Imbedded in the skin are some 3,000,000 to 4,000,000 structures sensitive to pain, 500,000 touch or pressure detectors, more than 200,000 temperature detectors. These tiny organs—plus the ears, eyes, nose and tongue— are some of your windows to the outside world. Reports about the state of things inside your body come from other built-in sense organs which give rise to sensations of muscular tension, hunger, thirst, nausea.

The brain has other sensory maps. On the cortex at the back of the head are visual maps, screens made up of a mosaic of nerve cells. Every pattern you see around you, every tree and building and face, produces patterns on these screens as various cells in the mosaic. Other sensory fibers lead to the smell areas of the cortex, which are buried deep down in the walls of the chasm between the cerebral hemispheres. Each sense thus has its map on the cortex, its exclusive zone in the highest center of the nervous system. In this way, the brain sorts the information upon which its activities are based.

In nerve messages, as in dot-dash telegraph codes, patterns of pulses stand for the items of information being sent. But the interpretation of nerve signals depends first of all on the place they arrive at. No matter how accurately senses have been coded, no matter how meaningful the signals are, they will be misinterpreted if they arrive at the wrong place. A happy-birthday telegram means just that, even if it should happen to reach the wrong person. But a slip-up in the nervous system is something else again.

Suppose you were listening to fast music—say, the Benny Goodman version of "Sing, Sing, Sing"—and the nerve signals somehow got switched to the wrong line, arriving at the visual areas of the cortex instead of the hearing areas. You'd "see" the music as a mad rush of flashing lights, moving forms, vivid colors. Such mix-ups actually occur, and may result from "cross talk" between nerve fibers. Cross talk is familiar to repair men of your local telephone company. If insulation wears off neighboring wires in a telephone cable, electricity leaks away and you may find yourself listening in on someone else's conversation.

Similar leaks in the nervous system may account for many peculiar sensory disorders. Current escaping from a touch fiber to a nearby sound fiber, for example, might make you hear crashing noises when you bumped your elbow. Somehow certain drugs increase cross talk among sensory fibers, and nerve injuries may produce the same effect. There is no reason to doubt that a certain amount of cross talk takes place in the normal nervous system; the nerve signals traveling through neighboring fibers interact in some way. We do not yet know the significance of this effect. But new evidence indicates that cross talk between fibers of the right and left eyes have something to do with the mechanism whereby we see objects as three-dimensional solids.

The brain is continually adjusting and readjusting the tensions of many muscles so that you maintain your posture and balance.

Simply standing up represents an acrobatic feat which is no less remarkable because it is performed automatically. Everyone naturally sways a bit in an upright position, and a failure in the balance-controlling centers of the brain would send you sprawling. There is one powerful muscle which, if uncontrolled, would snap your leg back at the knee, pressing your calf hard against your thigh. Another muscle would keep your leg stiff as a ramrod. The brain receives messages specifying the tensions of more than two hundred pairs of opposing muscles, every one of which must be properly adjusted to keep you standing.

Things become more complicated during a walk over uneven ground—and even more complicated when you dive from a high board, lower a sail in a storm or ride a surfboard. Every action, however simple, is made up of many individual muscle contractions and large-scale movements. These movements must follow one another at just the right time and in just the right order. The brain does the timing. It coördinates all sequences of movements so that we move smoothly and not in a series of jerks. When it comes to pursuing the activities of everyday life, we are thus reasonably sure of ourselves and our positions in the world.

The hand, working under the direction of the brain, is capable of an unlimited variety of skilled manipulations. A master pianist can play 120 notes a second, or a dozen notes a second with each finger. One famous surgeon used to put a piece of silk thread in a matchbox and impress reporters with the following trick. Working within the cramped space of the half-closed matchbox, he nonchalantly tied the thread into complicated surgical knots—using only the thumb, index and middle fingers of his left hand.

Every set of coördinated movements, from such highly skilled performances to routines like walking and driving a car, involve the integrating powers of the nervous system. All activities—direct or indirect, successful or unsuccessful—are attempts to keep the fire of life burning steadily and as long as possible. And this includes all our attempts to understand life itself.

Our adjustments are never perfect. Things are too complex and too uncertain for that. Still, we do not and cannot stop trying, and the brain coördinates our continuing efforts.

The Memory–

REMARKABLE STORAGE BATTERY

by Bruce Bliven

How are we able at will to summon up mental images of places seen years ago? What is the mysterious process involved? Because of brilliant laboratory work carried on in several countries in recent years we are beginning to find the answers to such questions. In essence, the physical process is electrical.

The human nervous system—brain, spinal cord and nerves—contains what is substantially a wet-cell electric battery, generating a direct current of about a tenth of a volt—roughly one twentieth as much as a flashlight battery. The electric charge is created by two body chemicals, sodium and potassium, operating on nerve tissues bathed in a fluid that is chiefly water. As each section of nerve fiber receives an electrical impulse, it triggers a reaction in the next section, so that impulses travel instantly to and from the marvelously intricate message centers of the brain.

To get a faint idea of what is going on continuously in the brain and the spinal cord, think of a thousand telephone switchboards, each big enough for a city like New York, going full tilt receiving and transmitting requests, questions, orders. Through its incredible ability to hook together thousands of reverberating circuits in a fraction of a second—each representing a memory or an idea—the brain is able to bring together into one grand circuit the data needed to think and make decisions.

Many scientists believe that every experience of our lives is recorded and preserved by these electrical circuits, including millions that we seem to have completely forgotten. Psychiatrists have found that when a patient tries day after day he can recall buried incidents of his childhood, even though he invariably begins by saying, "I don't remember a thing."

How the brain stores its memories is still not fully known. Some scientists believe that each item of memory is contained in a loop of cells connected by tiny tendrils with an electrical current going around and around the loop, which might be hundreds or thousands of cells in length. Other theories suggest that the memory is somehow impressed, or "etched" on the cell, or exists on a chain of cells like knots in a string. We do know that for the first thirty to sixty minutes after being received, any sensory impression is "floating around," so to speak, in the brain, not yet firmly registered. This may be why, after a sharp blow on the head, people often permanently forget what happened to them during the previous fifteen or twenty minutes.

Be that as it may, the number of items that can be remembered is far greater than the total number of brain cells. Dr. Ralph W. Gerard, a neurophysiologist at the University of Michigan, estimated that after seventy years of activity the brain may contain as many as fifteen *trillion* separate bits of information. Thus your memory is a treasure house whose size and strength are almost beyond human comprehension. It is a pity that so many of us store up so much less learning and experience than is possible.

Since our senses report, automatically and continuously, everything that we see, touch, hear, smell or taste, the avalanche of impressions would be overwhelming if there were not ways to screen them out. Fortunately at many points in the nervous system there are tiny gaps, called synapses, which prevent millions of minor signals, such as a one-degree change in temperature, from getting through. The electrical impression from any one nerve fiber is not strong enough to jump across one of these breaks, but the impression from a large bundle of fibers transmitting simultaneously can do so.

A good example of this protective mechanism is the retina of the eye, which has about 100,000,000 light-sensitive cells capable of transmitting an impression. But there are only about 1,000,000 nerve fibers leading back into the brain. Thus, before it can reach the brain, an impression has to be strong enough to command the response of at least 100 cells.

There are three main message centers in the brain. Each part receives and acts upon messages appropriate to its special functions. The medulla oblongata (see illustration) takes care of automatic functions like breathing and the pumping of the heart. The cerebrum with its covering of gray matter in turn is the seat of consciousness, memory, reason—in short, the human personality. The cerebellum controls the voluntary action of the muscles, partly on orders from the cerebrum. A reflex action, like with-

THE BRAIN

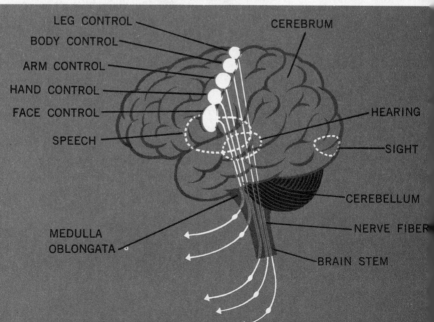

LEG CONTROL
BODY CONTROL
ARM CONTROL
HAND CONTROL
FACE CONTROL
SPEECH
CEREBRUM
HEARING
SIGHT
CEREBELLUM
NERVE FIBER
MEDULLA OBLONGATA
BRAIN STEM

drawing your foot when it is tickled, might be handled by the spinal cord alone.

The size of the brain area used by each part of the body is governed by the amount of conscious control the member requires—the more control, the larger the brain area. For example, the hands and fingers, which can perform highly complicated maneuvers, require a brain area much larger than that set aside for the legs. (The tongue and lips also require a proportionately big brain area.)

How are light, sound, temperature and the other aspects of the external world translated into seeing, hearing, feeling? All we know is that certain physical conditions cause our sense organs to transmit electrical messages to the appropriate receiving area in the brain, and that the quality of the sensation is determined by the pattern of impulses received.

While the brain is exposed during an operation, a small electrical charge applied to the nervous tissues where sight and hearing are recorded can make a patient see flashes of light or hear buzzing, ringing or knocking. Stimulation to a speech center will cause the individual to cry out like a baby but not to indulge in articulate speech, which is too complicated for such stimulation.

When these experiments are performed on individuals who are conscious (brain tissue is not sensitive to pain) they report that they do not feel as though some external force were causing the babylike cries to be uttered. On the contrary, they feel a strong but *inward* compulsion to cry out.

In many cases messages go simultaneously to more than one of the four main parts of the nervous system. Sometimes these centers are required to coöperate, sometimes not. You huddle deeper under a blanket on a cold night on orders from the cerebellum, but the message might also go up as high as the cerebrum and cause you to dream of the Arctic. But these are "low-priority" messages. An important signal, such as the smell of smoke in the night, alerts all the message centers, sets the electrical circuits flashing at a furious rate and leads to conscious action.

Many actions that require a great deal of conscious attention the first time they are performed can afterward be shunted down into a part of the brain functioning at a lower, less conscious level. Riding a bicycle, swimming and other skills which initially demand thought (cerebration) gradually become automatic or reflex actions. We also learn to discard from consciousness unwanted messages that are many times repeated. Thus a city dweller sleeps through the sound of traffic but is awakened in the country by the crowing of a distant rooster.

What causes mental disturbance? In both retarded mentality and certain types of insanity there is damage either to the brain cells themselves or to their electrical processes.

Excessive anxiety, ungovernable rage and other unreasonable states of mind evidently result from electrical circuits that get out of control. Some mental illnesses seem associated with the inability to bring together a sufficiently large number of the reverberating electrical circuits of the brain. The deluded individual who thinks he is Napoleon is able to use the circuits that contain the name of Napoleon and the fact that he was a general. But he is unable to connect with these circuits the ones that should tell him that Napoleon was somebody else who died many years ago.

What constitutes genius? Presumably the highly gifted person has some inborn capacity to coördinate his electrical circuits unusually well. The more we learn, the greater the store of memories on which we will be able to draw. The more we exercise the function of combining hundreds of circuits into larger ones, the easier it becomes and the more extensive these circuits will grow to be.

The late Sir Charles Sherrington, the great authority on the brain, after pointing out that man's brain is, in proportion to his weight, far larger than that of any of the animals, suggests that its evolution is still continuing: "Nor is the brain's present state, we may suppose, more than an interim phase, on the way to something else, something better, we may hope."

Can any more exciting prospect be held out to mankind?

Your Brain's Unrealized Powers

by Bruce Bliven

Here are seven important facts, some turned up by recent research, which can help you to use your brain more efficiently:

1. *There is no such thing as "brain fag."* Laymen often speak of "mental fatigue" or "brain fag," thinking that long, concentrated mental effort produces tiredness in the brain itself. Yet scientists believe that this state cannot exist. Your brain is not like your muscles. Its operations are not muscular but electrochemical in character.

When your brain appears tired after hours of mental work, the fatigue is almost certainly located in other parts of the body, your eyes or the muscles of your neck and back. The brain itself can go almost indefinitely.

A young woman undertook as an experiment to multiply in her head a series of two four-digit numbers, one after the other, as rapidly as possible. She went on doing this for twelve hours. During that time there was only a slight decrease in her efficiency, measured by speed and accuracy. At the end of twelve hours she stopped only because of bodily fatigue and hunger.

What seems like mental fatigue is often merely boredom. In

reading a difficult book, for example, you are torn between the desire to go on and the impulse to stop. According to Edgar J. Swift, psychologist of Washington University, it often is not fatigue that you feel but inattention and the inability to ignore distracting thoughts.

2. *The brain's capacity is almost inexhaustible.* That part of your brain involved in thinking and memory, and all your conscious activities, has as its most important part ten or twelve billion minute cells. Each of these has a set of tiny tendrils by means of which an electrochemical message can pass from one cell to another. Thinking and memory are associated with the passage of these electrical currents. The wisest man who ever lived came nowhere near using the full capacity of his wonderful mental storehouse. (Quite possibly, people in general employ only 10 to 15 percent of the capabilities of their brains.)

3. *Your IQ is less important than you probably think.* Many of us have an unnecessary inferiority complex about our IQs—the figure that represents native intelligence as compared to that of the average individual. It is easy to score *lower* in such a test than you deserve. This might result from temporary ill health or emotional disturbance. So, if you have ever seen your score on an IQ test, you can be reasonably sure that your IQ is *at least* that high.

What is the physical basis of high intelligence? Contrary to a common belief, it does not require an unusually large skull. It is likely to be associated with especially large numbers of surface convolutions in the cerebral cortex, the great top part of the brain. Highly intelligent people also have good blood circulation to the brain, bearing oxygen, glucose and certain other important chemicals. It is possible that a person with some very special talent—a mathematical or musical genius, for example—may have an unusually thick bundle of nerve fibers in one particular place in the brain.

But the physical endowment of your brain is far less important than what you do with it. The number of brain cells in an individual with an IQ of 100 (which is average) is large enough so that, used to the full, it could far exceed the record, so far as memory is concerned, of the greatest genius who ever lived. A person of average IQ who industriously stores up knowledge and skills year after year is better off than a person with a very high IQ who refuses to study. Research by the noted Yale psychologist, Dr. Catharine Cox Miles, indicated that some of the most important men in history had no more than ordinary IQs.

Among them, for example, are statesmen such as Cromwell, John Adams and Lincoln; military heroes like Drake, Napoleon and Nelson; writers like Goldsmith, Thackeray and Emerson. All these men, to be sure, were above the average in intelligence; yet they ranked far below the most brilliant of the individuals studied. What they possessed in high degree was *character*, and the ability to keep plodding ahead until they achieved what they had set out to do.

4. *Age need not prevent your learning.* One of the commonest misconceptions about the brain is that as you grow older something happens to it causing the learning process to become more difficult. This is true only to such a minute extent that for most of us it is of no practical importance.

Learning is associated with ability to create new reverberating electric circuits in the brain, and as long as that power remains you can continue to acquire new knowledge and skills—even at ninety.

It is true that all old people suffer impairment of their physical powers, and that some experience a decline of mental power. The best current medical opinion is that, in both cases, what happens is a series of minor "accidents" to various parts of our marvelously complicated physiological mechanism. None of these may be serious by itself, but the total effect can be severe.

Impairment of the brain in the aged is associated with decreased circulation of the blood and the precious substances it carries, especially oxygen and glucose. This is probably why old people remember happenings of their youth more vividly than those of the recent past; the youthful memories were implanted when blood circulation was better.

Yet severe mental impairment occurs only in some elderly people. Everyone knows of men and women who are vigorous and alert mentally into the ninth or even tenth decade of life. Their existence proves that impaired mental powers are not an inevitable accompaniment of passing years, but a result of disease processes.

Science knows of no reason why the average person cannot continue to learn with at least 85 to 90 percent efficiency through the seventh decade and beyond. It would be a fine thing if retired people went back to school or college or began to learn new skills and subjects. On the false notion that they are "too old to learn" millions of elderly people cut themselves off from exhilarating intellectual adventures.

5. *Your mental powers grow with use.* Like the muscular system of the body, the brain tends to atrophy with disuse, and to become better with exercise. This is proved by the fact that if the optic nerve is destroyed early in life, the brain cells in the corresponding visual area of the brain stay undeveloped.

As your brain matures, the nerve fibers are surrounded with a fatty substance called myelin, and they do not function properly until this has taken place. A newborn baby lacks most of its myelin, which is one reason why we cannot remember much that happened before we are two or three years old. Many physiologists believe that intensive exercise of any part of the brain encourages the growth of additional all-important myelin.

Anything you do with your brain exercises it, though obviously there is more exercise in doing something difficult than something easy. The more reasoning you do, the easier it is to go on to new reasoning. The ability to memorize also improves with practice. Robert S. Woodworth, professor emeritus of Columbia University, estimated that the time required to memorize anything can, with practice, be reduced as much as two thirds.

Every aspect of your personality is stored in your brain. This includes your willpower, which is also developed by practice. Each time you exert your will to drive yourself to the completion of an unpleasant or irksome task you make it a little easier next time to do what you need to do.

6. *The unconscious mind is a marvelous storehouse.* The most wonderful part of your mind is undoubtedly the unconscious, which lies below the recoverable memory and is thousands of times larger. We don't yet know very much about the unconscious mind, but we are learning fast and someday may know how to tap its great powers.

Your unconscious mind contains many millions of past experiences that, so far as your conscious mind knows, are lost forever. By means of several devices we now know how to bring back lost memories. One method is "free association," used by psychiatrists. If a patient lets his conscious mind wander at will, it can give him clues to forgotten things which, skillfully pursued by the doctor, will bring up whole networks of lost ideas and forgotten terrors. There are certain drugs which also help in this process; hypnotism, too, can be of tremendous value in exploring a patient's unconscious.

Many psychologists believe that we can make more use of our unconscious minds. Innumerable people have found that they can profitably "talk to" their unconscious. Some people find that they can bid themselves to wake up at a certain time in the morning. You can sometimes even improve your tomorrow's mood if you will say to yourself when you go to bed—and believe it—that you will be more cheerful in the morning.

7. *The "old" brain and the "new" can be kept in proper proportion.* Your brain may be described (with severe oversimplification) as having three parts: the upper, the middle and the lower. The lower section is where the automatic functions of the brain are performed—keeping the blood and lungs functioning, for instance. The midbrain participates in these operations but also serves as a bridge, to pass messages on to the upper brain or cerebral cortex. This top part of the brain is the single characteristic which most strongly separates man from animal.

The earliest living organisms on the earth had only a trace of the upper brain, or none at all; as we come down through evolution, the proportion steadily increases, which is why the upper is called the "new" brain. Even the highest of the primates, the chimpanzee and the gorilla, have at most only one third as much upper brain as a human being.

While we have been developing the new brain, we have, of course, retained all the characteristics of the "old" one. When certain areas inside your skull are electrically stimulated, you will bite and scratch like an animal. To some extent, the old brain represents ruthless egotism, while the new is the seat of elaborate abstract concepts like honor, *esprit de corps* and beauty. Growing up represents the triumph of the new brain over the old.

Deep emotion in the old brain can blot out the circuits in the new brain which represent reason and foresight. The man who commits a murder in a sudden rage knows, with his new brain, that he is likely to be caught and punished, but he does not think of these things until his passion has subsided.

We must not, of course, try to live by the intellect alone or reject the legitimate and important demands of the emotions. Pushing down into the unconscious a legitimate emotional impulse can only cause it to fester there. We must, however, try to keep the old brain and the new in proper proportion to each other, remembering that when either gets the upper hand too completely the human being cannot properly fulfill his destiny.

Suppose there should suddenly be dumped into man's conscious mind a small part of what he had forgotten: Out of all his past, ten million faces would surge up from darkness into a dreadful glare; a vast murmur of voices would gather out of silence and grow until it built pandemonium in his skull. In that sea of faces he would not find the few that had been dear to him; voices he had loved would be drowned in rapid chatter. The few good books he had read would be smothered under the ten thousand bad. Worst of all, he would search in vain among the trivialities, the broken purposes and the weak surrenders of his own past for that ideal self of which his weak memory had allowed him complacently to dream.

—Odell Shepard

Why Strokes Occur

Adapted from "Why Strokes Occur" *by Irvine H. Page, M.D., and* "What You Should Know about Strokes" *by Tom Mahoney*

❧

The stroke which President Eisenhower suffered was not caused, as some news stories suggested, by worries over Sputnik. It was a so-called "little stroke," one of the commonest ailments of men in their sixties the world over. In all likelihood the stroke would have occurred even if the President had been living a calm, uneventful existence on his Gettysburg farm.

The word "stroke"—literally a striking down—has frightening overtones for most people. A stroke can be very serious, even fatal. But it can also be quite mild. A "little stroke" does not necessarily shorten a person's life and may impair his faculties only temporarily. It most certainly should not be looked upon as the end of a man's productive life.

Strokes, which doctors term "cerebrovascular accidents," or apoplexy, have advanced from seventh to third place among the natural causes of death, and are now behind only heart disease and cancer. More than 140,000 people in the United States are killed by strokes each year, and at least four times this number suffer nonfatal strokes. Yet stroke receives less attention than many maladies that affect fewer persons.

Often called apoplexy, a stroke occurs when the blood supply to the brain, or to some portion of it, is cut off. To perform its

vital functions the brain needs an enormous quantity of oxygen—
20 percent of the total amount consumed by the body. It gets
this oxygen directly from the bloodstream. More than a pint and
a half of blood must be circulated through the brain every minute.
If brain cells are denied their quota of oxygen for even five
minutes, they die. Once killed, they cannot grow back. Though
this damage is irreparable, the brain's ability to perform all functions is often recovered. The area affected may be large or small.

A stroke usually takes place in the cerebrum, that part of the
brain where nerve centers controlling sight, hearing, speech and
bodily movements are located. These zones of nerve cells are on
the surface of the cerebrum, and nerve fibers run from them deep
into the brain and on down the spinal cord, carrying impulses
between the zones and the parts of the body they affect. If a
blockage stops blood flow to one of these control zones, or to
nerve fibers leading from the zones, then the activity controlled
by the zone will be impaired. For example, if the nerve center
controlling speech is damaged, the ability of the zone to coördinate ideas and words and to send correct signals through the
nerves to tongue and vocal cords is affected. The victim will
find his ability to speak impaired.

There are at least four ways in which a stroke can take place:

1. *Clotting.* In atherosclerosis, fatty substances like cholesterol
accumulate on the walls of the blood vessels, narrowing the space
through which the blood can pass. (Atherosclerosis is the most
serious form of hardening of the arteries.) As the blood flow slows
down, it may begin to stagnate. Tiny "platelets"—specks of
chemical "dust" in the bloodstream—may begin to cluster on
rough spots caused by atherosclerosis. Thus coagulation may
form the core of a clot, or thrombus, which blocks the further
flow of blood and produces a condition known as thrombosis.

Sometimes the artery seems to be closed by a nervous spasm.
Occasionally the spasm relaxes or the brain manages to establish
some circulation around the obstruction. When this happens,
many of the impaired brain abilities return and much of the
paralysis disappears.

Another form of clotting is called embolism. After surgery and under some other conditions, a blood clot, or embolus, may break away in the body and be carried through arteries to the brain, where it blocks a blood vessel. *Embolus* is from the Greek word meaning "a plug." When strokes occur in young persons, a cerebral embolism usually is responsible.

Once lodged in the brain, little can be done about an embolus. But administration of one of the "anticoagulant" drugs may prevent the formation of additional emboli or growth of the one already present. Anticoagulants also slow coagulation of the blood and prevent formation of emboli during surgery.

2. *Hemorrhage.* A brain artery may rupture. The blood escapes, damaging the surrounding tissue. Since the brain floats in cerebrospinal fluid and is encased by unyielding bone, much bleeding may also cause serious pressure on the brain. Cerebral hemorrhage—usually detectable by blood in the spinal fluid—is harder to recover from than any other type of stroke.

If the hemorrhage is massive, death may come swiftly. But most hemorrhages are small. There may be only a slow leakage of blood, only a few tiny arteries and capillaries broken down. The damage may not be enough to cause the patient to lose consciousness.

Some clots resulting from cerebral hemorrhage may be removed by surgery. Where the clot has not hardened, the surgeon may drill a small hole in the skull and drain the liquid clot through a hollow needle.

3. *Compression.* A tumor, swollen brain tissue or a large clot from a cerebral blood vessel may press hard enough upon an adjoining blood vessel to stop its flow.

4. *Spasm.* An artery of the brain may constrict and thus reduce or pinch off the blood passage, the damage depending upon how long it takes the affected artery to relax again. The specific role of spasms of the cerebral vessels and whether they actually occur in stroke are subjects of medical controversy.

The seriousness of a stroke depends upon which blood vessel is affected, the kind of blockage, how long the brain areas involved go without oxygen, plus a number of other considerations. In many cases, especially among younger persons, other blood vessels may take over the functions of the one blocked. Sometimes, even when certain brain centers have died, other areas of the brain are able gradually to take over.

On rare occasions the victim of a stroke may be a young person, even a child. In such cases the stroke results from some illness like rheumatic fever or extremely high blood pressure. It might also result from an aneurysm (a blood-filled pouch) of a blood vessel, which the child was born with. Surgery can often remove this difficulty and, if the rest of the circulatory system is healthy, the child can look forward to a normal life span.

The average age of a stroke victim is sixty-four. There has been a steady increase in the number of strokes among our people in recent years, because the number of elderly persons has been increasing. Elderly males seem to succumb more easily than elderly females. No reliable statistics are available on the frequency of recurrence of strokes, but it is generally agreed that, in most cases, a stroke victim is sooner or later stricken again.

If the stroke victim does not die—and he usually does not—a variety of things may happen to him. He may feel tired, numb, weak, stuporous or confused. He may show emotional or personality changes. He may have headaches and suffer disturbances of vision, speech or memory. He may lose sensation in certain parts of his body. He may not be able to walk. He may be stricken paralytically and have to lie in bed for years. There are about two million such incapacitated or handicapped stroke victims in the U.S.A. today. Many of them could be at least partially rehabilitated by properly supervised nursing care, adequate diet, massage and exercise.

What can you do to avoid a stroke? You can, first of all, have a thorough annual physical examination that will include checking your blood pressure and your heart action. Strokes usually do not come without warning signs.

Approximately one out of every four individuals with a blood pressure of over 200 eventually may have a stroke, reported Dr. Harry J. Johnson, medical director of the Life Extension Examiners, an organization of doctors which has made nearly three million health examinations. Early detection of high blood pressure gives you the opportunity to reduce it. In doing so, you reduce your chance of having heart attacks as well as strokes.

Additional premonitory symptoms of stroke include: severe aches in the back of the head and neck, dizziness or fainting, motor or sensory nerve disturbances, nosebleeds and certain hemorrhages in the retina of the eye. These symptoms, however, can be found with other diseases and are not necessarily indicative of high blood pressure or pending stroke.

The causes of high blood pressure remain in dispute, but doctors have come up with several methods of controlling it: (1) avoidance of overweight and strain of all kinds; (2) various diets; (3) surgery—the severing of nerves which constrict the arteries; (4) drugs which temporarily relax the blood vessels.

Happily the body is often capable of making its own repairs. Some physicians advocate anticoagulants as a preventive measure. But there is no unanimity about the worth of this treatment; there is no certain evidence that it might not in some cases be harmful. Going on a low-fat diet in the hope of preventing a stroke is futile once atherosclerosis has made its subversive inroads.

A stroke is obviously not to be brushed aside lightly. On the other hand, one should not get panicky when one occurs. A little stroke might do no more than make the victim feel a bit ill and cause some slight, momentary disturbance of his faculties. Even a more severe stroke is seldom as severe as it seems at first. In the shock of the initial impact a victim and his family may feel that he is hopelessly paralyzed or has gone out of his mind. This is hardly ever the case. And it does no one any good, least of all the victim, if everyone acts as though the funeral notices had gone out. Even the severest cases can recover with astonishing rapidity.

A stroke does not necessarily mean the end of a career. Louis Pasteur, the great French scientist who fathered microbiology, lived twenty-seven years and did his greatest work after suffering a stroke at forty-six. Sir Joshua Reynolds produced a hundred canvases after a stroke at fifty-nine. George Frederick Handel composed his immortal *Messiah* and lived for many years after a stroke.

Great advances have been made in the treatment and retraining of stroke patients by a number of hospitals, including those caring for war veterans. Special exercises, water therapy and electric devices are employed to restore function to limbs and teach undamaged brain centers to take over the tasks from those that have been injured.

Much, of course, depends on the patient's own courage and desire to regain his skills. It is humiliating for a man to have to learn to speak again, to have to teach his left hand to do what his right did, to have to learn to tie his shoes. He needs all the understanding that his friends and family can give him.

When Pasteur was stricken with a cerebral thrombosis, his condition seemed so hopeless that construction was stopped on a laboratory the government was building for him. Pasteur learned of this, and declined rapidly. His friends appealed to Emperor Napoleon III, who ordered construction resumed. Pasteur then began to recover and in the new laboratory conquered rabies and half a dozen other diseases.

∽

No ROBOT could come even close to duplicating the human brain. A machine even remotely like it would have to be about the size of Rockefeller Center, and it would take several lifetimes to wire it up. The electrical-power requirements would be about equal to the power used now to supply the greater part of New York City. And the necessary cooling system would be so enormous that you'd probably have to divert the Hudson to supply it.   —Dr. Norbert Wiener

PART 2 · THE HEART

Knowledge of the heart has become a very necessary part of our daily living. In a sense, each man has now become his own doctor, for it is not the wonders of heart surgery—marvelous though they are—but practicing good sense that preserves the human heart.

It is a wonderful machine. The following section reveals not only how it works but how you should keep it in working order.

The Heart—

WONDROUS, COURAGEOUS ORGAN

by Henry Morton Robinson

Don't worry too much about your heart, as so many healthy people seem to be doing nowadays; rejoice, rather, that nature has placed in your breast one of her most delicate yet durable marvels, an organ of surpassing patience, flexibility and strength. Rejoice, and try to understand how it works. It will work all the better for being understood.

Borrow a doctor's stethoscope, and listen to the beating of your own heart. In its steady rhythm—lubb-*dup*, lubb-*dup*—you will hear the sound of life itself as blood courses through the valves and chambers of this inimitable pump. For the heart, mechanically speaking, is just that—a pressure pump which forces the blood, with its freight of oxygen, food or waste, through the vessels of the body.

Driven by the heart, the approximately six quarts of blood in the average human body make a round trip about once every minute. In twenty-four hours the heart receives and pumps out again between seven and nine thousand quarts of blood. In a life span of the Biblical three score years and ten, the heart lubb-*dups* some two and a half billion times, without a single shutdown for repairs. And—so it seems to one listening through the stethoscope—without a rest.

Yet, without rest no muscle can endure, and the heart is a muscle. Though brief, the pauses between *dup* and the next lubb are rest enough. The normal heart, like man himself, spends twice as much time relaxing as it does at work. Besides, the heart draws extra rations. Though it weighs but 1/200 of the body's weight, it requires 1/20 of the blood in circulation for itself.

Your heart is about the size of your fist and is snugly enclosed in a tough protective covering called the pericardium. Attached to the body only by the great blood vessels stemming from its base, it hangs within your chest, pointing diagonally downward toward your left breast. It is divided into two parts, right and left, by a blood-tight wall. Each part forms a separate pump.

And each of these two pumps, in turn, has two interacting chambers: the auricle, which receives blood into the heart from the veins, and the ventricle, which forces it out again into the body through the arteries. The heart's specialized muscles are so cunningly layered and interwoven that they can squeeze, twist and literally wring out the contents of their chambers at every lubb—in other words, at every contraction of the pump.

What causes the heart to beat? This question, asked seventeen hundred years ago by the anatomist Galen, was not answered until about 1890, when investigators began to suspect electrochemical energy. They were right. We now know that a kind of electrical timing apparatus called the pacemaker normally generates, about seventy times a minute, a tiny electrical impulse which sweeps down and across the muscle fibers, causing them to contract.

The heart, then, is a kind of electromuscular pump, contrived by millions of years of evolution, for the purpose of keeping the blood circulating in two main circuits. One, starting from the left chamber of the heart, is the great systemic circuit, which the blood makes through the entire body for the purpose of maintaining its tissues. A shorter, independent circuit goes from the right chamber of the heart to the lungs, to let the blood discharge its freight of carbon dioxide and pick up life-renewing oxygen. This is the pulmonary circulation.

In order fully to understand the action of the heart, let us trace more precisely the course of the blood. Dark venous blood, laden with carbon dioxide and waste matter picked up in its progress through the body's veins, is drawn into the right auricle as the auricle lies momentarily relaxed. When the auricle is filled, the valve in its floor opens and the blood pours into the ventricle below.

When the ventricle is full, its smooth pumping pressure closes the valve, which bellies out like a parachute. This same pressure

THE HEART

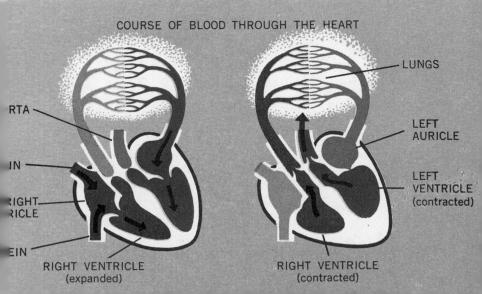

COURSE OF BLOOD THROUGH THE HEART

LUNGS

RTA

LEFT AURICLE

IN

LEFT VENTRICLE (contracted)

RIGHT RICLE

EIN

RIGHT VENTRICLE (expanded)

RIGHT VENTRICLE (contracted)

simultaneously *opens* another set of valves (half-moon-shaped) and forces blood out of the ventricle into the artery that leads directly to the lungs. In the thin-walled network of the lungs the dark blood is purified by exchanging its load of carbon dioxide for oxygen from the outer air. Thus freshened, the blood returns bright crimson to the heart—and the marvel of pulmonary circulation has been accomplished in less than ten seconds.

Meanwhile, the left chamber of the heart, more powerful than the right, carries on the next phase in rhythmic unison with the first. Fresh from the lungs, the blood enters the left auricle. When the auricle is full, the valve opens and the ventricle begins to fill. A fraction of a second later the ventricle contracts, pushing its cupful of blood into the aorta, the huge artery that leads out from the base of the heart. When the pressure in the aorta exceeds that from the ventricle, the half-moon valves between them close. The brisk *dup* that you hear is the sound of the valves as they slam shut.

From the aorta, widest of the rivers of life, the red flood branches out, ever more slowly, through arteries and arterioles and tiny capillaries, to every cell in the body.

The heart repeats this process of contracting and relaxing, of systole and diastole, lubb-*dup*, lubb-*dup*, day after day, year in, year out, in disease and health, through sleep, love and battle, with the enduring constancy of time itself, with an efficiency not equaled by any of man's inventions, and a courage that passes all understanding.

In 1816 in Paris, a physician, René Laënnec, was consulted by a young and buxom female suffering from a heart ailment. Being too modest to put his ear against her bosom to listen to her heart, he tried a rolled-up piece of paper and found it conveyed the sound distinctly. This led to his famous invention—the stethoscope.   —Freling Foster

Steady Pace or Heartbreak?

Adapted from "The World's Most Efficient Pump" *by G. A. Skinner and* "Stop Breaking Your Heart" *by Howard Whitman*

❧

There is no man-made pump that compares in efficiency with the human heart. It is able to run a hundred years and more without the loss of even a few minutes for repairs.

Even this efficient machine needs care, for the causes operating to induce heart trouble are many. Probably among the first is rheumatic fever, found often among young people. This is very likely to leave the heart damaged, although the patient may seem completely recovered and may even indulge in quite heavy athletics for some years. But trouble develops in the thirties, as a rule, and in the fifties or earlier the person with this sort of heart may break down.

Then there is the rapid pace of present-day life, to which some ascribe much of the increase in the death rate from heart disease of recent years. Hearts today are as good as those of yesterday, except for the changed conditions under which they are forced to labor. Years of constant tension may lead to high blood pressure, increasing materially the burden on the heart. In time permanent damage is done which, if nothing more, restricts considerably the physical activities of the possessor.

Certain methods of exercise use up the reserves of the heart with undue rapidity. One of the most serious is the common custom, indulged in by many men who spend most of their time at desks, of trying to get a month's exercise, very strenuously, in a single day. Especially dangerous is it for such a man on a fishing or hunting trip to go into competition with guides and others who are physically active much of the time. His pride insists that he keep up with them and he does—but often at the cost of a serious heart strain. Youth withstands much more of this sort of strain than do middle or late life, as the elastic limit of the circulatory system is in youth much higher.

The same sort of strain takes place in comparatively young men who, splendidly trained athletes in college, have then let all training go. In the course of ten years or so they acquire a fine income, a family and probably thirty or forty pounds of surplus weight. They decide that something must be done. If exercise is taken in moderation and gradually increased as the body becomes accustomed to it, the results usually will be excellent. Often, however, the same vigor is used right at the start that was the habit of college days, and trouble is almost certain.

In order to remain at the greatest efficiency, the heart, like all other muscles, should be used not only reasonably, but regularly. Otherwise, the reserve built up in active days is gradually lost, and the heart gets "soft," unable to withstand sudden or prolonged strains. If, however, the individual takes a fair amount of exercise daily he is always in training and the heart will withstand astonishing loads, even in late life. It is the man playing often for short periods throughout his career who can play tennis in the late sixties, apparently without harm.

There is no set time that a man becomes old, but long observation has set fifty as the age to commence to slow down in every way, particularly in strenuous physical exertions. A man may boast that he is as good as he was at twenty-five, but he is not, no matter how much he may feel that way.

The greatest protection against heart attack, suggests Dr. Irvine H. Page, famed heart specialist of the Cleveland Clinic, is the "achievement of equanimity." "Some men can achieve this intellectually," he comments. "They ask themselves, 'What kind of philosophy do I intend to live by?' And they find one which nurtures life instead of destroying it. Others achieve equanimity emotionally, through a belief in beauty, in ideals, in unselfishness. They let the annoyances of life pass in one side and out the other."

This does not mean that you should deliberately repress your emotions, however. When you get angry—and all of us do, at times—most doctors believe there is greater danger in holding your anger back than in expressing it. Dr. Henry I. Russek comments, "That's why we need 'gripe sessions' in our daily lives. Easy release of angry feelings not only lessens the danger of continuing inner pressure but makes violent blow-offs less necessary."

Uↄ

The Why and How of Heart Attacks

Adapted from "Stop Breaking Your Heart!" by Howard Whitman and "Candidates for Heart Attack" by George Dock

Many people have thanked God for their heart attacks. They have recovered to find a new life with greater satisfactions, more peace. But why do so many of us have to wait until we come within an inch of death to learn this lesson? Can't we learn how to live *before* the heart attack?

I put the question to a famous coronary victim, Kentucky author and poet Jesse Stuart, who suffered a heart attack some years ago. "People just won't listen," he said. "I wouldn't listen myself until the good Lord gave me a heart attack."

Just what is the lesson life is trying to teach? What is the truth to which people won't listen? It is this: A person's attitudes toward life, his emotions, are strongly linked to heart attacks. There are indications that they may be as important as such better-defined factors as overweight, diet and heredity.

The heart and the emotions are tied together in language we use daily: *heartbroken, heavyhearted, heartfelt, heartache.* Physicians in ancient times considered the heart the seat of the emotions but could not prove it. Modern physicians are at last proving the effect that emotions have on the heart's behavior.

A study by Dr. Henry I. Russek, U.S. Public Health Service consultant in cardiovascular research, and Professor Burton L. Zohman, of the State University of New York College of Medicine, found emotional stress four and a half times more prevalent in coronary victims than in people with healthy hearts. The coronary victim, they report, "commonly possesses an ambitious, driving nature and exhibits a consistent tendency toward compulsive striving, self-discipline and hard work. He frequently sets herculean tasks for himself, exceeding his normal capacity and tempo, minimizing warning signals and neglecting prudent rules of health."

Drs. Meyer Friedman and Ray H. Rosenman, of San Francisco, made a study of two specially selected groups of men. Group A consisted of highly competitive, ambitious men who were constantly fighting deadlines. Group B men were easygoing, with far less drive. Seven hundred percent more heart disease was discovered in Group A!

In a study of coronary patients at Temple University Hospital, Philadelphia, Dr. Edward Weiss and his colleagues found "gradually mounting tension" prior to the attack in 49 percent of the cases and "acute emotional stress" just before the attack in 37 percent. They checked an equal number of noncoronary patients and found no instances of gradually mounting tension, and acute emotional stress in only 9 percent.

One of the patients was a forty-three-year-old machinist in charge of a number of machines in a large shop, who took pride in keeping them in perfect working order. Here's how he described his own "gradually mounting tension": "Everything was okay until the last few weeks. Then the boss started a speedup. The equipment broke down, and as fast as we could rebuild it something else would break. Work used to be enjoyable, but now I hated to get up in the morning. All the knocks I've had in life couldn't add up to this. When I saw my work being smashed to pieces, it broke my heart."

How can emotions break the heart?

"Under stress of emotion, adrenalin is poured into the bloodstream from the adrenal glands," explains Dr. Herbert Pollack of New York University Postgraduate Medical School. "This causes the smaller arteries to contract. The heart, in an effort to maintain full circulation in the face of this resistance, steps up the pulse rate and blood pressure. When the adrenalin secretion causes the *coronary* blood vessels to contract, the heart muscle is deprived of its full blood supply and the result is pain which we call angina pectoris. This type of adrenalin response may predispose an individual to actual permanent blocking of a coronary blood vessel—coronary occlusion."

Nature intends that shot of adrenalin to provide extra strength and alertness to meet whatever threat brought on the emotional surge. Primitive man found it useful in encounters with wild beasts. So does modern man when he fights a fire in his basement or snatches his child from the path of a car. But continual tension, repeated emotional emergencies—as though all of life were a crisis—is more than nature bargained for.

The damage usually begins long before a heart attack—in the narrowing of the arteries by the formation of fatty deposits in their linings. The process (atherosclerosis) which thickens the inner arterial wall also roughens it, and blood clots form more readily in contact with the rough surface.

Today there is evidence that emotional tension, in addition to its direct effect on the blood vessels as described above, hastens the process of narrowing the coronary blood vessels by interfering with the metabolism of fats and overloading the bloodstream with the fatty substance—cholesterol—which thickens the arteries.

Cholesterol is an essential element of the blood. It is manufactured within the liver and is also absorbed from the cholesterol contained in certain foods—including animal fats, egg yolk, butter, cream and milk—the most valuable of all foods for infants, growing children and undernourished adults. Cholesterol is not found in fruit, vegetables, cereals or nuts. Lean meat and fish contain a little of it, and provide large amounts of protein, which seems to give the body the power to burn up some of the excess cholesterol in our blood.

Postmortems made upon thousands of Chinese revealed astonishingly few cases of coronary illness or the atheromata (fatty deposits in the walls of arteries) which are its forerunners. In China, rice and protein-rich millet and soybeans are the mainstay of millions. Eggs, milk and animal fats are almost unknown luxuries to them. The blood-cholesterol level of the average Chinese is little more than half as high as that of most Americans.

U.S. Army medical officers have been disturbed by the high death rate from coronary disease among American troops (especially in the lower age brackets) in training camps in the United States, where the per capita consumption of eggs, milk and fatty foods was far above the average peacetime intake.

British troops, who drank more tea than milk, and ate more bread and beef than ice cream and eggs, incurred a considerably lower death rate from coronary attack. So there seems to be a definite relationship between high-cholesterol diet and high coronary mortality.

Resistance to coronary disease is very much a matter of heredity, because of the importance of the inborn thickness of the arterial lining, which varies so widely among people of any age group. But the rate at which that lining takes on greater thickness and a rough surface is the deadliest factor in laying the individual open to coronary attack. Some experts believe it can be slowed down through dietary measures.

People vary in their ability to deal with cholesterol. Many persons keep their blood cholesterol at safe levels even on food containing a great deal of that substance. Others develop fatally high cholesterol on diets practically free from it.

It is well to remember that the problem of human diet is complex, that individuals vary greatly in their needs. We all know families whose members live to a vigorous old age on diets that fairly sag with cream and eggs and fats. But they may owe their long lives to a rare combination of congenitally thin coronary linings, some inherited mechanism for burning up surplus cholesterol and a healthy supply of protein in their fare.

A U.S. Air Force doctor, Colonel Marshall E. Groover, tested the blood-cholesterol levels in a group of Air Force officers under emotionally placid conditions and later under stressful circumstances. In some, emotional stress caused a remarkable rise. One officer had a cholesterol level, when calm, of 190 (milligrams per 100 milliliters of blood serum). After he got news that his son had quit school to be married, it spurted to 380.

Drs. Friedman and Rosenman checked the cholesterol levels of a group of accountants: the average was 210. But just before April 15, when the emotional stress of a tax deadline was upon them, their cholesterol level averaged 252.

What are the outward signs of the man who is building toward a heart attack? (It *is* most frequently a man. Statistics indicate that the death rate from heart disease in middle age is almost three times as high in men as in women.) Can we identify him in advance? Some doctors think we *can* select the men among whom coronary disease may develop.

"When one has studied 'younger' patients with coronary disease, one knows that they exhibit rather telltale characteristics," say Dr. Friedman and Dr. Rosenman, who have encountered many such individuals at Mount Zion Hospital and Medical Center. "For example, these men frequently use emphatic gestures, particularly the clenched fist, to accompany their talking. They scan each day in advance to see how much activity they can squeeze into it, and how they can accelerate any project's pace. They hate to waste time.

"When you talk to the coronary-prone man, he often believes he knows what you're going to say before you've actually said it. He will sometimes finish your sentence for you, or his lips will silently finish it, or he may urge you on by saying 'Yes, yes,' at intervals."

In addition to the usually recommended regime of low-fat diet and moderate exercise, Drs. Friedman and Rosenman try to put such patients on a deceleration program. "Get up early enough so you won't have to rush," they say. "Cut out unnecessary activities, delegate duties that you don't *have* to do yourself."

The doctors use a timepiece as a symbol of their patients' trouble. Dr. Rosenman keeps track of the number of times his patients look at their watches during an interview—it may be as many as sixteen times in an hour. When he brings this to their attention, they get the point.

Most men can reduce the emotional stress in their lives without sacrificing mental creativeness and the enjoyment of full living. In my home town, for example, forty-nine-year-old Bill Torno runs a lumberyard. He had a heart attack on March 28. Now he calls it his "birthday." "That's when I learned how to live for the first time," he says. "Before the coronary I was always on the go. I felt that I had to be on top of *every* detail in the business—and every aggravation, too. Now I get to the yard at 8:30 instead of 7:30. If I see an aggravating argument building up, I just walk away from it. And you know something? The business runs better! I have time to think of the really important things."

Bill Leonard, CBS television and radio broadcaster, who had a heart attack at forty, observed: "Before it happened, I thought there was no excuse for not taking on more work. When a fellow got older, okay; but up to forty-five or fifty he ought to take on anything. Being tired certainly was no excuse."

When Leonard's coronary struck, he was doing nineteen radio and TV programs a week. The industry knew him as indefatigable. After the attack he said: "I simply don't try as hard, as much or as often. I'm lazier—and it doesn't bother me. I spend more time just doing things I like to do—playing bridge, taking long walks, playing golf."

Life is almost always sweeter for the man who has survived a heart attack. There are now many "Coronary Clubs" of happy men, but unfortunately thousands don't live to join them.

Can't we have a "*No Coronary* Club" for those who are smart enough to understand their peril before death makes them forever ineligible?

How to Live After An Attack

by Peter F. Steincrohn, M.D.

Many a man might be saved after a heart attack if he were fortunate enough to break a leg also. The enforced rest would give his heart the opportunity to recover. But that isn't the whole story. Treating the heart properly doesn't depend entirely upon what you do for it those first few weeks after the attack. It's how you live forever after that matters.

Most people do not realize that the heart patient often lives with his disease for many years. Many cardiacs who have dreaded being shuffled off in a matter of days have lived twenty, thirty or forty years longer than they thought possible. Much needless illness and suffering can be avoided when the patient knows what the doctor is trying to accomplish.

All heart trouble isn't serious. Three out of four fearful persons who walk into the doctor's office have normal hearts. A fleeting pain in the left chest ("It's right over my heart"); the recent loss of a relative or friend ("Why, I saw Jack only yesterday and he looked perfectly healthy"); the desire for reassurance ("There's so much heart trouble around, Doctor")—these are only a few of the things that strike fear into healthy people.

On the other hand, many people who actually have heart disease don't visit their physicians for a checkup. John Jones refuses to chance "hearing the bad news." John Brown uses these excuses: "It's just because I'm slowing up," or "It's only indigestion." Yet the "acute indigestion" reported in former years was often heart disease.

Here is a simple formula, for the healthy as well as for the heartsick, that guarantees a smoother trip along the road to longevity:

First. Visit your doctor for a physical checkup if you have any of the following symptoms: chronic cough, spitting up of blood, fainting spells, asthmatic attacks, swelling of the ankles, gas pressure, tiredness, indigestion, palpitation, rapid pulse, shortness of breath, chest pain, dizziness or the inability to lie flat in bed.

Second. Listen only to what the *doctor* says. Specific advice for the individual should not come from sympathetic but untrained friends, from papers, periodicals or books.

Third. Get plenty of rest—rest—and more rest. This is the prescription *par excellence* for the tired heart. In no other disease is it so true that he who knows how to rest lives longest.

There are many kinds of heart disease: congenital, rheumatic, syphilitic, atherosclerotic, bacterial, among others. They are in many ways similar, but in more ways different. Medicine has appropriate drugs for each, but there is only one basic treatment. Call it a Way of Life. Without it most other treatment is useless.

Some years ago Dr. Charles Miner Cooper, a well-known San Francisco physician, wrote the following letter to a patient who had suffered a heart attack. Now practically a West Coast classic through wide circulation and reprinting, it contains sound advice even for those who are in good health.

Dear Mr. Blank:
You have evidently made an excellent recovery from your recent heart attack. That attack should have warned you to live a life which would lessen the work of your heart. However, you have continued to be overweight; you have been eating and drinking as much as you desire. You have carried on strenuous business activities, working long hours and often at top speed. You have not curbed your quick and, at times, rather violent emotional reactions. The load on your heart has been too heavy. Hence you now are incommoded by shortness of breath and other disturbing symptoms.

You come to me for advice, as you have gone to other doctors, perhaps hoping that I can give you a drug which will enable you to carry on as you have been doing. Unfortunately there is no such drug. But let me outline a regime which will help you immensely if, after a period of almost complete physical, mental and emotional rest, you will follow it very conscientiously:

1. You should bring your weight down to what is normal for your height, build and age. This reduction must be brought about slowly, by modifying your diet and by graduated exercises—not by reducing drugs. Refrain permanently from overloading your stomach on any occasion.

2. You must cut down the extent and speed of your physical activities. Do not run to catch a train, hurry up stairs, attempt to park an automobile in a closed-in space, or use any set of muscles to the limit of your vigor. Refrain from physical effort immediately after eating, and do nothing that will make you short of breath. If at any time you begin to breathe fast, or experience a constricting chest pain, lie down and rest.

3. You must indulge in mental tasks only when your mind is fresh, and cease them when you become weary. Thus you will be able to give your best consideration to business problems with the least strain to yourself.

4. You must curb your emotional reactions. When I tell you that I have known a patient's blood pressure to jump 60 points

almost instantaneously in response to an outburst of anger, you can understand what strain such reactions can throw upon the heart. I realize that you are quick on the trigger and inclined to blame those whose behavior incites you, rather than to consider yourself foolish for letting them disturb you. Such a viewpoint is not uncommon. The great Scottish surgeon John Hunter, suffering from much the same condition as you, and appreciating the effect of such emotional reactions upon his heart, said his life was in the hands of any rascal who chose to annoy him. Even he forgot that he should discipline himself, and he had a fatal attack during a fit of anger.

Whenever a business problem starts to vex you, or you begin to get angry, let yourself go limp all over. This will dissipate your mounting inner turmoil.

5. Try to be cheerful under all circumstances. Unfortunately, you are a moody man, given at times to considerable sadness. Such a state does not lend itself to the proper energization of the heart and blood vessels. It may seem to you that to be cheerful when you are inclined to sadness is easier said than done. Let me make a suggestion: Whenever you are feeling down in the dumps, think of some particularly pleasing worthwhile experience you have had. Your mood will often respond to the thought.

If you were a smoker, I should have to tell you to refrain entirely, as I believe tobacco to be injurious to those afflicted with degenerative cardiovascular lesions.

Your heart is calling for a complete change in your ways. It is further asking that it be permanently housed in a lean, cheerful, placid man who will intelligently curb his physical, mental and emotional activities.

I have a number of patients who years ago had the same thing happen to their hearts as has happened to yours. Today they are still enjoying a sense of well-being and are doing valuable work. You may similarly respond if you will seriously follow the foregoing regime.

Magic in Breathing

by W. P. Knowles

During the past thirty years Captain William P. Knowles has been consulted by more than 60,000 sufferers from respiratory complaints. At the Institute of Breathing in London, which he founded, some 500 persons a year study correct breathing practice. In World War II Captain Knowles instructed RAF and Army personnel on ways to achieve physical fitness.

I have a theory that famous work songs, ranging from those of the Volga boatmen to the cadent melodies of the Negro, offered more than just a rhythmic beat to help in hauling that barge, or toting that bale. It's my belief that the songs encourage men to *breathe out* while they worked, to release air from the lungs in a moderate and orderly manner. You can't sing without exhaling gradually, and when you exhale you expel impurities and empty the lungs for a fresh and involuntary intake of air.

Real breath control means learning to control the way we *exhale*, not the way we *inhale*. Energy is best renewed by the orderly release of breath, not by strenuously pumping the lungs full of air. Thus in sustained physical exertion—carrying a heavy bag, walking rapidly, wielding a garden shovel—your power is enhanced when you concentrate on the slow expulsion of air from the lungs.

Speakers, singers, swimmers and runners know this. The rest of us can find it out by simple tests. When you step into a cold shower, for example, the tendency is to gasp and tense the muscles. This only increases the torture. If, instead, you try breathing out in a steady purring breath, you will be amazed at how slightly the temperature of the water affects you. Exhaling helps the body accommodate itself to change.

The next time you have something heavy to lift—whether it be a large pot of soup, a typewriter or a suitcase—try taking a full, deep breath and holding the breath while you lift. Much of the weight oddly disappears. The effect is like picking up a box expecting it to be full, only to find it empty.

Those who have played the game of levitation have found that a person or a table can be hoisted by the mere finger action of a group if all present breathe deeply and simultaneously as they lift. This illustrates the mysterious aid that comes from conscious and calculated use of breathing.

Careful breath control, with emphasis on exhaling, helps us to relax under any kind of tension or stress. Most of us are only half-breathers: we breathe in because we can't help it but we fail to breathe out completely. The result is that we sigh a lot— a sign of our need to exhale. The sigh is nature's way of deflating the lungs when we have neglected the breathing apparatus long enough. The sensible thing is to learn to sigh in a systematic and organized fashion. We know that any interference with breathing causes acute distress. It follows, as common sense and science show, that any improvement in our breathing can bring exhilaration to mind and body.

Normally we do breathe without apparent effort—about 18 times a minute, 1080 times an hour, 25,920 times a day. The more air we exhale, the more we can breathe in. The amount we take in, which can be measured by a watch-size instrument called a spirometer, is known as our vital capacity.

A thoughtful management and husbanding of breath can be

of practical daily aid, can tone us up and contribute visibly to our health and vitality. To increase our vital capacity is the object of all breath discipline. Thus consciousness of breathing out becomes the most important factor of all.

But the main thing is to cultivate the habit. Breathe out before you begin any task. Once you grasp the idea of correct breathing you will find rewards in a dozen different ways. Even in a day of escalators and elevators there are still stairs to climb—usually by puffing and panting. But try this: As you climb the first two steps, keeping the shoulder blades in position, breathe in. On the next two, breathe out. With a rhythm of two in and two out, two in and two out, you can glide up flights of stairs and arrive at the top without gasping for breath.

What happens is this: By quickening the breath rhythmically as we climb we expel a greater amount of carbon dioxide and take in a greater supply of oxygen.

The principle can be illustrated and confirmed further if we shorten our rhythm when we walk up a hill or long slope. In this case, breathe in while you take three paces and breathe out as you take the next three—three in, three out, keeping the shoulder blades in position. A hill that otherwise would leave you clutching for breath can be easily accomplished by this simple change in breathing tempo.

If some strenuous exertion without the right alteration in your breathing leaves you "out of breath," there is a simple way to get your breath back. Breathe faster. Pant like a dog for a few seconds. Then take a couple of full, easy breaths. Again pant and follow with a few full breaths. This will quiet your breathing much more rapidly than the forced effort to breathe naturally.

When a runner gets what we call his "second wind" it means that, at a certain point, he has unconsciously assessed his increased needs and countered the faster accumulation of carbon dioxide by a deeper and steadier intake of oxygen.

During World War II, I was asked to suggest a series of exercises for early-morning use by the Royal Air Force. Hangars and mess hall were cold; fuel was short. To warm up the men, I prescribed the following routine: they were to inhale and exhale through the nostrils, rapidly at first, then slowly; quick, short breathing for thirty seconds, then slow and full breathing for thirty seconds. Repeated several times, the exercise makes the body glow with warmth.

What the unfortunate majority of us need these days is a breathing program that can help us at our desks or stoves or machines. Tenseness and even depression may be overcome by the following exercise: Place the shoulder blades as nearly together as you can without strain, then breathe out gently and fully. Pause, then inhale with a deep, slow, gentle breath until the lungs are comfortably filled. Breathe out slowly through the nose with a long sigh and without altering the position of the shoulder blades. Do this a dozen times and your depression should disappear. Why? Because you have stimulated and inspired your brain and eased the nerve tension with a fuller supply of life-giving oxygen.

In what is known as stage fright a person often seems to suffer from a mild form of suffocation. Actors and experienced public speakers know the benefits of breath control. Any of us can profit from the actor's practice of stopping in the wings and fortifying himself with several full breaths before entering a scene.

One of the best exercises to establish the habit of proper exhaling involves reading aloud. From a newspaper, read aloud on one breath as many words as you can without effort. Now count the number of words you covered. Tomorrow try again. See how much you can increase the length of your exhalation.

Practice with some favorite passage of literature or Scripture which you have memorized, such as the First Psalm. You probably won't get beyond "the seat of the scornful" on the first attempt, but after a dozen daily efforts you may get through the whole psalm on one breath.

Another effective way to practice controlled outbreathing is counting. Sit down comfortably in an upright position, breathe in gently and steadily to the count of 4. Pause a second and then breathe out to the count of 12. Next time breathe in to the count of 5 and out to the count of 15. Continue this practice until you see notable progress. By the time you are able to breathe out to the count of 21 you will find that humming helps immensely to limit the amount of air you release. Humming as you breathe out gives you your own form of work song.

Many are the by-products of breathing out consistently, but the greatest of these is awareness. It introduces a sharp change in our regular habits and, in a sense, makes us repossess our bodies. Conscious breathing brings with it a consciousness of posture. You begin to realize that you cannot sit all hunched up and breathe well either in or out.

The average person goes around with his shoulder blades wide apart. By drawing the shoulder blades close together he accomplishes the incidental result of squaring his shoulders. But he also accomplishes far more: he frees the whole abdominal region of unnecessary weight and pressure and sets up arrangements for proper movement of the diaphragm. He is relieved immediately of some of the burden of breathing, for ordinarily we use part of our breath intake to lift the weight of our ribs and chest. Pulling the shoulder blades close together gives us a feeling of lightness in the abdominal region and prompts us to breathe deeply.

By practice we can make our breathing involuntarily good just as it is likely now to be involuntarily bad. The body responds to wise treatment, and a consistent effort to enlarge vital capacity by learning to breathe out will pay off. Good habits will take over and in turn become second nature.

In the strained circumstances of modern life automatic breathing is not sufficient for our needs. Sedentary or monotonous work habits call for new and consciously controlled rhythms. It will pay to test daily some of the suggestions offered here. Experience will demonstrate the constructive use we can make of a power we now overlook.

Our Lungs—

THOSE WONDERFUL WINDBAGS

by J. D. Ratcliff

W̶e cramp them with poor posture and subject them to smog, dust and industrial fumes. We inflate them half a *billion* times in an average lifetime—wear and tear that would destroy any man-made material. Despite such punishment these remarkable organs—our lungs—give most of us long and trouble-free service.

Wherever we live—frigid North, arid desert, sooty city—our lungs require air much like that found in a tropical swamp: hot, moist, dirt-free. If the smoke and dust we breathe ever reached the lungs' minute air passages, they would be clogged within hours. If bacteria gained admittance freely, we would die of flaming infections. To guard against such disasters, nature has devised an incredibly complex air-conditioning system.

Its wonders begin with the nose, whose special construction is a measure of its importance. Made mostly of pliable cartilage, it can be mashed and pummeled and still continue to function. Hairs in the lining of the nose screen out large dust particles, and its passages help warm the air. Most of this warming task, however, is accomplished in deeper nasal passages, where the bones are covered by tissues with an enormously rich blood supply. Air passing over these tissues is warmed like air passing over a radiator. On cold days the blood vessels dilate to produce more heat; on warm days they shrink.

As part of the elaborate humidifying system, glands leak fluid into the nasal passages—as much as a quart a day. Added moisture comes from tears that constantly bathe the eyes and spill over into the nasal passages through tear ducts. Here, too, the war on bacteria, which we breathe by the millions each day, gets underway. A remarkable enzyme called lysozyme, one of the most powerful bacteria-destroyers known, turns up in tears and mucous secretions.

The inspired air still contains a potentially lethal burden of dust particles. To help get rid of them, airways are lined with glands which secrete a sticky film of mucus. It acts much like flypaper in trapping dust particles. This "flypaper" would be hopelessly clogged with dirt in a short time but for another remarkable mechanism: air passages have their own sweeping system. Microscopic cilia—hairs—cover the entire route, and flail back and forth twelve times a second. Moving faster in one direction than the other, they sweep debris *upward*—toward the throat. Swallowed, it will be harmless in the digestive tract.

The incredible energy of the cilia can be demonstrated by snipping a bit of tissue from a frog's throat. If placed on a table, the cilia will "walk" the tissue off the table. If placed in a bottle, the tissue will climb out!

At times we tax the capacity of these cleaning mechanisms— for example, when we smoke too much. In a futile effort to trap countless millions of smoke particles, the throat secretes excess mucus. The mucus itself becomes an irritant and must be coughed up. In a cough, air is trapped in the lungs by the glottis, the valve at the upper end of the windpipe, or trachea, which carries air to the lungs. When the valve opens suddenly, air rushes out with explosive force. Thus the cough, which we may consider a nuisance, is actually essential to life—as an emergency cleaning measure.

Normally we take eighteen to twenty breaths a minute, using

only about one eighth of our lung capacity. With each breath we inhale about a pint of air. Since resting lungs hold six pints, only a sixth of the air is changed at a time. During violent exercise, when cells are hungry for oxygen, deeper and more rapid breathing can bring into the lungs ten or more times the oxygen supplied during rest.

The lungs are not simply inflatable bladders; they are among the most complex structures in the body. Cut through, they look something like the cross section of a rubber bath sponge. Each lung has its own duct from the windpipe; it enters near the top and starts branching like a tree. The branches are the bronchial tubes. Their job: to deliver air to the *functioning* part of the lung, those 750,000,000 microscopic air sacs called alveoli. All together

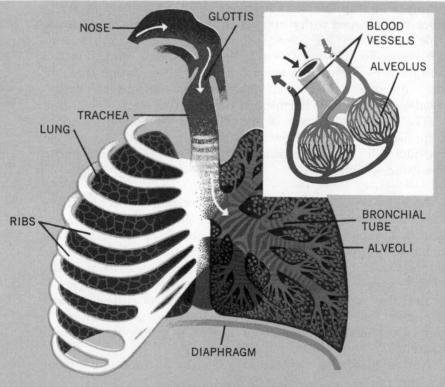

THE RESPIRATORY SYSTEM

they have a surface area 25 times that of the skin; spread flat, they would cover 600 square feet.

Each alveolus has a cobwebby covering of capillaries, so tiny that red blood cells must pass through them single file. Through their gossamer walls the blood gives up waste carbon dioxide and takes on refreshing oxygen. Every few minutes the body's entire supply of blood must pass through these minute blood vessels— *in* one end a dark blue-black, *out* the other a bright cherry-red. Day and night this all-important work must proceed without interruption.

Breathing itself is an intricate process. The lungs hang loosely in the chest, each in a separate compartment. (The heart is between them, in its own compartment.) Around them is a partial vacuum. Therefore, when the chest is enlarged, the vacuum tugs the lungs outward, thus sucking in air. Expansion of the chest is brought about by either—or both—of two methods. The diaphragm, the sheet of muscular tissue which divides chest from abdomen, may drop downward. Or the ribs, which are hinged to the spine, may swing outward. Expiration is simply a recoil mechanism.

Until the 1930s the chest was generally taboo territory for the surgeon, for once it was opened the lungs, no longer in a partial vacuum, would collapse and breathing would cease. Then came improvements in anesthesiology—chiefly the increased use of tubes which can be slipped down the windpipe so that the anesthetist can rhythmically force air and oxygen into the lungs. With this innovation a brilliant new day dawned for chest surgery.

❧

SMOKING two cigarettes is enough to impair a person's night vision, according to Dr. Charles Sheard of the Mayo Clinic. A vasoconstrictor, the nicotine cuts the flow of blood to the retina, causing a 15- to 30-minute delay in the time eyes require to adjust themselves to dim light. It is because of this that Army Air Forces training manuals advise against smoking before night flights.   —*Science Digest*

How Harmful Is Smoking?

Adapted from "How Harmful are Cigarettes?" *by Roger William Riis*
and "Lung Cancer and Cigarettes" *Lois Mattox Miller*

In all the history of human habit, there have been few changes
so remarkable as the tidal-wave increase in cigarette smoking.
Within our lifetime a new habit has taken hold to an extent we
do not begin to realize, and with effects that we certainly do
not understand.

In the United States, in 1961, 61 million people consumed 488
billion cigarettes. Two out of three men, two out of every five
women, one out of every five boys at the end of their freshman
year in high school smoke cigarettes. The average consumption is
eleven cigarettes a day. Some 7.1 billion dollars a year are spent
on tobacco products, considerably more than are paid to all the
public-school teachers in the United States.

Up and up runs the graph at a towering angle, with no sign of
leveling off. Americans are, at a lively pace, being engulfed in
one giant nationwide cloud of cigarette smoke.

What is this substance which we breathe into our mouths and
lungs in such stupendous clouds? It contains a number of
ominous-sounding chemicals. Two of the chemicals are under

grave suspicion: benzopyrene, which chiefly affects the respiratory tract, and nicotine.

Nicotine

Nicotine is the essential ingredient of tobacco. It is what makes tobacco tobacco and not just another weed. When one smokes, most of the nicotine escapes into the air. About a third gets into the mouth, where a little is absorbed. Of what goes into the lungs, perhaps a fifth is absorbed. A pipe gives one a trifle more nicotine than does a cigar.

The hotter the burning surface, the more nicotine is taken into the system. Thus, the faster one smokes, the more nicotine one gets; smoking twice as fast results in ten times as much nicotine. And the closer to the end of a cigarette one smokes, the more nicotine also, because the butt, having filtered the first part of the cigarette, has more than its share of nicotine.

In pure form nicotine is a violent poison. One drop on a rabbit's skin throws the rabbit into instant shock. The nicotine content of a trifle more than two cigarettes, if injected into the bloodstream, would kill a smoker swiftly. If you smoke a pack a day, you inhale 400 milligrams of nicotine a week, which in a single injection would kill you quick as a bullet.

In factories which make nicotine insecticides, cases of acute poisoning occur now and then. One worker sat on a stool the concave seat of which held a little spilled nicotine. In less than two minutes he fell to the floor, blue in the face, apparently dead. Rushed to the hospital, he recovered quickly, as one does from light nicotine poisoning. But when he returned to the shop and put on those nicotine-soaked trousers again, again he fell headlong on the ground, and had to be revived a second time.

In the 488 billion cigarettes we smoke each year there are nearly twenty-eight million gallons of nicotine. Administered with precision, this is enough to kill a thousand times the population of the United States—a wild idea, of course, but nevertheless suggestive of nicotine's lethal power.

If nicotine is such a poison, then why doesn't smoking kill us?

Partly because the remarkably adjustable human body can gradually build up a tolerance for larger and larger doses of poison; partly because, in smoke, it is not accumulated in sufficient quantities. Just what the harmful effects of smoking are, the reader will judge for himself from the following evidence.

Smoking and Health

First, no doctor claims that smoking *soothes* the throat. The argument, as an editorial in *The Journal of the American Medical Association* put it, hinges on "the extent to which cigarettes irritate the throat." If you smoke a pack a day, you take in 840 cubic centimeters of tobacco tar in a year. That means that you have drenched your throat and lungs with 27 fluid ounces, or 15 full cocktail glasses, of tobacco tar containing benzopyrene.

The brown stain in filters or on your handkerchief when you blow smoke through it is not nicotine, for nicotine is colorless; it is incompletely burned tar products, like the soot in a chimney. Many physicians suspect that its main constituent, benzopyrene, though an irritant rather than a poison, is a greater threat to heavy smokers than nicotine.

In the matter of irritation, it is far more important how you smoke than what you smoke, whether you puff briskly or gently, how far down the butt you smoke, how long you hold the smoke in the mouth and lungs. Rapid smoking increases the irritation because it brings the smoke into the mouth at temperatures up to 135° Fahrenheit.

Do cigarettes affect the stomach and digestion? Every smoker has noticed that a cigarette seems able to still the pangs of hunger for a while. This is not a delusion. The sensation of hunger is caused by contractions of the stomach walls, and smoking can suppress these contractions. By the same process, smoking interferes with the appetite and thereby with good nutrition. Excessive smoking may also cause gastritis. By favoring an accumulation of acid secretions, it brings about heartburn. Relief comes in a matter of hours after the smoking stops.

Excess acidity of the stomach provides the kind of climate

ulcers like. The most recent work in this field, done by New York University, showed that patients who continued to smoke during treatment for their peptic ulcers had more relapses than those who did not, or those who had never smoked at all. In Boston, doctors had an interesting case some years ago, a man who had all the symptoms of duodenal ulcer. Even the X ray showed it. But an operation found no ulcer at all. The patient stopped smoking, under orders, and his "ulcer" left him. Three months later, feeling quite well, he took up smoking again, and back came the "ulcer." This time the doctors ordered him off cigarettes completely. Since he stopped smoking, he has had no more "ulcers."

Antitobacco crusaders assert that pregnant women should never smoke. Doctors have worked on this point for years and are clearer about it than about almost any other aspect of smoking. The conclusion: Smoking does not do pregnant women any more harm, or any different harm, than it does anyone else.

Two pediatricians in Philadelphia analyzed mothers' milk for nicotine content. They found 1.4 parts in ten million among moderate smokers, 4.7 parts among heavy smokers. But they could detect no effect whatsoever on the babies.

Where staying power is demanded, tobacco lowers athletic performance. At the Aldershot Army School in England a three-mile cross-country run is a required event. Over seven years the performance of almost 2000 men was analyzed, in groups of heavy smokers, moderate smokers, nonsmokers.

The heavy smokers, 8 percent of the total, drew 9 percent of the last ten places, but only 5 percent of the first ten. The moderate smokers, 73 percent of the total, got 62 percent of the first places and 83 percent of the last places. The nonsmokers, 18 percent of the total, took 32 percent of the firsts and only 7 percent of the lasts.

Nonsmokers, in four years at Yale and at Amherst, grew more in height and weight and lung capacity than did their smoking colleagues. At Yale the increase in chest development of the abstainers was 77 percent better, their increase in height 24 percent greater.

At Wisconsin students were asked to hold a small metal point in a small hole, trying not to let it touch the sides. Electrical connections registered the number of times it did touch. Regular smokers were 60 percent more unsteady than nonsmokers.

Coaches are almost unanimous in saying that muscular power is lowered and fatigue begins earlier in smokers. Nowhere is there any medical evidence—despite the advertisements—that smoking improves an athlete's abilities.

What does tobacco do to the heart? As to the long-run effects, medical opinions differ. As to the immediate effects of cigarette smoking upon the mechanism of the heart and upon the arteries and veins, there is no difference of opinion, for these effects are easy to observe and measure.

Smoking speeds the pulse by as much as 28 beats per minute. In this respect individuals vary, and the same individual varies at different times. The average increase in pulse due to smoking is ten beats. Smoking can produce arrhythmia, an irregular stop and jump of the heart which often thoroughly frightens its owner. Habitual smokers have a 50 percent higher incidence of palpitation of the heart than nonsmokers.

Smoking raises the blood pressure, markedly and quickly. The higher your blood pressure is, the more sharply does tobacco lift it. Apparently the blood pressure does not develop any tolerance for tobacco, as does the digestive system. Nevertheless, smoking does not *cause* permanent high blood pressure. When the smoking stops, the pressure falls slowly to normal.

Smoking constricts the blood vessels, especially those of the feet and hands. The smaller the blood vessel the tighter is it constricted, and often smoking closes the tiny vessels under the fingernails entirely. As soon as one starts a cigarette, the rate of blood flow in the hands decreases to less than half normal, and it stays down for about an hour. The temperature of hands and feet drops.

Nicotine constricts the veins; alcohol dilates them. When we drink and smoke at the same time, we are in effect prodding ourselves with a pitchfork to get a lift and beating ourselves on the head with a club to offset it. Hence the popular belief that taking a highball offsets the effect of taking a cigarette. Doctors at

Rochester, Minnesota, went into this interesting possibility, making 121 tests on 65 persons. The winner was nicotine; it was more potent than alcohol: "the constricting effects of smoking cannot be prevented by alcohol."

. There is no proof that smoking causes heart disease. But there is evidence that heart disease is more prevalent among smokers than among nonsmokers, and that smoking may intensify existing heart disease. Virginia doctors, in an article on angina pectoris, point out that "coronary disease develops before the seventh decade significantly more often in smokers than in nonsmokers." The chief difference of opinion among doctors is as to *how much* damage smoking does to the heart. All doctors agree it can damage sick hearts. It is, in short, never a help and often a menace. It seems reasonable at present to agree with the recent statement of the committee on smoking and cardiovascular disease of the American Heart Association, that present evidence "strongly suggests that heavy cigarette smoking may contribute to or accelerate the development of coronary disease or its complications, at least in men under the age of fifty-five."

Lung Cancer: The Royal College Report

Will cigarettes induce cancer? The increase in lung-cancer mortality shows a suspicious parallel to the enormous increase in cigarette consumption in the United States. From 1930 to 1959, lung-cancer death rates increased nine times. At the present time cancer of the mouth and respiratory tract kills 37,000 men and 7000 women annually in the United States.

"It is probable that lung cancer soon will become more frequent than any other cancer of the body unless something is done to prevent its increase," declares Dr. Alton Ochsner, former president of the American Cancer Society and director of the famous Ochsner Clinic in New Orleans. "It is frightening to speculate on the possible number of [lung] cancers that might develop as a result of the tremendous number of cigarettes consumed in the decades from 1930 to 1960."

Out of London in March, 1962, came a chill blast which

sobered cigarette smokers and jolted the tobacco industry on both sides of the Atlantic. The venerable 444-year-old Royal College of Physicians, which never deals with trivia or sensationalism, completed an exhaustive study and published a fact-filled report, *Smoking and Health*, "intended to give, to doctors and others, evidence on the hazards of smoking so that they may decide what should be done." The Royal College report stated unequivocally:

• "Cigarette smoking is a cause of lung cancer and bronchitis, and probably contributes to the development of coronary heart disease and various less common diseases."

• "Cigarette smokers have the greatest risk of dying from these diseases, and the risk is greater for the heavier smokers."

• "The many deaths from these diseases present a challenge to medicine; insofar as they are due to smoking they should be preventable."

• "The harmful effects of cigarette smoking might be reduced by efficient filters, by leaving longer cigarette stubs, or by changing from cigarette to pipe or cigar smoking."

The report had immediate repercussions in Parliament. It also stirred some nervous activity in Washington, where bureaucrats and Congressmen had dodged or pigeonholed the smoking-health issue for the past ten years. Tobacco-industry spokesmen issued the standard rejoinder that the evidence was merely "old data without new research findings," but the statement sounded weaker and more pathetic than ever.

Sir Robert Platt, president of the Royal College of Physicians, commented: "Naturally every possible opposition has been raised to the idea that these diseases are due to cigarette smoking. But not one of the opposing theories will hold water, whereas everything confirms the evidence against cigarettes."

"During the past forty-five years," the report explained, "lung cancer has changed from an infrequent to a major cause of death in many countries. To account for this increase, it is necessary to postulate some causative agent to which human lungs have been newly and increasingly exposed during the present century. Cigarette smoke is such an agent and there is now a great deal of evidence that it is an important cause of this disease."

Since 1953 at least twenty-three investigations in nine different countries have reported on the relationship between lung cancer and smoking. "All these studies," the report states, "have shown that death rates from lung cancer increase steeply with increasing consumption of cigarettes. Heavy cigarette smokers may have thirty times the death rate of non-smokers. They also have shown that cigarette smokers are much more affected than pipe or cigar smokers (who do not inhale) and that the group which had given up smoking at the start of the survey had a lower death rate than those who had continued to smoke."

This strong statistical association between cigarette smoking and lung cancer "is supported by compatible, though not conclusive, laboratory and pathological evidence." Some sixteen substances capable of initiating cancer in animals have been identified in tobacco smoke. In addition to these carcinogens, the smoke contains a variety of irritants which cause "precancerous" changes. These have been noted in the lungs and bronchial tissues of smokers who have died of causes other than lung cancer.

The Royal College report devotes a full section to the theories advanced by those who doubt the cause-and-effect relationship. "None of these explanations fits all the facts as well as the obvious one that smoking is a cause of lung cancer."

How about air pollution, onto which the tobacco propagandists try desperately to shift the blame? In *Smoking and Health*, the investigators point to the lung-cancer death rates of smokers and nonsmokers who live in cities, in rural areas and even in countries where air pollution is virtually unknown.

Finland, for example, which has the second highest lung-cancer death rate in Europe is essentially a rural country which has little air pollution but a population of heavy smokers. "This suggests that smoking is more important than air pollution," the report concludes. Moreover, "it is clear that at all levels of air pollution cigarette smokers suffer a risk of lung cancer which increases with the number of cigarettes smoked, and even in the most rural areas of the United Kingdom heavy cigarette smokers develop lung cancer fifteen to twenty times as frequently as non-smokers."

"Patients with bronchitis, peptic ulcer and arterial disease should be advised to stop smoking," the Royal College suggests to doctors. "Even a smoker's cough may be an indication that the habit should be given up."

The report observed that the proportion of nonsmoking British doctors has doubled in recent years from 24 percent in 1951 to 50 percent in 1961. "The doctor who smokes cigarettes must, like any other individual, balance these risks against the pleasures he derives from smoking and make his choice. But the doctor who smokes will lessen the effect of public education concerning the consequences of the habit and will find it harder to help his patients who need to stop smoking."

The Royal College report is not the first comprehensive analysis to be made of the smoking-health problem. But it is probably the best factual statement, buttressed by over 200 citations of scientific sources, to be written in the plain English which the average layman can understand. (Besides being widely summarized in the British press, the first 15,000 copies of *Smoking and Health* were sold out on publication and it since has become a best seller.)

Smoking and Health is also the first report to spell out a practical program of preventive measures for the individual and the government. Some specific recommendations:

• More public education, and especially of school children, concerning the hazards of smoking. "The Central Council for Health Education and local authorities spent less than £5000 [$14,000] in 1956–60, while the Tobacco Manufacturers spent £38 million [$107 million] on advertising their goods during this period. Such public education might advise safer smoking habits (filter tips, longer stubs, preference for pipes or cigars) for those whose addiction is too strong to be broken."

• More effective restrictions on the sale of tobacco to children ("cigarettes are freely available in slot machines"). Wider restrictions on smoking in public places.

• Raising the tax on cigarettes, and perhaps lowering taxes on pipe tobacco and cigars. ("Pipe smokers incur a considerably smaller risk than cigarette smokers. The risk in those who smoke only cigars is even smaller and may be no greater than that for non-smokers.")

•"Since filters vary in efficiency, it would be desirable to have them tested by some official agency and have the results indicated on the packet."

The Royal College report was immediately subjected to full Parliamentary discussion, and Enoch Powell, the Minister of Health, informed the House of Commons: "The Government certainly does accept that this demonstrates authoritatively and unquestionably the causal connection between smoking and lung cancer and the more general hazards to health of smoking." The report's recommendations, he said, "are under consideration by the Government."

Whither Washington?

The forthright British approach was in sharp contrast to the timidity with which the health services, regulatory agencies and legislators in Washington, D.C., had up to then shied away from the clearly defined issue of smoking and health. In 1959 the Surgeon General of the U.S. Public Health Service published in the *Journal of the American Medical Association* a lengthy report which covered much the same ground as the current Royal College report, and accepted the causative role of cigarettes in lung cancer. But, unfortunately, some of the Surgeon General's colleagues had written into the report a brief paragraph which downgraded and dismissed filter tips even as partial health protection, and the Federal Trade Commission seized upon this convenient excuse to sweep the whole issue of the tar and nicotine content of American cigarettes under the carpet.

There have recently been, however, encouraging signs of a change of heart. Dr. Michael B. Shimkin of the National Cancer Institute has come out publicly in support of the American Cancer Society's proposal for a federal ruling that packages be clearly labeled with the tar and nicotine content of the cigarettes.

Following the publication of the Royal College report (but

only then), it was disclosed that a House Appropriations subcom-
mittee had heard the testimony, in closed sessions a month earlier,
of physicians from the National Institutes of Health. They
stressed the overwhelming evidence linking cigarette smoking
with lung cancer and other diseases, and urged an educational
campaign on the hazards of smoking.

The FTC, apparently, has been holding its own closed-door
meetings to find some way out of its quandary. The trade paper
Advertising Age quoted Byron H. Jacques, head of the FTC bureau
of trade-practice conferences and industry guides, as admitting:
"If there is really a significant difference in the health hazards
involved in filter tips compared with nonfilters, some change in
our attitude might be necessary."

The FTC has long argued that it needs scientific authority and
new legislation to handle the job properly. But many well-
informed Washington lawyers maintain that the federal government (Food and Drug Administration, FTC, or USPHS) has all
the authority it needs under present laws, including the broad
Federal Hazardous Substances Act, which went into effect in
July, 1960. Many cigarette manufacturers state, privately, that
they would welcome package labeling and standardized testing—
but (for sound legal reasons) only if the government takes the
initiative and tells them what to do.

On June 7, 1962, the U.S. Government at last took a significant step—but a first step only—when Surgeon General Luther
Terry announced that he was about to appoint an advisory committee of experts to study the effect of cigarette smoking on
health. The committee's study, said President Kennedy, would
take several months and "go into '63." Meanwhile, this observation in a well-known British medical journal, *The Lancet*, should
be pondered in Washington: "Future historians will have views
on our failure to find even a partial solution to the problem of
smoking during the first ten years after its dangers were revealed.
The enormous and increasing number of deaths from smoker's
cancer may go down in history as a strong indictment of our political and economic ways of life."

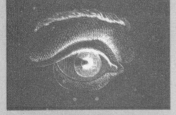

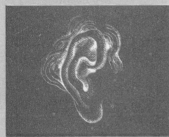

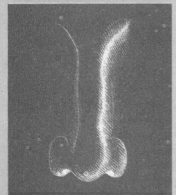

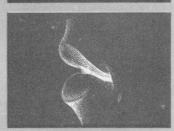

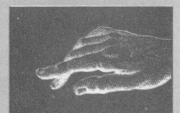

CHAPTER 5

Our Sentinels

STANDING by, night and day, the remarkable sentinels of the body—eyes, ears, nose, throat and skin— keep us in constant contact with the world around us, introduce us to its delights, protect us from its dangers. To know the structure and function of these amazing organs is to marvel anew at the complexity and precision of nature's master plan.

❦

What Your Skin Does for You

by Ruth and Edward Brecher

❦

Have you ever wondered, after bruising or cutting yourself, why nature didn't supply you with a tougher hide? Scientists have an answer. Your tender skin, they report, is far more than a protective covering: it is an organ ranking with the brain, heart and lungs in its importance to human life. It performs services of which you are hardly aware—services which would be hampered if it were a tough, thick hide.

Consider what happens when you cut your finger. At once blood gushes from the tiny blood vessels in the skin, washing out dirt and germs. Then the blood vessels constrict so that the flow diminishes, and soon a clot of rapidly hardening blood fills the gash. Like glue it attaches itself firmly to the two sides of the cut, then gradually shrinks, drawing the sides closer together.

As the hours pass, threadlike connective-tissue cells called fibroblasts invade the clot from all sides, gradually building up new tissues. Once the gap has been solidly filled in, surface skin cells begin to grow from the two edges until they meet in the center, leaving only a hairline scar or none at all.

Each step in this process occurs at just the right time. Remember this when next you cut or burn yourself, and don't try to scrape off the scab. You might interrupt important steps in the healing process, and be left with an unnecessary scar.

Your skin is a storehouse—and a remarkably roomy one, too. If you weigh 150 pounds, you are carrying about 25 of those pounds in your skin, mostly as fats and water. When your body takes in more of these than it requires, some of the excess is deposited in your skin. Later on, the skin can return stored materials to the bloodstream for transportation to organs which need them. Salts, sugars and other essentials are similarly deposited in your skin.

Your skin can also provide emergency blood rations to vital organs. Suppose that while walking down the street you are unexpectedly assaulted. Your muscles and internal organs immediately demand more blood for fight or flight. It comes partly from your skin, where small blood vessels shrink or collapse and bigger emergency channels open up to provide a rapid shortcut for blood hurrying to the regions of need. As this blood leaves your skin you "turn pale with fear," or with anger.

The blood vessels of the skin help keep your temperature normal. When your body gets too hot, they expand so that more blood flows to the surface of the skin and is cooled. When you go out in the cold, the skin's blood vessels contract, less blood enters the skin and internal heat is conserved.

The sweat glands in your skin are also temperature-regulating devices. When you get too hot, these glands secrete sweat, which evaporates and cools you.

Your skin is studded with nerve endings, some of which respond to warmth, some to cold, some to pressure, some to pain, itching or tickling. The nerve endings provide your "sense of touch," which works in a remarkable way. From early infancy until your skin becomes wrinkled in old age, it is generally a bit too small for you, and is therefore gently stretched. If the degree to which it is stretched changes, you feel that you have been "touched."

Thus when you rub a pencil gently along your skin, it is not really the pencil you feel but the change in stretch which the pencil produces in your skin. You may "feel" the pencil even when it only touches the hairs of your forearm, for each hair touched disturbs *some* nerve endings ever so slightly.

The skin you wear today isn't the same skin you wore last year; invisible shedding goes on from hour to hour. Your skin has three major levels: an outer collection of layers (the epidermis), a middle layer (the dermis) and an inner (or subdermal) layer. In the lower part of the epidermis is a thin sheet of cells where most skin growth occurs. Each cell in this sheet divides from time to time, forming new cells which are crowded slowly upward to the surface. The trip may take weeks. On the way, each cell dies, and its exterior disintegrates into microscopic specks of scale.

Some twenty or more layers of scale form the surface of your skin. These invisible fragments of dead cells are constantly being rubbed off and replaced. If the skin surface is scraped so that it loses its tiny scales more rapidly than is normal, the rate at which new cells are formed is trebled or quadrupled.

The outer layer of scales is thickest on the fingertips, palms

CROSS SECTION OF THE SKIN

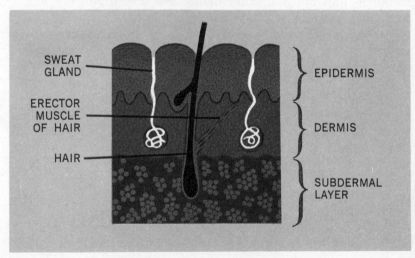

and soles. If one spot is rubbed too often, the skin there forms a corn or callus, an accumulation of hard, dead scales. Severe sunburn hastens the skin-shedding process and produces a visible peeling.

The varieties of human skin color depend mostly on the amount of a single pigment called melanin. Ordinarily, darker skin has more melanin. Only about ⅟₂₅ of an ounce of melanin separates the blackest human skin from the skin of an albino, which lacks pigment entirely.

Chemicals are already available which will inhibit melanin production in the laboratory. It is conceivable that, in time, human beings may be able to select the shade of skin they prefer.

Human skin maintains its health by means of a fatty substance called sebum, secreted from millions of glands located near the roots of the hairs. Oozing to the skin surface, sebum forms a protective mixture with sweat to keep your skin moist and pliable. In very cold weather the sebum congeals on its way to the surface, and your skin becomes dry and chapped. In some people, overproduction or underproduction of sebum causes excessively oily or excessively dry skin.

Have you ever remarked, "I was so frightened that my hair stood on end"? Perhaps it actually did. Attached to the fine hairs growing over most of your body are miniature muscles which, by contracting, can "erect" the hairs. This rising and bristling of the hairs was no doubt originally a device for making fur-bearing animals look bigger and more ferocious to their enemies. We no longer have enough fur to frighten our enemies, but bristling, paling, blushing and other skin changes contribute much to the rich patterns of feeling which we consciously recognize as emotions. When you say that you "felt frightened all over," or "mad all over," a large part of what you felt was an awareness of these subtle skin changes.

Aging produces marked changes in the skin. The newborn baby is wrinkled because his skin is still too big for him. As his body fills out, the wrinkles vanish. From then on, countless elastic fibers embedded in the skin keep it smooth and properly tight.

At puberty, sex hormones stimulate a rapid increase in sebum production which may clog the pores, causing skin eruptions during adolescence. Later, the sebaceous glands quiet down again, and the skin clears. In old age, sebum production drops very low, and the skin fibers lose much of their elasticity. Loose, wrinkled, dry skin results.

Your skin is peculiarly your own; no other person's is quite like it. One illustration of this uniqueness is your fingerprint pattern, which never duplicates that of anyone else. Another: Skin from one part of your body can be successfully transplanted to another part, but will survive only temporarily if transplanted to someone else, unless that person is your identical twin.

If you should suffer a large burn, skin taken from another person *can* be helpful in the healing process, however. This borrowed skin survives only a few weeks—but that's long enough to protect the underlying tissues from infection and fluid loss during the period of greatest danger. Skin can be frozen and stored, so that any hospital can maintain a skin bank with a modest supply continuously on hand for emergencies.

Marvelous indeed is nature's way of packaging our bodies. But marvelous also are the ways in which man has been learning to understand nature's methods—and to make intelligent use of them.

How Much Sun Is Too Much ?

Some authorities say that to start a safe sun-tan, you should stay out no more than twenty minutes — about long enough to turn untanned skin a faint pink. The next day, you can stay in the sun an additional ten minutes and continue adding ten minutes a day for the week it will take to develop a tan. Others insist that *any* exposure adequate to produce a tan probably damages the skin.   —William Barry Furlong

The Evolution of Eyes

by Thomas Hall Shastid

Ages ago, when earth had cooled and life had begun to appear in its tepid waters, one of the first things developed was eyes. Even the amoeba, the lowliest of all known animals, of which countless trillions exist today precisely as they were when life originated on this planet, may be said to possess eyes. Or rather, the amoeba's body is all eye—every portion of the amoeba can perceive light. But while in the process of evolution some eyes, like this generalized light sense of the amoeba, have stood quite still, others, like the literally superhuman eyes of birds, have moved forward incredible distances.

When we come to the insects we find that they have two kinds of eyes: simple and compound. If one looks at a common housefly one can see that its head consists almost entirely of two large, dark-brown lobes, the compound eyes, each made up of more than 4000 eye units. From each compound eye a mosaic picture—of more than 4000 minute picture fragments—is conveyed to the fly's central nervous system. The fly also has three single eyes, situated, in the form of a triangle with its sharpest point downward, in the space above and between the two compound eyes.

The compound eyes of the fly are used for distance (from three to four yards) and the single eyes for near vision (from one to two inches). Some insects have only compound eyes, some only single, but most of them have both. None of these insect eyes have any movement—the eyes are set on the fly's head as solidly as so many jewels in a watch.

Leaving the insects, the fishes are the first of the great back-boned class of animals. In fishes, nature produced the first true focusing arrangements and muscles with which to move eyes in their sockets. But fish are color-blind. Tell this to a fisherman with his brightly colored flies and he will laugh derisively, but it is a demonstrable fact. Fish can distinguish between different colors, but do not see them as colors—only as various shades of gray, precisely as a color-blind person would. Fish have also a very restricted visual field, seeing scarcely anything below the level of the head.

The reptilia added little to eyes. In general snakes have very poor sight. Most of them see only objects in motion and are nearly deaf too, so that their knowledge of the world reaches them largely by way of the little forked tongue, probably the most wonderful tactile organ in existence. This feels myriads of vibrations in the atmosphere which to our coarse sense of touch are nonexistent.

Birds' eyes are the most remarkable of all earthly eyes, being often both telescopic and microscopic. In birds the visual acuteness is almost incredible, in some instances 100 times as great as that in men. A bit of grain that human eyes can barely see at a distance of one yard, a bird can see distinctly at a distance of 100 yards. This remarkable sight is almost a necessity because the sense of smell in birds is exceedingly poor. Even vultures, contrary to popular superstition, do not smell their food, even though it be carrion, but see it.

Mammals may be classified as nonprimates and primates, the primates including monkeys, apes and men. In nearly all the nonprimates the eyes are set out not on the front of the face but at the side of the head. Scarcely any of the nonprimates have any overlapping of the visual fields of the two eyes and those which do have some overlapping have no true stereoscopic vision—vision with depth and relief to it. Hares and rabbits actually have the fields overlapping behind their heads (behind because these animals are not hunters but those hunted), yet they have no stereoscopic vision.

Among mammals a very great difference exists in the shape of the pupil when in contracted condition. The domestic cat has a narrow vertical pupil, which it needs for the purpose of hunting its prey up and down trees. (This is not true of all the cat family; lions and all the larger *Felidae* have round pupils.) The horse has pupils which are wide horizontally in order that the animal, when grazing, can see sidewise, both to right and to left, over a wide expanse of ground. A horse's eyes, also, are placed prominently up and out on the corners of its head so that it can aim a kick at a wolf—the horse's natural enemy—without turning the head.

All eyes that shine in the dark do so by virtue of a concave reflector behind the retina. The purpose is to enable the animal to see better in the dark. The little light that is stirring in the outer world enters the pupil, passes through the transparent retina, which utilizes this light for vision, and on to the reflector, which sends it back to the same object from which it came. Here it is joined to the fresh, original light from the object, and the same process is repeated. Thus the carnivora and some other animals, whose vision is very much poorer than ours by day, see much better at night. And that is why primitive man lived in great terror of the dark. He was eater by day, eaten at night.

All the primates have strong focusing muscles. In all the monkeys and apes the eyes, just as in men, can both be converged on the same point, and stereoscopic vision thus obtained—but not very long maintained. Only in man, of all the mammals, does there seem to be continuous binocular and stereoscopic vision. Even in the human child, however, the eyes do not as a rule move in perfect unison with each other till about three months after birth, because stereoscopic vision, in the history of life, is of extremely recent appearance. This explains the ready loss-of-binocularity (cross-eyes) in many persons as the result of eyestrain.

Whenever our eyes are in motion they are stone-blind, excepting only when they move without changing the point at which they look. Anyone can easily convince himself of the truth of this statement. Let him stand before a mirror and look at the image of one of his eyes. Let him look first at the right side of that eye, then at the left side of the same eye, and then back again. Never, so long as he lives, will he see his eye in motion. The reason is that, just so soon as an eye begins to move, it is blind. We are never conscious of the blind interval partly because the picture which is last seen before the eye begins moving persists in the sight center of the brain and thus laps a little over the interval during which the retina is blind. But the chief fact is that the retina, by means of its motion blindness, gets minute intervals of rest with very great frequency all through our waking hours. In this way, too, the blurry and therefore useless pictures which we should receive if the eyes saw while in motion are avoided.

One peculiar thing about man's eyes is not found in the eyes of animals. In all mammals the eyes are *two* little cameras, each producing a tiny picture, but in the brain of man only one composite or stereoscopic picture is seen.

Glance casually at any picture in a magazine. Isn't it a fact that whatever object happens to be in the lower left-hand corner is the first thing you see? Eye movements have been studied by means of motion pictures and as a result artists know that we instinctively look at the lower left-hand corner of a picture first and then at the upper right. This knowledge may be applied in other fields than art. If you have a room where the door opens almost in the center, and if you want your guests to see a new chair or piece of bric-a-brac of which you are particularly proud, place it on their left as they enter. But if there is a worn place in the rug, put that on the right side.

Large department stores have found that merchandise displayed in the left side of a window and fairly low will attract more shoppers than if displayed with equal prominence in the right-hand side.   —Carl J. Warden

The Mysterious Power of Human Sight

Adapted from "The Mysterious Power of Human Sight"
by Sir Charles Scott Sherrington
and "You Can Learn to See More" by Wolfgang Langewiesche

How does a pin's-head ball of cells in the course of so many
weeks become a child? Consider the story of the making of
just one individual part: the eye.

The many cells which make the human eye have first executed
correctly a multitudinous dance engaging millions of performers
in hundreds of sequences of different steps. To picture the complexity and the precision of this performance beggars any imag-
ery I have. It suggests purposive behavior—not only by individual
cells but by colonies of cells. And the impression of concerted
endeavor comes, it is no exaggeration to say, with the force of a
self-evident truth.

The eyeball is a little camera. Its smallness is part of its perfection. But this is a spheroid camera which focuses itself automatically, according to the distance of the picture interesting it.
It turns itself in the direction of the view required. Indeed it is

two cameras finished to one standard so that the mind can read their two pictures as one. And it is contrived as though with forethought of self-preservation. Should danger threaten, in a trice its skin shutters close, protecting its transparent window.

The biconvex lens is made of cells like those of the skin but modified to be glass-clear. It is delicately slung with accurate centering across the path of the light which enters the eye. In front of it a circular screen controls, like the iris stop of a camera, the width of the beam and is adjustable, so that in a poor light more is taken for the image. In a camera, this adjustment is made by the observer working the instrument. The observer supplies the actual motor power. In the eye this adjustment is automatic, *worked by the image itself!*

Not only must the lens be glass-clear but its shape must be optically right. The optician obtains glass of the desired refractive index and skillfully grinds its curvatures in accordance with mathematical formulae. With the lens of the eye, a batch of granular skin cells are told to travel from the skin, to which they strictly belong, and to settle down in the mouth of the optic cup and arrange themselves in a compact and suitable ball. Next they are told to turn into transparent fibers, and to make themselves into a subsphere—a lens of the right size, set at the right distance between the transparent window of the eye in front and the sensitive seeing screen of the retina behind. In short, they behave as if fairly possessed.

Furthermore, the lens of the eye compassing what no glass lens can, changes its curvature to focus on near objects, as well as on distant ones, when required—for instance, when we read. And not merely the lens but the pupil—the camera stop—is self-adjusting. All this without our having even to wish it; without even our knowing anything about it, beyond the fact that we are seeing satisfactorily.

The lens and screen cut the chamber of the eye into a front half and a back half, both filled with clear humor, practically water, kept under a certain pressure to maintain the eyeball's right shape. The front chamber is completed by a layer of skin specialized to be glass-clear. The **skin** above and below this window grows into movable flaps, dry **outside** like ordinary skin, but moist inside, which wipe the window clean every minute or so by painting fresh tear water over it.

The eye's key structure is the light-sensitive screen at the back. It receives, takes and records a continually changing moving picture, lifelong and not requiring a change of "plate," through every waking day. And it signals its shifting exposures to the brain. It is a ninefold layer of great complexity. It is, strictly speaking, a piece of the brain lying within the eyeball.

The cells that are at the bottom of the cup become a photosensitive layer—the sensitive film of the camera. The nerve lines connecting the photosensitive layer with the brain are not simple. The human eye has about 137,000,000 separate "seeing" elements spread out in the sheet of the retina. The number of nerve lines leading from them to the brain gradually condenses down to little over 1,000,000. They are in series of relays, each resembling a little brain, and each so shaped and connected as to transmit duly to the right points of the brain itself each light

STRUCTURE OF THE EYE

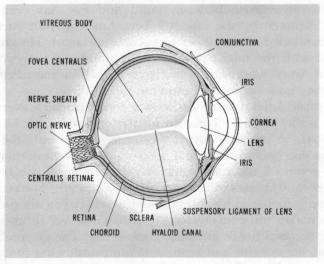

picture momentarily formed and "taken." On the sense-cell
layer the image has, picturelike, two dimensions. But the step
from this to the mental experience is a mystery. For it is the mind
which adds the third dimension when interpreting the two-
dimensional picture! And it is the mind which adds color.

The chief wonder of all we have not touched on yet. The eye
sends into the cell-and-fiber forest of the brain throughout the
waking day continual rhythmic streams of tiny, individually
evanescent electrical potentials. This throbbing, streaming crowd
of electrified shifting points in the spongework of the brain bears
no obvious semblance in space pattern to the tiny two-dimen-
sional upside-down picture of the outside world which the eyeball
paints on the beginnings of its nerve fibers to the brain. But that
little picture sets up an electrical storm. And that electrical
storm affects a whole population of brain cells. Electrical charges
have in themselves not the faintest elements of the visual—have
nothing of "distance," nor "vertical," nor "horizontal," nor
"color," nor "brightness," nor "shadow," nor "contour," nor
"near," nor "far" nor visual anything—yet they conjure up
all these.

The twilight zone between mind and eye has been most
deeply explored by the late Adelbert Ames, Jr., an American
who abandoned a law career to become an artist. He grew en-
thralled with the mind: how does the mind use the eye? One
phase of Ames' work was the study of optical illusions. Princeton
University now has a small museum full of these.

A typical Ames demonstration is a room in which everything
slopes: walls, ceiling, floor. But all the distortions are so calculated that, to the eye, they cancel each other out; the room
looks, as you peer in through a peephole, just like a normal four-
square room. A tall man walks from one part of the room to
another—and shrinks to a dwarf before your eyes. The ceiling of
the room is higher in his corner than it is where you are standing,
and this makes him seem shorter. What does it prove? It proves how
heavily our experience influences our seeing. The eye really sees
only patches of color and light. The mind says what that is and

the mind has nothing to go on but past performance. Rooms are four-square: that has been true in your experience. When the tall man walks across the room, you are more willing to see him grow short than to see a room of such devilishly ingenious craziness.

Just looking is not enough. A little boy who touches everything he sees gets to know the world. A tourist traveling in foreign countries, on the other hand, too often sees only his own preconceptions. We should act like little boys and not tourists.

How explain, then, the building and shaping of the eyeball, and the establishing of its nerve connections with the right points of the brain? And how explain not the eye but the "seeing" by the brain behind the eye? This is the wonder of wonders, familiar even to boredom, so much with us that we forget it all our time.

Hear Ye! Hear Ye!

Dull as the human ear is—and we moderns do not hear nearly so well as savages—it is, if trained, capable of adding immeasurable richness to the world of our senses. One must learn to hear. The rewards of perseverance are exemplified in the experiences of the blind, whose acute hearing nearly compensates for loss of sight. On one occasion the late blind Justice Fielding, walking into a room for the first time, said: "This room is about 22 feet long, 18 wide, and 12 high." He guessed this by ear with great accuracy, thanks to his ability to detect the special resonance of a room and to judge its size thereby. Similar sensitivity was illustrated by the blind Sir Arthur Pearson who, walking home in earnest conversation with a friend, stopped at the right house, though his friend had nearly passed it by in his absorption. Sir Arthur's ear had detected the familiar sound of the slight echo resulting from the fact that the house had a porch unlike that of any other near it.

—Adapted from Sir William Bragg, *The World of Sound*,
and Sir Arthur Pearson, *Victory Over Blindness*

The Ear—

A WONDERFUL MACHINE

by Robert O'Brien

A forty-seven-year-old housewife had been mildly hard-of-hearing since the age of fourteen. Suddenly her hearing got worse. Cut off from normal communication, she lived in a world where people's lips moved, and no sound came forth, where a glass broke silently, where children's laughter was a noiseless grimace.

Then an otologist, or ear specialist, diagnosed her trouble: otosclerosis, a common cause of deafness among women that hardens the middle ear and prevents it from conducting sound waves to the brain. A few days later, he gave the patient a local anesthetic and performed a simple operation called a stapedectomy. Deftly, he worked loose a tiny bone that the disease had "frozen" solid in the middle ear. Then he removed it, fixing in its place a stainless-steel filament one fifth of an inch long, to restore sound conduction. The operation—as in nearly 90 percent of all stapedectomies—was a success.

"I feel reborn," she told me. "The first sound I remember hearing again was rain, falling softly on the roof at night. I lay in bed, listening. I awoke my husband, and made him listen. It was music—the most beautiful I ever heard."

This occurred in 1960. The stapedectomy represents a brilliant combination of recent research and technical skill in the fight against otosclerotic deafness.

Of all our sense organs, only the eye is as complex, as finely balanced as the ear.

Our hearing mechanism consists of three parts: the outer, middle and inner ear. The outer ear comprises the curled shell on the side of the head—for collecting sound waves—and an ear canal—a little tunnel about an inch long that ends at the eardrum. Tissue-thin and the diameter of a pencil eraser, this membrane is stretched tight, like a drumhead, between the outer and middle ear.

The middle ear occupies a hollow cavity large enough to hold four or five drops of water. Arching across the air space is a chain of three tiny bones: the hammer (*malleus*), anvil (*incus*), and stirrup (*stapes*), so named because they resemble these articles in miniature. At the outer end of the chain, the handle of the hammer is fastened to the eardrum. The chain's inner end, formed by the footplate of the stirrup, is fastened to another membrane.

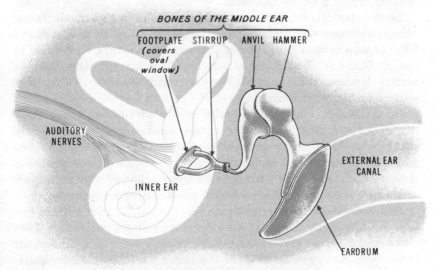

BONES OF THE MIDDLE EAR

FOOTPLATE STIRRUP ANVIL HAMMER
(covers oval window)

AUDITORY NERVES

EXTERNAL EAR CANAL

INNER EAR

EARDRUM

STRUCTURE OF THE EAR

This membrane, the oval window, is the diameter of a pinhead. It separates the middle-ear cavity from the fluids and spiral canals that form the inner ear and control our sense of balance.

In the hearing process, sound waves funnel into the ear canal, strike the eardrum and make it vibrate. The vibrations travel along the bony chain to the oval window, which transmits the vibrations to the inner ear. There, by nerve endings whose magic is as yet little understood, the vibrations are translated into impulses and flashed along the 30,000 fibers of the auditory nerve to the brain.

With such an intricate and delicately wrought organ, many things can go wrong. The two major types of impairment are conductive deafness, and perceptive (or nerve) deafness. A combination of the two is called mixed deafness.

Conductive deafness occurs when sound waves are unable to reach the inner ear. It may be caused by foreign objects, excessive wax or liquid, otosclerotic bone growth, breaks in the chain of bones, infectious swelling of middle-ear tissue. One otologist says that conductive deafness is like trying to hear a piano being played under a heavy blanket.

Such interference, however, seldom causes complete deafness. (Far less than one percent of the population is *totally* deaf.) One reason is that skull bones themselves conduct vibrations to the middle ear. Test it for yourself. Close an ear, then hold a watch against the mastoid bone behind that ear. The ticks will come through clearly.

Bone conduction explains why many victims of conductive deafness hear their own voices quite loudly, and consequently speak so softly. They frequently hear well over the telephone, because the receiver is clamped to the big temporal bone encasing the ear; but they have trouble hearing television or a church sermon, whose sound waves travel to them through the air.

In perceptive (or nerve) deafness, the outer and middle ear function normally, but certain vibrations can go no farther. Circuits to the brain are out of order. What's wrong? Damage, in most cases, to nerve endings of the inner ear, fibers of the auditory nerve, or hearing centers of the brain itself. Causes vary.

They include loud noises, head injuries, tumors and some diseases.

Nerve deafness generally results in impaired hearing of high-frequency sounds—sounds formed by a relatively high number of cycles, or vibrations, a second. In conversation, speech tones frequently missed by the nerve-deaf are *p*s, *k*s, *t*s, hard *c*s and *g*s, and *d*s. They may, for instance, hear *gain* as "-ain," *call* as "-all," *down* as "-own." They complain that their friends or relatives mumble. "I can hear you all right," they say, "but you're not making sense."

And to them, you aren't. Secretaries in early stages of nerve deafness begin to falter in dictation. Because bone conduction is of little help, victims hear poorly over the telephone and may miss vital words and phrases. Their own voices sound faint; unconsciously, they speak too loudly.

Since nerve damage cannot be repaired, nerve deafness presents serious obstacles to successful medical or surgical treatment. But Army and Navy specialists worked near wonders in rehabilitation with servicemen deafened by shellfire and explosions during World War II. As a result of their new techniques in speech reading (lipreading), speech analysis and auditory training, the nerve-deaf today, particularly children, stand a better-than-even chance of overcoming their handicap. Says a leading California orthodontist, stricken with nerve deafness in infancy, "I was told from earliest childhood that I couldn't talk, but I do. I was told I couldn't drive, fly, go to college, become a doctor. But I have done all of these."

What about hearing aids? Tiny transistorized devices—hidden behind a necktie, built into eyeglass frames or worn inconspicuously over the ear, and priced at $50 and up—are an indispensable help to thousands with impaired hearing. But experts urge the handicapped to consult an ear specialist before buying one, and to be realistic in their expectations. "Hearing aids can be a great boon, and are a major means of coping with hearing loss, but they're not perfect," says Dr. Raymond Carhart, noted Northwestern University audiologist. "They remain, after all, an 'aid.' They will amplify sound so you can use it, but don't expect them to restore normal hearing." If fitted early enough, most handicapped children of average intelligence can learn to use hearing aids. How early? Experts recommend, "As early as possible." Two- and three-year-olds have used them successfully.

Even more dramatic, however, have been advances in microsurgery. Today, working freely in the cramped galleries of the ear, surgeons restore hearing to patients whose impairments a few years ago were written off as hopeless.

The ear specialist can build a new eardrum with a graft of skin from the ear canal. If the hammer, anvil or stirrup—or any combination of them—has been destroyed, he can reconstruct the drum and middle-ear lining with mucous-membrane grafts from cheek or lip, and restore transmission of sound vibration. In extreme cases where the entire chain has been destroyed, he can sometimes fashion a middle-ear chamber that gets along without one.

These developments are encouraging otologists to step up the attack on other questions of vital concern: What causes otosclerosis? How does the inner ear transform sound vibrations into nerve impulses? What is the significance of the electrical signals, or potentials, emitted by the inner ear?

Researchers in medical centers across the nation are tackling these problems with high hopes of success. One development has been the creation of the Deafness Research Foundation in New York City. Organized in 1958 by Mrs. Hobart C. Ramsey, an otosclerosis victim whose hearing was restored by surgery after twenty years of partial deafness, the foundation's annual grants have risen from $15,000 to over $105,000. It has recently launched a project of exciting significance: the establishment of a nationwide chain of temporal bone "banks"—medical centers or laboratories to which people may bequeath their middle- and inner-ear structures for research.

What the University of Chicago's Dr. John R. Lindsay calls "the terrible barrier of silence" is being crossed in new and wonderful ways. As researchers probe more deeply into the mysteries of hearing and the mechanism of the ear, it is certain that still greater triumphs lie ahead.

Your Educated Nose

Adapted from "Have You an Educated Nose?" *by Roy Bedichek*
and "How Your Nose Knows" *by Ruth and Edward Brecher*

Most school systems have art teachers educating the eye and music teachers educating the ear, but none so far has attempted to tutor the nose. Yet the nose holds the key to distinctions no other sense can unlock, and to esthetic pleasures as great for some as music and pictures are for others.

Not vision, not hearing, not touch nor even taste, so nearly kin to smell, can call up memories with such verity. The odor of new-mown hay, burning leaves in the fall, bluebonnets, stable manure, ham and eggs cooking, new leather—or many another aroma—may suddenly bring back a magic moment, alive and unimpaired by lapse of time.

The sense of smell has few words which belong to it exclusively. Just in from an early-morning ramble through a grove of sycamores, I search in vain for a word to describe the pleasing odor that lingers in my nostrils. This paucity of odor words—common to most languages—is all the more remarkable when we consider that smell is the most experienced of the senses.

The newborn calf, shaky on its spindly legs, with wide-open but unseeing eyes, searches along the vast underside of its mother, guided by smell to the distended udder. Cows, sows, ewes and nanny goats, bitches, mares—all identify their young by odor, even after the infant has found its voice.

The sense of taste tells you only whether a substance is sweet, sour, salty or bitter. It is your sense of smell that reveals the true savor of food.

Try sipping onion soup while holding your nose, or when you have a head cold. The characteristic flavor vanishes. All that is left is a hot, somewhat salty liquid. By means of taste alone, you can barely distinguish between a food you love and one you detest.

In the human face the outside nose is obvious, but another nose, in the upper nostrils, is a hidden mechanism of unimaginable delicacy. On each side of the upper nostrils, a spot about the size of a dime contains special nerve cells. Odor molecules, which in the form of gases travel even in the stillest air or water, are carried to these cells and produce chemical reactions.

Flavors reach the nose "through the back door": they travel from the mouth down the throat and then up again along the air passages which lead to the nasal cavities. You "smell" when you inhale; you sense flavors when you exhale; otherwise the

NASAL CAVITY

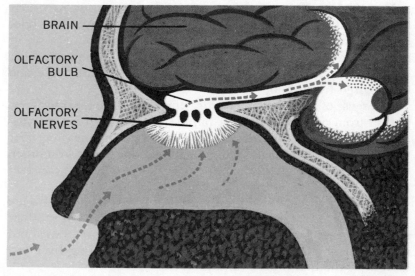

BRAIN

OLFACTORY
BULB

OLFACTORY
NERVES

two processes are the same. Both depend upon your olfactory tracts—the nerve-rich surfaces which form the ceilings of your two nasal cavities.

Each olfactory area is about the size of a postage stamp and located so high in the nasal passages that, during ordinary inhaling, moderately odorous air may pass under it without arousing any decided smell sensations. When you see something whose odor you wish to sample, you sniff—and this carries the odor-laden air upward to the olfactory tract. There is no need to sniff while you eat, though. As you chew your food, warm vapors are released from it; the act of swallowing and the related act of exhaling pump these flavor-laden vapors upward toward the nose.

In general, the higher the temperature of a substance, the more molecules are given off and the more intense is the odor. This explains why good cooks insist on serving dishes piping hot.

Unlike the eye and the ear, which respond to only a limited and precise range of vibration, the mechanism in this inner nose is able to receive a virtually unlimited number of odor stimuli.

In certain respects, smell is the subtlest of our senses. A scientist can, with the help of costly laboratory aids, identify one drop of a chemical mixed with a million drops of something else. But with his unaided nose the same scientist, or anyone else, can instantly identify a highly odorous mercaptan—for example, that responsible for the stench of the skunk—even though each molecule of it is diluted with billions of molecules of air.

Why are some smells pleasant and some unpleasant? The answer seems to lie partly in the distant past of mankind and partly in each individual's experience. The stenches of rotting and of excrement are almost universally detested; they are warnings of possible contamination. And the odor of the skunk is nauseating not only to humans but to animals as well.

On a spring-morning stroll in the country, or a walk in the woods, there are fresh and delightful nasal experiences at every turn. Some people have the bad habit of picking a flower or a spray from a fragrant shrub and holding it to the nose. They will learn from experience that one odor in the bush is worth two in the hand. Nature anticipated the perfumery trade by mixing odors indiscriminately in the wind, and the sniffer abroad is in for delightful surprises. Unique blends are bound to occur; mixtures never before sensed by mortal man may come casually into his nostrils.

Though in our Western civilization the sense of smell has fallen from its great estate as dispenser of sensuous delights, it is a sense that can be developed. The Japanese, who perfume many things that come into daily use about the household, have a game of competitive identification of odors. Helen Keller, through her blindness, has acquired an exquisite sense of smell. Often she knows without being told what occupations people are engaged in, through the odors of wood, iron, paint or drugs clinging to their garments. "When a person passes by," she wrote, "I get a scent impression of where he has been—the kitchen, the garden or the sickroom." In short, she can smell a way of life.

We are only at the threshold of discovering the linkage of smells with the emotions, and the still unexplained physiology of the transmission of sensory data to the brain. Perhaps one day, when we come to understand this delicate sense, we will give it the education it deserves. Then we may be able to restore to the human nose the full power and acuteness it once had, before neglect and the violent affront upon it of burning gasoline, smoke and the thousands of other products of civilization disrupted the marvelous mechanism of olfaction.

SMELLS are surer than sound or sights
To make your heartstrings crack.
—Rudyard Kipling

All about Your Throat

by Evan McLeod Wylie

Any morning in winter more than a million North Americans wake up with sore throats. No other ailment save its frequent companion, the ordinary cold, is so much with us. Yet because its victims are so numerous and their misery so familiar, there is a tendency to regard it as a pesky but trivial illness. The truth is that the sore throat is perhaps the most important alarm signal in the human body—a warning that carriers of disease have penetrated the body's outer defenses and are gathering strength to press their assault farther.

The word "throat" covers several separate structures linked by a system of valves—raising and lowering and squeezing devices—that permit us to breathe, talk, eat and drink. Clog one of these for an instant and life is jeopardized. Alter their amazing anatomical arrangement by a fraction of an inch and the world would be reduced to sign language.

The tissues of the throat are delicate but remarkably durable. Protected by only a thin sheet of mucus and saliva, they endure temperatures ranging from ice cream at 8° Fahrenheit to coffee at 160°. Every fifteen seconds air swishes past them at ten miles per hour; a sneeze or cough rips through at a speed as high as

200 miles per hour. In one day they are exposed to around 3000 gallons of oxygen and carbon dioxide and some billion dust particles. In addition to the auto-exhaust fumes that permeate the air most of us breathe, a heavy smoker's tissues must face the onslaught of parching, tar-laden smoke. The complex chain of events we call the swallow, which requires the split-second teamwork of dozens of pairs of muscles, takes place around 3000 times a day. And unless the throat's owner is a hermit, it will also be called on daily to carry out the rapid-fire muscular expansions and contractions necessary to form more than 25,000 words of talk.

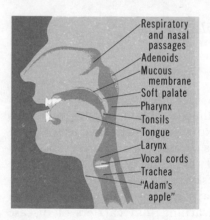

Respiratory and nasal passages
Adenoids
Mucous membrane
Soft palate
Pharynx
Tonsils
Tongue
Larynx
Vocal cords
Trachea
"Adam's apple"

Let's look at the chronically overworked structure. Open wide in front of a mirror and the most you will see is the tip of the soft palate hanging from the roof of the mouth. But if you had a physician's tongue depressor, you could flatten out your tongue long enough to glimpse a bit of the middle portion of the throat, called the pharynx—a sort of crossroads of the windpipe, nose, mouth and esophagus. On each side of the pharynx you might see twin beds of soft tissue called the tonsils. With a specialist's long, slender mirror and forehead light, you could see a reflected view of the larynx (Adam's apple) with its two taut, ivory-white vocal cords.

It is in the hollow larynx, or voice box, that the column of air pressed upward from the lungs is transformed by the cords, vibrating like rubber bands, into high- and low-frequency sound waves. These vibrations, in turn, are molded into words by the rapid muscular actions of the walls of the throat, the soft palate, tongue, lips and teeth.

Because the larynx is constantly exposed to germ-laden air and smoke and because many of us abuse our voices, the larynx tissues and vocal cords often become so inflamed that the voice is reduced to a hoarse whisper or is lost altogether, a condition known as laryngitis. But hoarseness does not necessarily imply infection. It may be due to emotional problems which cause a tightening of the throat muscles and disturb the delicate vibrations of the vocal cords, thus altering the volume and pitch of their sound waves. Suppressed rage and tension may cause the voice to become harsh and shrill; deep-seated fear or guilt may make it thin, shaky and high-pitched. Even total loss of voice can occur in a perfectly normal larynx that is paralyzed by acute anxiety.

The throat is not only overworked, it is also crowded, becoming within a few hours after birth the domain of millions of germs which swarm in the air we breathe and in the food we eat. Here the skirmishes with most internal infections are fought out, and the result determines whether or not the attacking organisms will succeed in reaching other parts of the body. Among diseases ushered in with a mildly inflamed throat are influenza, infantile paralysis, meningitis, scarlet fever, whooping cough and measles. And the dangerous acute inflammation known as "strep throat," if unchecked, may progress to rheumatic fever, which sometimes leads to crippling damage to the heart and kidneys.

The throat's passageways also offer choice routes for invading microbes to spread into the upper nasal passages to cause acute sinusitis, into the middle ear and mastoid bones to cause abscesses and deafness, and down the trachea into the lungs to bring on pneumonia and pleurisy. When the throat is attacked by the virus that causes the common cold, the growth of bacteria already residing in it immediately increases and may bring on attacks of bronchitis, tonsillitis or laryngitis. This explains the popular misconception that the sore throat is a symptom of the common cold; actually it may be a separate disease.

To counter germs, however, the throat has a highly effective ring of defense traps. Known as Waldeyer's ring, this consists of islands of lymphoid tissue whose function is to attract the germs and then overwhelm them with large numbers of white corpuscles and antibodies rushed to the site via the bloodstream.

The tonsils and adenoids are masses of this spongy lymphoid tissue. They are particularly large during childhood and are often inflamed as they do battle with infectious organisms. Through them most children gain lifetime immunities to many diseases which might cause more dangerous illnesses in adult life. Sometimes, however, the tonsils, weakened by germ wars, become chronically diseased, and a physician may recommend surgical removal.

The other key defense mechanism of the throat, particularly important in adult life, is a lining of delicate, reddish mucous membranes which manufacture the watery secretions that keep the throat moist and shield the body tissues from bacteria. The mucus flows as an elastic but continuous sheet, carrying away the invading germs. Many factors in modern living, however, tend to interfere with this normal secretion. Tobacco smoke, industrial smog, exhaust fumes and heavy alcohol consumption all irritate the membranes, constrict their blood vessels, dry up the flow of mucus and decrease its effectiveness. Air-conditioning and central-heating systems can wring too much moisture from the atmosphere.

The mucous membranes can also be weakened by faulty diet, chronic fatigue and constant mental stress, which drain the body's defenses. All that is needed then is the triggering action of a sudden change in temperature, or of a wetting or chilling. As this draws the blood to other parts of the body, the blood vessels of the throat constrict, the temperature of the membranes drops and the ever-present bacteria seize their opportunity to attack the tissues.

Sore-throat sufferers have through the years swabbed, sprayed, irrigated and painted their throats. They have sucked on cracked ice, gargled with scalding hot solutions, downed hot toddies, inhaled the dizzying fumes of pine oil and quinine and girdled the neck in rubber ice-collars. Americans seeking relief from sore throats and from the colds that often accompany them spend millions of dollars a year for soothing medicaments, syrups, drops, sprays and lozenges.

Most physicians admit that the old home remedies and patent

medicines can be useful to *relieve the symptoms* of the sore throat. The chief ingredient in most syrups and drops, they explain, is sugar, a soothing agent which promotes the flow of saliva. Some contain codeine or its derivatives, which help suppress unnecessary coughing and give the throat's inflamed tissues a rest. The neck ointments and oils, acting as mild counterirritants, draw increased amounts of blood to the throat region, which is in itself a help.

The principal objection among medical men to the patent remedies is that they encourage a tendency to seek relief at the drug counter instead of in the one place where it can be quickly and cheaply obtained—at home. For it is the consensus of throat experts that the best remedy for the sore-throat victim is simply to stay in bed for forty-eight hours, consume generous portions of a high-protein diet and plenty of fruit juices, stop smoking and keep his mouth shut. In the occasional case of a stubborn infection or an acute inflammation, such as the strep throat, a house visit by the family doctor should do the trick.

If you have a sore throat, said the late Dr. Alfred Schattner, specialist at the Manhattan Eye, Ear and Throat Hospital, to adults, "You probably have only yourself to blame for abusing your throat or permitting your body's resistance to fall below normal. Nature favors neither man nor microbe, and he who is best able to protect himself will survive."

Though she'd never had much truck with doctors, Aunt Maisie got through the examination and treatment pretty well. As she was leaving, the physician said, "I'd like to see you again in two weeks." She kept the appointment, but was indignant at the end of the month to find the doctor had charged her for both visits.

"The second one was your idea," she told him over the phone. "*You* wanted to see *me*."
                                                            —Thora Eigenmann

The Myth of
the "Terrible Tonsils"

by Lois Mattox Miller

For many years parents and doctors considered tonsils useless, disease-breeding things. We embarked on a surgical crusade, and at its peak more than two million people yearly in the U.S. and Canada—mostly young children—had their tonsils out. Today many physicians are urging a "closed season" on tonsils, until parents and family doctors catch up with the modern concept. *The Journal of the American Medical Association* sums it up this way: "Tonsils when functioning normally are protective organs and should not be removed. Definitely infected tonsils and especially tonsil stumps should be removed under general anesthesia and with adequate surgical technique and skill."

Swollen and inflamed tonsils, however, are by no means "definitely infected." In this angry state they are merely doing the job nature intended for them: trapping and draining off infection, and helping to build up immunity for the future. "More often than not," says one specialist, "swollen tonsils deserve a medal for valor instead of condemnation."

The tonsils are now recognized as part of the lymphatic system, which has the important job of trapping, destroying and draining off infection before it can penetrate deeper into the system. They belong to the first line of defense in the upper respiratory tract—the favorite invasion site for most germs.

The traplike function of the tonsils has been demonstrated by a number of investigators. One doctor injected India ink into the nasal membranes of patients scheduled for tonsillectomy. When the tonsils were removed, he found the ink particles trapped within the spongy capsules. Vaccine virus, inoculated on the arms of infants, turned up in the tonsils three days later.

Tonsil flare-ups occur most frequently in children under ten years of age. This is the time when the body is waging a constant fight against a host of infections, building up immunities that will last a lifetime. In the latest evaluations of tonsil function, doctors warn that the tonsils are intended by nature to play an important part in the development of "autoimmunization" in the young child.

At the age of five or six years this immunization is far from complete. Repeated infections are necessary to build it. Immunization will increase steadily if the tonsils are left intact, even though the tonsils themselves occasionally become swollen and inflamed in the process. But if the tonsils and adenoids are removed before immunization is complete, the doctors say, "the child will remain unprotected and may be endangered later in his lifetime."

Formerly, tonsillitis attacks usually prompted the doctors to say: "Let's have those tonsils out in the spring." School nurses and medical examiners were even more adamant: any child with "enlarged" tonsils was likely to be sent home with a note ordering tonsillectomy.

Tonsil flare-ups are often warning signals, indicating some other trouble. The extraction of bad teeth or treatment of sinus infection puts an end to tonsillitis attacks in a surprising number of cases. Allergies also can cause the tonsils to become enlarged. Treat the allergy or remove the infection, the doctors advise—

don't just remove the tonsils. Tonsil surgery in such cases is like trying to put out the fire by silencing the alarm bell!

The old idea that tonsillectomy "prevented" colds and respiratory diseases was thoroughly debunked a few years ago by a ten-year study of 4400 children who, according to former standards, "should" have had their tonsils removed. For various reasons only half that number had the operation performed. But the entire group remained under study for the next ten years.

Comparison showed that removal of tonsils failed to reduce the incidence of colds, ear infections, sinusitis, laryngitis, bronchitis, pneumonia or tuberculosis. Indeed, there seemed to be more colds and respiratory diseases among the children whose tonsils and adenoids had been removed.

Pediatricians point out that most childhood diseases now can be either prevented or controlled by the use of antibiotics. With these drugs available, tonsil surgery is clearly obsolete as a preventive measure.

When the tonsils are definitely diseased, or the adenoids so enlarged that they interfere with breathing, surgery is obviously in order. Then the operation should be performed by an experienced surgeon. The common belief that tonsillectomy is always "simple and safe" is now tempered with caution.

"We regard tonsillectomy as a major operation and not without danger," say doctors. "The more skilled the tonsil surgeon, the greater is his respect for this supposedly simple and minor procedure."

All doctors agree upon one safe rule: Because respiratory ills are more common during the winter months, tonsillectomies should be performed in the spring or summer, *but never when there is polio around.*

Simply stated, the current view of tonsils is this: Have them removed only if they are definitely infected, enlarged to the point of obstruction or the *cause* of repeated attacks of tonsillitis. That is something for the doctor to decide. Otherwise you can count them among nature's blessings and forget the old wives' tales about the "terrible tonsils."

CHAPTER 6

The Marvelous Teamwork of Command and Control

OUR NERVOUS system, in its efficiency and complexity, dwarfs anything that man has so far devised in the field of communications. The work of our muscles is so complicated that science has not yet discovered all the secrets of human movement. The bone structure, outranking steel in strength, provides also, as few of us know, a manufacturing plant and storehouse for the body. Together, the nerves, muscles and bones give man the controls he needs to carry out the incredibly complex commands of his brain.

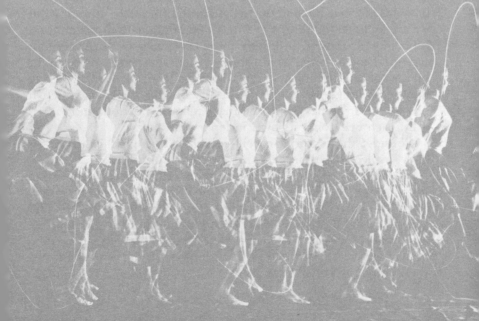

How Your Nervous System Works

by J. D. Ratcliff

We are awed by the complicated tangle of wires in a large telephone cable; wonder-struck by the efficiency of a communications system that completes a call from Melbourne, Florida, to Melbourne, Australia, in a few minutes. But we are inclined to take for granted a communications system that is far more extensive, infinitely more complex—our own nervous system. Day and night millions of messages pour through its billions of cells, telling the heart when to beat, the limbs when to move, the lungs when to suck in air. But for the links which it provides, our bodies would be mere masses of chaotic individual cells, each cell going its own independent way.

Consider the sensory nerves—which tell us whether a steak is tasty, a piece of music pleasing, a view inspiring.

The tongue has 3000 taste buds, each with its nerve connection to the brain. No one knows exactly how these taste-bud receptors work, but current thinking suggests that particles of food fit into them like light plugs into sockets, closing circuits and sending electrical impulses to the brain. The brain interprets them, then arrives at a judgment: the potatoes need salt, the orange is sour, the lamb chop is delicious.

The ears have 100,000 auditory cells. Minute nerve ends in the inner ear pick up a particular sound frequency and start vibrating—waving like wheat in the wind. A current is generated. It may be so feeble that it must be amplified thousands of times before it can be detected; fed into the brain, it is identified as a musical note. Or a medley of sounds may feed in at the same time, to be instantly recognized as a friend's voice, a train's whistle, the bark of a dog. Thus we hear *with* our ears but *in* the brain.

Each eye has 130,000,000 light receptors which send group impressions to the brain. We see the lovely spring foliage *with* our eyes, but it is the brain that gives us a feeling of joy and appreciation. Sometimes the eye nerves play strange tricks on us. We bump our head in a dark room and there is a blinding flash of light—we "see stars." What has happened is this: the bump has stimulated the optic nerve to send electrical impulses which the brain interprets as a flash of light.

The skin contains a vast network of receptors. If a hot object is pressed against the skin, some of the 30,000 "heat spots" will warn of danger. It has 250,000 cold receptors, and something like half a million tactile (touch) spots.

The brain pays little attention to messages from only a few receptors. A hot needle can be pressed against the skin with no great discomfort. But press an equally hot iron against it and a general alarm goes out. That's why it's dangerous to test a baby's bath water with only your fingertips. The water may not be too hot for your fingers, but it can be highly uncomfortable for the baby when receptors all over his body spring into action.

In the main, the function of nerves is to prod muscles into action. But they also have a mysterious ability to dampen or inhibit motion. Otherwise when we moved a leg to take a step it might continue to rise as if we were kicking a football. During sleep, apparently, this dampening effect becomes dominant, pervading the entire brain. This accounts for the occasional paralysis of terror in dreams: we want to cry out but cannot; we want to run, but our leaden legs refuse to move.

Nerve cells have characteristics which set them apart from all others. Most body cells reproduce themselves by simple division: a cut fingertip heals itself; hair, fingernails and toenails push themselves out constantly as cell division progresses. Nerve cells follow no such pattern. We have our lifetime supply at birth, and once a nerve cell is destroyed it is destroyed for good—although subsidiary nerve channels may establish pathways around the damage.

Individual nerve cells look somewhat like pollywogs, with large cellular heads and long filamentous tails. The cellular head is the critical, nonreplaceable part of a nerve; the tail can regenerate itself if cut or injured. Most of the heads are located in the brain or spinal cord. The tails, or nerve fibers—which may be of microscopic length or as long as three feet—are bundled together, often by the thousands, into nerve trunks which can be as big around as your thumb. From the brain and spinal cord these nerve trunks branch out into the farthest reaches of the body.

There are several main divisions of the nervous system. The autonomic branch governs such "automatic" functions as digestion, breathing and the heartbeat. It is divided into two parts: the sympathetic system, which generally stimulates activity, and the parasympathetic, which generally retards it. If the body were entirely under the control of the sympathetic system, the heart, for example, would race itself to death. If entirely under the parasympathetic, the heart would stop. The two must be in perfect coördination. When quick energy is needed in times of stress, the sympathetic gains the ascendency, speeding up heart and lung activity. In sleep, the parasympathetic lays a calming hand on all bodily activity.

Motor nerves—the nerves which govern such voluntary actions as walking, talking, chewing—appear to work in another manner. When the brain sends out a message ordering an arm to be lifted, a tiny electric "shiver" starts out from the brain through motor nerves. The impulse is so small that it would never reach the arm but for the fact that every few centimeters along the nerve fiber there is a "relay station" which recharges the dying current, so that the impulse arrives at its destination with exactly the same value it had when it left the brain. This elaborate sequence also takes place in a twinkling: messages are transmitted through nerves at over 200 miles an hour.

People sometimes complain of "frayed" or "shot" nerves. Actually, nerves aren't responsible for feelings of tension. Emotional conflicts in the brain are the cause. A troubled brain may send out electrical impulses which result in too large a secretion of stomach acids, leading to ulcers. Or it may order the tightening of muscles in blood-vessel walls, which leads to high blood pressure. In these situations the nerves, like telephone wires carrying bad news, are simply acting as a communications system.

Occasionally, however, nerves *do* get out of whack. One of the causes of hiccups, for example, is irritation of the respiratory nerves. Shingles, an acute inflammatory skin disease, is the result of irritation or infection of the sensory nerves.

As research men have gathered more and more facts about the nervous system, physicians and surgeons have put this new knowledge to work. Nerve repair is perhaps the most exacting of all surgical arts. In accidents, nerves are often severed and must be rejoined if a hand, arm or leg is again to be useful. The nerves to be sewn may be no larger than a hair and must be sewn with still finer suture materials. Working with a magnifying glass and filamentous silk or linen, skilled surgeons are often able to do this job.

When injury is so extensive that nerve ends cannot be pulled together, the answer is a graft, borrowed either from the patient's body or from a "bank." Such grafts do not grow; they merely form a bed on which the nerve fibers regenerate themselves. One of surgery's most rewarding sights is to see life return gradually, over a period of months, to a limb thus repaired.

Nerve researchers still face a host of unanswered questions. They are unable, for instance, to explain what a tickle is. Nor do they clearly understand some of the remarkable reflexes with which we are born: how the newborn puckers his lips, ready to feed; or how he curls his fingers to grasp objects.

When we reach a complete understanding of the nervous system, we shall be close to understanding a supreme riddle of the universe: how that mass of cells known as man manages to behave like a human being.

The
Miracle of Muscle

by J. D. Ratcliff

❧

Events that take place when a dog wags its tail, a baby toddles across the floor or you scratch your nose with your forefinger dwarf in complexity the workings of a hydrogen bomb. All are examples of muscular contraction—so commonplace we pay it no heed, yet so mysterious that it has baffled the most gifted scientists.

More than half the human body is muscle—"the most remarkable stuff in nature's curiosity shop," as one scientist has said. From birth to death, muscles play a critical role in everything we do. They propel us into the world in the first place—when the womb suddenly empties itself. They provide nearly all our internal heat. They push food along the digestive tract, suck air into lungs, squeeze tears from lachrymal glands. And *finis* is written for us when the heart muscle, after beating two and a half billion times in a seventy-year life span, falters and fails.

We speak of "muscles of iron." Yet the working, or contractile, element in muscle is a soft jelly. How this jelly contracts to lift a thousand times its own weight is one of the supreme miracles of the universe. An elaborate series of chemical and electrical events, which would require hours or days to duplicate in the laboratory, occurs almost instantaneously when a muscle contracts—in the twitch of an eyelid, for example.

There are three types of muscle in the human body. One is the striated muscle, which looks like a sheaf of hair-sized filaments. These are the muscles of motion—that propel us when we walk, that lift a forkful of food, that nod our heads. Next come the "smooth" muscles. These control such involuntary actions as the churning of intestines during digestion, the dilation of the pupil. A third type is found in the heart. In structure, it is midway between the other two. All types of muscles are startlingly efficient machines for converting chemical energy (food) into mechanical energy (work).

Hundreds of books and scientific papers have been written on muscles—but none explains fully the process by which muscles contract, *how* you wiggle a toe. "It is essential that we understand these puzzles," says Dr. Albert Szent-Györgyi, of the Institute for Muscle Research, Woods Hole, Massachusetts, and a Nobel Prize winner. "In one way or another, failure of muscles to contract properly accounts for the vast majority of deaths—from heart failure, high blood pressure and other diseases."

Two proteins, Dr. Szent-Györgyi has found, are mainly responsible for the contraction—actin and myosin. Alone, neither is contractile. But when an electrical impulse from the brain orders the batting of an eye, or the wrinkling of a nose, actin and myosin combine to form actomyosin, which *is* contractile.

In a sense actomyosin is the muscular "engine." Its fuel is a remarkable chemical substance, adenosine triphosphate—ATP for short. ATP is a submicroscopic bombshell of energy. Actomyosin fibers contract violently on contact with it. At death, ATP disintegrates rapidly and muscles become hard, inelastic. This is rigor mortis.

To demonstrate the critical importance of ATP, Dr. Szent-Györgyi has stored rabbit muscles, which had been washed free of the chemical, in freezers for periods up to a year. Taken out, thawed and touched with ATP, the hard, brittle muscles spring to life; once again they show the elasticity they had when they propelled a rabbit in its hopping gait.

Creating "living" tissue in the laboratory has been something of a scientific will-o'-the-wisp. But muscle researchers have come close to it. At Woods Hole, Dr. Szent-Györgyi mixed jellylike actin with jellylike myosin. Then, with the aid of a tiny glass nozzle, he spun this material into gossamer filaments. Watching through a microscope, he added a droplet of ATP to the fluid surrounding the filament. There was violent contraction! He had created artificially perhaps the most fundamental of all life processes—muscular contraction. "It was," he says, "the most exciting moment of my life."

Where are such experiments leading? They may open a new frontier of attack on some of mankind's greatest ills. There is no logical reason why the human heart should beat two billion times during a lifetime, then suddenly fail. Almost nothing is known about the cruel crippling of muscular dystrophy; or why muscles in blood-vessel walls should tighten to produce the misery of hypertension; or why the uterine muscles of many women become crampily contracted each month to cause painful distress. Once the mechanics of muscular action are thoroughly understood, Dr. Szent-Györgyi thinks, "we will be at the beginning of a new biology, a new medicine."

Meanwhile, there is a great deal all of us can do to keep our muscles functioning well. First, they must be properly fed. Generally speaking, the average diet includes all the protein needed for muscle repair, and all the carbohydrate required for muscle fuel. But muscles can starve through lack of exercise—witness hospital patients who eat perfectly balanced meals and get out of bed too weak to walk. Reason: Muscles are nourished by thousands of miles of hairlike capillaries, which transport food and carry off wastes. In the sedentary adult, large numbers of these capillaries are collapsed, out of business, nearly all the time. Exercise alone can open them up and provide better muscle nutrition.

Often, muscles become unduly fatigued when required to work at too fast a rate. One housewife rushes at her chores and is worn out by noon, while her more leisurely sister accomplishes just as much and finishes the day still fresh. A series of treadmill experiments tells why. In one, subjects were paced at 140 steps a minute. Gradually the speed was increased to 280. At the doubled rate, the oxygen requirements of muscles increased eightfold! Supplying such demands is fatiguing in itself. All work and exercise should be paced to get the most out of our muscles.

Like all other body organs and tissues, muscles must have rest. Millions of people sleep the traditional eight hours, then get up exhausted. The most likely explanation: One set of muscles has been cramped, tensed all night—wearing out the rest of the body. The best way to avoid this is to lie quietly in bed, legs straight, arms at the side. Contract one set of muscles at a time, and consciously relax them.

Overburdened or weakened muscles sometimes require additional support. This is particularly true of the back muscles, whose chief function is to hold the body erect. Most low-back pain traces to weakness of these muscles. Every physician has his favorite set of exercises to provide new strength. But until exercises are well underway, extra support is sometimes necessary. A polo belt is useful for this purpose.

It is best, of course, not to wait until muscles are weakened before giving them the care and consideration they deserve. For, to a great degree, we are what our muscles make us—sick or well, vigorous or droopy, alive or dead.

PHYSIOLOGISTS have shown that one reason people are touchy, easily insulted or grieved, is that they go through life with jaws set, faces strained and muscles tense. This causes them to jump at the slightest noise, or the slightest insult to their egos. They say their nerves are on edge, but it is mainly their muscles, from eyelids to toes, that are jumping. When all your muscles are relaxed and at ease, your nerves and ego will also be at ease.   —Albert Edward Wiggam

RECENTLY I charged a businessman what I thought was a reasonable fee for my services as an anesthesiologist during a major operation. Apparently he didn't agree. Pinned to his check was this note: "I saw your mask, but I didn't see your gun."   —Floyd F. Marchi, M.D.

Muscular Aches and Pains

An Interview with Janet Travell, M.D.

Dr. Janet Travell was selected by President John F. Kennedy as White House physician. She is the first woman to hold this post. Dr. Travell has successfully treated thousands of persons with disabling back pains, including the President.

Q *Dr. Travell, what types of pain grow out of muscular troubles?*

A Most frequently it is simple muscle "tension"—generalized contraction of muscles in the neck and the back, for instance, in people who are under pressures of anxiety. We call this tension "muscle spasm."

Q *Would you explain muscle spasm?*

A Spasm is the state of shortening of a skeletal muscle in which its owner loses the ability to relax the muscle voluntarily. Usually, if you say to your arm, "Relax," your wrist will drop and the muscles will lengthen. The person who has muscle spasm cannot do this.

Q *And this causes pain?*

A Muscle spasm usually creates some pain. When the muscle shortens far beyond its physiological limit, the contraction might be called a "cramp," and this is extremely painful. In addition, when only part of a muscle shortens, distortion occurs and shearing stresses are placed on the blood vessels and nerve structures within the muscle; this sets up a great deal of pain.

Q *How widespread is muscle spasm?*

A It is probably the most common complaint that affects the human race. We see it in such ailments as stiff neck, muscular headaches, the atypical facial neuralgias.

Q *Can a person tell that it is a muscle that is hurting him?*

A Curiously, he usually doesn't know this. When a muscle is in fixed spasm, it probably shuts down its own blood supply. In this condition, it frequently sets off "referred pain"—pain perceived at a distance from the muscle that is its source. This is analogous to the pain of a coronary thrombosis, or heart attack. When a section of heart muscle has an inadequate supply of blood owing to spasm of the coronaries, or to a thrombus—clot—in the coronary arteries, the heart gives rise to referred pain. The pain is felt up and down the breastbone or it may be perceived in the neck, or in the back or down the arm to the fingers. Similarly, if the gallbladder goes into spasm, you may have "referred pain" in the tip of the shoulder.

Q *How do you trace such pain?*

A Each muscle has its own pattern or distribution of referred pain. When you have accumulated experience with these muscle-pain syndromes [groups of symptoms which occur together], you recognize the referred-pain pattern. There are several guides. One: When the muscle is used, it not only produces referred pain but is accompanied by limitation of motion at the joint that it crosses. Another: Spontaneous pain is produced if one palpates the muscle that is the source of pain.

Q *Is arthritis linked with muscle spasm?*

A Arthritis, which affects the joints, is usually accompanied by muscle spasm, but the spasm is secondary to the inflammation of the joint itself. That is, the muscle around the joint will splint— harden—and tighten to try to protect the joint. Pain in a given region may be partly arthritic and partly muscular; so you may be able to do quite a lot to relieve arthritic pain by treating the muscles, recognizing full well that they are not the primary cause.

Q *What about "tennis elbow" and "Charley horse"?*

A "Charley horse" is a muscular pain. "Tennis elbow" is often a muscular problem.

When there is muscle spasm, the trigger area in the muscle gives rise not only to referred pain but also to referred tenderness. The place where the person feels pain becomes sensitive to touch. Thus, in the "tennis elbow" of muscular origin, the outer side of the elbow is very sore to the touch. And in the big muscle that swings the arm across and tightens the wrist—the action involved in one of the main tennis strokes—you will find a tender, firm "knot." If you inject that with procaine—Novocain—not only the pain in the elbow disappears, but the tenderness will also disappear within five minutes.

Q *What sets off muscle spasms?*

A Many kinds of stresses can be placed on muscles. One of the commonest is chilling, at a time when the muscle is fatigued from overuse or exercise. Or sudden overstretching of a muscle in a fall may result in its overcontraction—causing stiffness later, which may be so extreme as to result in a state of spasm.

Q *Does sleeping in a draft cause stiff neck?*

A This is extremely common. There may be times, of course, when you can sleep in a draft and not get a stiff neck. But if some kind of nutritional reserve in the muscle has been drained through overuse or exercise of the muscle, then, during the postexercise stiffness period, chilling can result in protracted spasm.

Q *To avoid this, what do you advise?*

A Take care of your muscles and don't sit in a draft.

Q *How do you "take care of your muscles"?*

A One of the most important things is this: Immediately after vigorous exercise, take a hot shower or a hot bath and get warm. I'm speaking now of such activities as tennis or golf or gardening. But exercise comes in many forms. I have told people who are doing a lot of typing, for example, that if they will run hot water over their arms or soak them in a sink of hot water for three minutes twice during the day they can avoid a lot of trouble.

Q *Can lack of sleep lead to muscle pain?*

A It leads to muscle fatigue, because the muscles don't relax at night if you don't rest properly; they don't recover from strain or work. (When we say "tension" we mean actually that the muscles are working all the time.) From muscle fatigue comes susceptibility to chilling and susceptibility to injury by ordinary physical activities.

Q *When you find a source of muscle spasm, what do you do?*

A First, I try to eliminate the basic cause. Second, I treat the muscle directly, and there are many ways to do that. You can use hot, moist packs, or massage, or procaine injections, or vapocoolant sprays, any of which may be effective. Whatever treatment you select is applied, not to the place where the person feels the pain, but to the place where the pain originates. Once you begin to do that, the results are remarkable.

Q *What are coolant sprays? You once called them "cold in a bottle."*

A Actually, a coolant spray is a liquid at room temperature and a gas at body temperature. If it's applied to your skin, it cools by evaporation. I use a nonproprietary mixture that is not flammable and doesn't explode and is relatively nontoxic. It's not generally available, but some medical centers are making it. There's a tremendous need for it.

Q *How does a vapor spray work?*

A Its mechanism is akin to that of counterirritation. It is not so much a means of freezing the skin as it is an intermittent "make-and-break" stimulus—of both touch and cold. Applied over a muscle, vapor spray changes the reflex control in the muscle.

Q *How quickly does it relieve pain?*

A It doesn't relieve pain at all unless you get the muscle to lengthen normally again. So, in combination with the application of the spray, it's necessary to put a gentle stretch on the muscle. The spray will permit you to move the part of the body that is hurting—the head, or the neck, or the shoulder, or the arm—in such a way that you can coax the muscle to lengthen. You very gently stretch out the spasm.

Q *Is early treatment important in dealing with muscle pain?*

A The longer the pain lasts, the more muscles you have to deal with. Pain may start in one muscle and after a while, neighboring parallel lines of muscles will shorten and tighten to protect the first one from carrying a load. The problem then is to get all the guy ropes back to normal resting length. That becomes much more difficult.

Q *Can your methods give relief to people who have a slipped disc in the back?*

A In the "acute" disc—the inflammatory stage of disc injury [an injury to the cushion of cartilage and fibrous tissue between two vertebrae]—relieving the muscle spasm doesn't help. After the disc has got well, my methods might help a great deal in dealing with what is sometimes called a "postdisc syndrome." Here the situation in the disc, or in the spine, is fine, but the patient continues to have the same pain in the legs and back—which is now entirely the result of the residual muscle spasm. This spasm may respond well to treatment.

Q *Why is it that doctors who are skillful enough to repair a slipped disc seem unable to cure the muscle spasms that persist afterward?*

A The doctor who repairs the slipped disc is primarily a surgeon. The medical follow-up treatment after slipped-disc surgery involves painstaking attention to the total medical and mechanical problems of the muscles over a period of time. There is no reason why a top surgeon should be doing this kind of job. It is unfortunate that we do not have a medical specialty devoted to the skeletal muscle system.

Q *Are more and more aches and pains inevitable as one gets older and the muscles age?*

A No, I don't believe they are inevitable. People tend to accept their pains. They think, "Well, I'm just getting older, and I've got a lame leg—I've got rheumatism." But I have rehabilitated many people in their seventies and eighties who thought they were being laid on the shelf permanently simply because they couldn't do the physical things they needed to do.

Q *Are these techniques being taught in medical schools?*

A Medical students are so busy learning about acute illness and life and death that they do not necessarily appreciate the importance of muscular pain. There isn't time for it in our current medical curriculum.

Our Busy Bones

Adapted from "Our Busy Bones" by J. D. Ratcliff,
"Our Living Bones" by Elsie McCormick
and "The Skeleton Speaks" by Wilton Marion Krogman

❧

"Lazybones?" There is no such thing. We may think that our bones are inert, dead, the body's structural steel. Actually, they are among the busiest living organs in the body. They are thriving manufacturing plants which make red and white blood cells twenty-four hours a day. Every minute about 180,000,000 red cells die. Your bones must replace them with healthy young cells, or you face anemic death. It takes six to eight weeks for the marrow to restore the red blood cells after a pint of blood has been removed.

Bones have other major responsibilities: they produce the white blood cells which fight off infection as well as the platelets which are essential for blood clotting, and they act as one of the body's storehouses for reserve nourishment. In their marrow they husband fats and proteins for time of need. And they contain nearly all the body's vital calcium and phosphorus. Calcium is necessary for the clotting of blood, the beating of the heart, the contraction of muscles and the functioning of the nervous system. By an intricate self-regulating system, calcium from milk drunk today is deposited in the bones, and calcium deposited last week or last year is withdrawn. If the calcium supply for the blood, nerves and muscles is lower than normal, the body withdraws some from the skeleton bank. Children on a poor, milkless diet have so much calcium taken away that their bones become soft and even crooked.

If you spend your days in an armchair, your system assumes that you have no need for strong bones, and proceeds to remove part of the precious minerals. Thus, people who fail to exercise are much more likely to suffer disabling fractures in their later years.

The human body has about 206 bones; the number varies. A child, for example, usually has 33 vertebral segments in his spine. In adults the lower segments fuse to make the sacrum and the coccyx, leaving 26. The number of ribs also varies. As a rule there are 12 pairs, but many people have only 11, some 13.

Bones range in size from the large femur, in the upper part of the leg, to the tiny stirrup bone that lies in the depths of the middle ear. They are among the most durable objects on earth. Human bones have been found that are nearly a million years old. Bones do not dissolve in water; if they did, they would soon be washed away by the body fluids. Hence they can outlast iron and other metals affected by dampness.

The human skeleton represents a masterpiece of engineering design, with each component part tailored to a specific job. The brain is protected by the skull, which is harder and denser where exposed to danger, as on top. The spinal cord, a highly sensitive and vital nerve center, is protected by vertebrae. The spine even has its own built-in shock absorbers—the discs of cushioning cartilage between segments.

The leg bones are hollow, in keeping with the engineering principle that a hollow column is stronger than a solid one of equal weight. On a weight-for-weight basis bones are stronger than steel. Bone construction is comparable to reinforced concrete.

There are two kinds of bony substance: spongy and compact. Any given bone, such as a rib, has both kinds. The compact bone forms a hard outer layer; inside lies the spongy bone, which in turn houses the weak tissue of the bone marrow, the nerves and the blood vessels. Bones contains thousands of small blood vessels and are quite as much alive as one's stomach. Active little cells

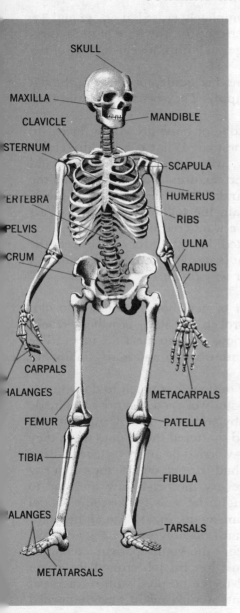

SKULL

MAXILLA

CLAVICLE

STERNUM

MANDIBLE

'ERTEBRA

SCAPULA

HUMERUS

RIBS

PELVIS

ULNA

CRUM

RADIUS

CARPALS

1ALANGES

METACARPALS

FEMUR

PATELLA

TIBIA

FIBULA

ALANGES

TARSALS

METATARSALS

called osteo*blasts* work night and day creating new bone, while house-wrecking cells known as osteo*clasts* labor just as hard tearing down material tagged for the scrap heap.

Sex shows itself plainly in a skeleton, the skull alone determining the factor in nine out of ten cases, while the pelvis will do it 98 percent of the time. The female skull capacity is some 200 cubic centimeters less than that of the male; the eyebrow ridges and mastoids are less prominent. Woman's pelvic bone is wider, and her whole skeleton finer and more graceful.

All the long bones grow from maturation areas, or "centers," by the addition of calcium and other materials. From birth to the age of 5 years these centers appear in order. From 5 to 12 years they grow in size. From 12 to 21, they unite with each other.

The 23 bones of the skull are separated by divisions called "sutures." As age advances, these sutures disappear one after the other, according to a rigorous schedule. The 3 on top of the head begin to fuse, the first at 22 years, the second at

24, the third at 26. They are completely erased at 35, 42 and 47, respectively. During this quarter century, the state of the sutures in a normal skull reveals the age, to within a year or less, of the normally developed skeleton.

The texture of the bones is another guide, for after 30, the flat ones begin to lose their blood supply. They become dry and brittle; sometimes they shrink.

Today the scientist's knowledge of bone growth is turned to answering the all-important question: What is a healthy child? He can tell, almost to the day, when this bone or that should increase in size, change shape and texture; he can tell whether the bones are absorbing minerals and salts as they should. If the X ray shows that the bones contain the telltale white lines of arrested growth, or that they have wandered from the norm, then the danger signal has been hoisted. Health history is checked, the diet is remodeled and treatment is started. Thus the skeleton is a telltale index of our health, our way of life.

Bones grow by the addition of new bony substance to old. When a bone is broken, each broken end starts growing—reaching out, in some magic, mysterious way, to meet the other. The connective-tissue cells become mineralized and hard, finally are changed into true bone.

Surveys indicate that mental outlook has much to do with the incidence of broken bones. In a study of 1500 fracture cases made at New York's Columbia-Presbyterian Medical Center, it was found that about 80 percent had shattered their bones when they were under emotional tension—worried or angry or faced with a difficult decision. One woman had tripped on a living-room rug and broken her leg just before her mother-in-law was due to arrive for a visit. A girl, about to be sent to boarding school because her mother was marrying again, had shattered her knee in a football game. "Mother can't possibly send me away now, when I may be crippled for life," the young patient exclaimed with relief. A man who had just lost his job crossed the street against a red light and landed in the hospital with a fractured thighbone. Some of the accidents studied might have happened anyway, but the pattern of emotional upset was far too prevalent to have been merely coincidental.

Thus, by watching your step, particularly when you are anxious or angry, you can help keep your faithful skeleton from something it doesn't deserve—a bad break.

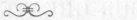

THE ANATOMIST is able to compute the stature of a dead person by a formula based on the length of the thigh bone. Statistics show that the height of a man will be 1.88 times the length of this bone, plus 813.06 millimeters; of a female, 1.945 times the length, plus 728.44 millimeters. Similar formulae may be applied to the human structure from the Ice Age down. The Neanderthal Man of 100,000 years ago, for example, was only 5 feet 4 inches tall, while Cro-Magnon Man, 75,000 years later, had achieved a full 6 feet. Shortly afterward an adverse environment must have overtaken him, for he dropped back to 5 feet 7 inches.

The skeleton of a normal human being, alive or dead, reveals infallibly to the scientist a personal physical history. Race, sex, age, height, serious illnesses and sometimes the cause of death are recorded in skull, pelvis and the "long" bones of the arms and legs—even though the bones may have been buried for centuries. The method of extracting this story is so accurate today that it is of prime importance to the criminologist, the historian and the archaeologist, and is even applied to the living skeleton by X rays as a check on growth and health.   —Wilton Marion Krogman

The Human Hand:

OUR GREATEST TOOL

by Evan McLeod Wylie

In the darkness of a mother's womb a tiny, ivory-colored human embryo enters its fifth week of life. Within the tightly curled, motionless little body, scarcely two inches long, millions of new cells are growing at an enormous rate. From just behind the neck region sprouts a pair of "buds." Rapidly they elongate into three segmented pieces. The extreme outer segment assumes a paddle shape. Five lobes appear on the edges of the paddle. Muscles, tendons and nerve fibers spread throughout it. By the third month of pregnancy, the miniature fingers of the little flipper flex spasmodically. A human hand has been formed.

Months later, when this baby is delivered from its mother's body, these little fingers will clutch and pluck at the hands of the obstetrician with startling determination. From this momentous hour of birth until the day when its fingers finally relax in the repose of death, the hands of this human being, directed by its brain, will chiefly determine what makes its life on this earth different from that of all other living creatures.

The hand is man's unique instrument of expression and sensation. With it, over a million years, we have shaped the world we live in. With it, many now fear, we may destroy this world overnight. No other part of the body is so intimately associated with human behavior.

With our hands we work, play, love, heal, learn, communicate, express our deepest feelings, construct our civilizations and create our greatest works of art. The hand and our emotions are linked together in our literature, music, fine arts, religious teachings. Among most of the world's peoples clasped hands are the symbol of faith, love and friendship, and the clenched fist the most forceful expression of human strength and determination.

Hands often reveal more than we intended them to. Fingers and palms, clenching, stroking, twisting, scratching, nail-biting and drumming, unconsciously complement the emotions. Instinctively, we watch how another person fingers a glass, lights a cigarette or shuffles papers for clues to his innermost thoughts and feelings.

In the portion of the human brain devoted to nervous tissue that controls the muscular portions of the body, your hands are allotted the largest territory of all. As the busiest, most complex instruments of the entire body, they require that much extra brain space. Anthropologists are fond of pointing out that if the most gifted scientists cudgeled their brains they probably could not come up with a stronger and more perfect tool for grasping and delicate manipulation than the human hand. And seen from an engineering standpoint, the loveliest hand actually is a highly complex mechanical device composed of muscle, bone, tendon, fat and highly sensitive nerve fibers, capable of performing thousands of jobs with scientific precision.

For your hand to act in the simplest sort of movement—such as grasping a pencil—an array of muscles, joints and tendons all the way from shoulder to fingertips springs into action. When you take a spoonful of soup—which also means adjusting wrist, arm and shoulder—more than thirty joints and fifty muscles are brought into play.

Because the shoulder is equipped with a ball-and-socket joint, the hand can rotate through a complete circle, palm up or palm down. At the same time, the palm of your hand can be moved around to cover any part of your body except a tiny spot between your shoulder blades. Because of its attachment to the wrist, it can spin, twist or grab and push when it is flat against the body or at arm's length.

All our finger movements are controlled by a tough set of fibers called tendons, which run like a system of pulley cords from finger, hand and wrist bones to the muscles that operate them. Some of these finger muscles are in the palm of the hand itself but *most* of them are in the forearm. That is why tight wrist cuffs or tight sleeves will make your fingers clumsy and tire your whole hand.

The thumb, operating independently from the other four fingers, is the busiest and most important of all the digits. Because of the thumb's unique ability to cross over and link up with any one of the other fingers for a pinch, grab or squeeze, we can get along with one thumb and one other finger, or even just the stump of another finger. In a serious hand injury, surgeons place greatest importance on saving the thumb. Some life insurance policies pay a quarter of their entire value for just the loss of a thumb and forefinger.

The rest of the fingers are markedly different in strength. In the average person, the middle finger is the strongest, followed in order by the index finger, the fourth finger and the little finger. Fingers two and three are the fastest of the five. The little finger is the slowest, but finger four is considered by teachers of music and typewriting to be the least responsive to training because of an innate muscular weakness.

The size of one's hand is not significantly related to the strength of its grip or whether it will be fast or slow or deft or clumsy in its skills. Among musicians, physicians, artists, athletes and all others who depend on their hands to earn a living there is an infinite variety of stubby fingers, slender fingers, large hands and small hands.

Nor do nimble fingers necessarily accompany ability in the more intellectual pursuits. Exceptionally gifted magicians, athletes and entertainers are not usually also pre-eminent in science, art or politics. But one thing is certain: Most of us make use of only a fraction of our hands' potential skills. Directed by a disciplined, determined brain, human fingers can be trained to perform astonishing feats. The flying fingers of a master pianist can strike 120 notes per second—or a dozen notes per second with each finger. A skilled surgeon can tie strands of silk thread into tight knots inside the human heart with two fingers.

The skin of the hand is not like the skin of any other part of the body. While extraordinarily tough, it is also wonderfully elastic and incredibly sensitive. The skin of the back of your hand actually stretches by almost half an inch when you grip or squeeze something; simultaneously, the palm side is shortened by half an inch. Beneath the thick skin of the palm is a buffer layer of fat which protects the hand's vital tendons and blood vessels while the outer surface is being subjected to the tremendous friction created by scraping, twisting, gripping and clenching motions.

The palms of the hands, and particularly the fingertips, are equipped with special sensory apparatus. A piece of finger skin smaller than a postage stamp contains several million nerve cells. On the surface of the skin are ridges called rugae, dotted with myriads of gland openings, pores and nerve endings which detect the temperature and texture of anything we touch. Then, buried beneath the skin is another group of special sense organs—yellow oval-shaped bodies called pacian corpuscles—which detect pressure. About one quarter of all these corpuscles in the entire body are located in the fingers and palms of the hands.

Whenever we touch or grasp any object, the combined sensory systems of the rugae ridges and the pacian perceptors send a steady stream of signals to the brain, telling us the object's size, its shape, its texture and its temperature. Stored in the memory portions of our brains are thousands of impressions built up since infancy of how familiar objects "feel." Thus do blind people learn to read braille type and move about easily in utter darkness while the rest of us, fumbling in our pockets for house keys and coins and matches, also feel our way through life, though to a lesser degree.

As might be expected, the most sensitive rugae and sensory corpuscles are found in the tips of the fingers, the index finger being the most sensitive of all. The worldwide system of fingerprint identification is based on the fact that the whorl patterns created by these rugae ridges are never identical in two people. In a microscopic analysis the differences or similarities in two specimens of fingerprints are quickly recognizable.

Just recently there have been new medical discoveries about fingerprints. Doctors at Tulane University who have been studying the microscopic patterns of the whorls on human fingers and palms reported that the victims of certain inherited heart ailments, rare eye diseases and mental disorders all had distinctive patterns. They speculate that perhaps the patterns of the skin of the hand may be inherited just as are the color of our hair and eyes. If, with the aid of electronic computers, combinations of such patterns could be found to be related to other ailments, fingerprints might be used to track disease as well as criminals.

Most people think that the tips of the fingers do the work of gripping and examining an object, but actually they would be useless without the fingernails to back them up. The nails provide the necessary firmness in pinching and holding an object while the brain analyzes it and decides what to do with it.

Although they appear to grow rapidly, fingernails require about four months to grow their own length. If they are dry and seem to split easily, proper food elements may be missing from your diet. A balanced diet frequently clears up the condition quickly.

The hand feels bony because it is packed full of bones. There are 16 bones in the wrist, 10 bones in the palm and 28 bones in the fingers of one hand. Cords of stringy material called ligaments hold all these bony joints together. A peculiarity about the bones of your hand is that they keep right on growing from infancy up to the age of sixteen in women and up to the age of nineteen in men. This is one of the factors which make it possible to determine age, or rather "bone age"—normal age for a particular bone development—by the study of a skeleton. Under the stimulation of sex hormones, bone development speeds up greatly during puberty. Occasionally, the premature onset of menstruation may affect the hand development of a young girl.

Cold is the greatest natural enemy of the human hand, because most of your finger's length is taken up by bloodless joints in which the temperature drops much more quickly than it does in blood-filled muscles. That is why you can skate or ski all day long in zero temperatures without covering your face, which is full of muscles richly supplied by warm blood, while without gloves your fingers grow painfully numb in a few minutes. Finger joints, like all body joints, are bathed in a colorless, viscous lubricating fluid called synovial fluid, which provides a smooth, gliding action when we bend an elbow or flex a finger. When this fluid gets cold, as it does most often in our exposed hands, it thickens; finger joints stiffen and won't operate.

In an emergency where gloves are not available, fingers can be kept operating most effectively if the whole hand is kept inside a windproof covering. Antarctic expert Dr. Paul Siple discovered that he could make fine adjustments on instruments in temperatures of 65° below zero by keeping his bare hands inside a feather-lined pillow and manipulating the instruments through the fabric.

When multitudes began to write, the world became aware that muscular coördination of fingers is so sensitive that the chances of two people having the same handwriting are calculated at one in sixty-eight trillion. The delicate pressures applied to fingers and arm muscles in handwriting varies so greatly in individuals that a given person's writing is difficult to imitate, but even more difficult to disguise. The legal and economic systems of all civilized societies are based on the validity of the handwritten signature.

Work, play and curiosity are constantly getting our hands into trouble. In the mechanized age in which we live, the hand is injured more often and more severely than any other part of the human body. The wrists, fingers and hands account for one third of the total casualties in the millions of annual industrial accidents. Around the home, the power tools in hobby workshops, such as high-speed electric saws, drills and lathes, may reduce a hand's intricate arrangement of bones, tissues, tendons and nerves to mangled wreckage in a fraction of a second.

Formerly, the dangerous infections that inevitably resulted from these accidents and the futility of attempting to repair the complex physical structures often left doctors little choice but to amputate the whole hand. Today, antibiotics and new operative techniques save many hands. Surgeons implant fine wires, metal splints and springs within the hand and perform intricate skin grafts, ligament shifts and tendon transfers. Plastic materials produce amazingly lifelike artificial hands and fingers.

Despite antibiotics, all hand lacerations are still extremely dangerous because, no matter how often we wash them, our hands pick up millions of germs daily. If a scratch or puncture permits them to gain entrance to the body, infection follows swiftly. "It's impossible to overemphasize," says one hand surgeon, "how much serious disability that results from hand injuries can be spared by early correct treatment."

Our hands deserve careful treatment. As tools of learning, working and communicating, they can be considered the fundamental vehicle of human thought—partner with the brain in forever separating man from the rest of the animal kingdom.

꙳꙳꙳꙳

GLEEFUL PATIENT with foot in traction, to visitor: "The doctor says I'm a natural skier—I have the kind of bones that knit fast."

—Reamer Keller cartoon

What You Should Know about Your Back

by C. Lester Walker

"Sure we'll win today," boasted the big varsity crew captain. "We're trained to the peak. Look at me: best shape I've ever been in."

Then he stepped over to open the window. It stuck. So he pushed up hard, twisting at the same time to shove a rug from underfoot. Suddenly he gave a sharp cry. "My back—something *went!*" he gasped, white-faced with pain.

"Ruptured intervertebral disc," pronounced the surgeon at the hospital. "Cushion between the vertebrae snapped out. No more rowing for you, boy."

The crew captain's case wasn't unusual. Bad backs, most of them similarly "self-inflicted," are second only to headaches as a source of bodily misery. There are many different kinds of back troubles: ruptured discs, sacroiliacs, slipped vertebrae, wrenched muscles, torn ligaments.

The difficulty is almost always brought about by misuse of the back. Records show that back injuries caused by lifting are three times as numerous as any other kind. Pushing, pulling and all forms of stooping and twisting account for their share. Poor posture in standing, sitting or sleeping often results in a chronic bad back.

The human spine sustains all the weight of the upper body—arms, head, trunk. Instead of being a simple arch like the backbone of four-footed animals, man's spine is a chain of bones with *four* arches, four in-and-out curves. It is like an S spring standing on end, and it takes four hundred muscles and scores of ligaments to hold it erect and in place. This spring takes all the jolt and jar of your footfalls. When the spring is taxed beyond its strength—a quick torque put on tired muscles, or an overstrained ligament stretched too far—you may get a sharp stabbing pain which means you are in for a siege of back trouble.

Almost any type of lifting can bring it on. You lift your small child from the crib—you have done it hundreds of times before, yet this time something "goes" in your back. Unaccustomed heavy work—the lift-twist-and-heave of shoveling snow—can wrench the joints of the vertebrae and rip ligaments away from their attachments to the bones.

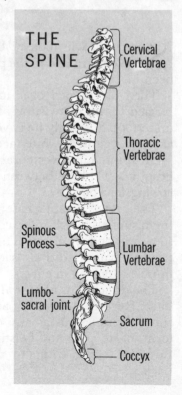

THE SPINE

Cervical Vertebrae

Thoracic Vertebrae

Spinous Process

Lumbar Vertebrae

Lumbo-sacral joint

Sacrum

Coccyx

A housewife lifts a basket of wash, wet and almost half as heavy as herself; she carries it—bent way back—up the laundry stairs. The muscles in the low (lumbar) section, the most vulnerable part of her back, try to do more than they are able. The result is severe muscle strain, and plenty of pain.

Jud Ford, a lawyer who took little regular exercise, wrecked his back while on vacation, as so many folks do. He lifted a small boat dock and carried it a few feet. He wasn't aware of anything happening then. But at dawn he was waked up by the pain, not only in his back but cutting down behind his thighs—sciatica. X rays showed that he had snapped out one of the cartilage-and-fibrous-tissue discs from between his vertebrae.

Another source of trouble is the sacrum—the big "keystone" bone at the base of the spine. The sacrum joints into the two bones of the pelvis—the ilia, which make your hips and the point where you sit down. This joint supports the whole weight of the trunk above; it is tough and strong, and powerful ligaments hold it in place. But sudden, abnormal and unreasonable stress can force the ligaments to relax their hold on the big bones. Then the joint relaxes, there is a sharp pain, usually in the hip and lower back, and you have an unhappy state of trouble known as a "sacroiliac." You can give yourself a sacroiliac by twisting yourself off balance—to reach over from your chair and raise a heavy lamp from the side table to bring it nearer to you, for example. Raising something from a lower level than you're standing on, say a big rock from a hole in your garden, can do it beautifully. Trying to release locked-together auto bumpers has produced many a sacroiliac.

Again, the trouble often is just above, in the lumbosacral—the first movable joint of the spine. This is the region our grandparents complained about when they said they had "lumbago." It's in this lumbosacral joint that you can most easily get what you have probably heard called a "slipped vertebra." If you jump suddenly, or carry a too heavy weight too far, your lowest lumbar vertebra may slide off the forward edge of your sacrum. This gives you a dislocation, straining the ligaments and muscles, which produces the aching back and the pain.

"But I never had a back injury in my life," you say, "and I've got a nagging backache most of the time." This may be due to "mechanical difficulties," by which the specialists usually mean *posture*. You'd be amazed at what the way you stand, sit and lie can do to a back.

Take a horrible example: Librarian Homer Titus, forty-five, has a bad back—with nagging, chronic pain—daily. Mr. Titus doesn't stand the way he ought to—chin up, chest erect, stomach flat (but not the exaggerated "suck-in" of West Point), feet and knees pointing straight ahead. Titus is a sloucher. He's round-shouldered, flat-chested. His abdomen sticks out. His back "sways" in. This atrocious and unnatural posture gives Mr. Titus a distorted spinal column; the strained muscles and ligaments furnish Cause A for his chronic bad back.

Some orthopedists assert you can get a bad back while you sleep. Is your bed one that sags deeply? Then you lie with a curvature of the spine. Years of that may make a good back into a bad one. To correct this condition, specialists often recommend a bed board between spring and mattress.

Depending on what *your* back trouble is, the physician will use everything from simple rest in bed to a combination of heat therapy, massage, diathermy and manipulation. He may use traction—stretching the spine so that the vertebrae, or their discs, will slip back into proper place; he may strap your back with adhesive tape, or put it into a belt, brace or corset to give it support.

There are some back troubles, such as the worst of the ruptured discs, for which surgery is the best method. Highly successful in many cases, these operations cure the bad back which in times past would often have been termed arthritis or sciatica and gone on laming and hurting indefinitely.

Most bad backs are preventable. Orthopedists offer a few cardinal rules:

1. Stand right, sit right, sleep right.

2. Don't (ladies) wear too high heels or sling-back pumps. They strain the spine and back muscles.

3. Don't make your back do strenuous things that it is not accustomed to.

4. Don't subject it to sudden, erratic motions—especially if you're not "warmed up."

5. If you must lift something heavy, lift it the right way. Don't lean over from the waist. Squat down, back straight; lift with your legs.

6. Don't habitually work at anything in an awkward, cramped or stooped position. Get that kitchen sink raised if it's too low.

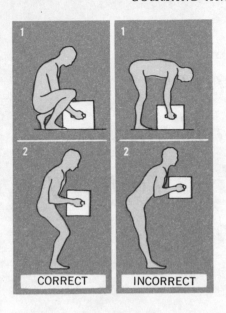

CORRECT INCORRECT

7. Use a cushion or backboard if auto driving "kills" your back.

8. Never try to lift, push or pull anything difficult or heavy when off balance or when you have to put in a turning or twisting motion at the same time.

9. Keep your back muscles in good condition by adequate and sensible exercise (swimming is best of all).

If, in spite of everything, you do find yourself with a bothersome back don't "let it go." Don't try self-treatment. Keep away from quack manipulators. Get expert medical attention quickly and see an orthopedic physician if possible.

THE ABILITY of science to determine the *race* of a skeleton meant a fortune to a half-breed Indian in Oklahoma not long ago. His son had disappeared at the age of eighteen, leaving behind a tract on which oil was later found. The father's claim to the royalties was contested because it could not be proved that the boy was dead. It was known, however, that a youth answering the general description had been killed riding a freight in Arkansas, and the court ordered the body exhumed. After three days, anthropologists established that the skeleton had belonged to a Negro-Indian male, about 5 feet 7 inches tall, between eighteen and nineteen years old. Other bone measurements corresponded so closely with the description of the missing youth that the court accepted the proof of his death. A fortune in oil was turned over to the father.

—Wilton Marion Krogman

Ladies and Gentlemen, Be Seated—Properly

by Janet Travell, M.D.

You wouldn't dream of buying shoes that don't fit. You wouldn't sleep in a bed that's too short. But have you considered the chairs you sit in? One can go into most homes and not find a single chair that's properly designed to support the person sitting in it. And this poor design, which violates the principles of human physiology, is one of the major reasons for the muscular pain which afflicts vast numbers of people.

Most people think that comfort in a chair implies something soft and yielding. The truth is that the more a chair is used for relaxing, the more important it is to have the bony framework of your body held up by that chair. When you sit in a chair that is not right for you, your muscles are compelled to do the work the chair should do. If the natural body weight that keeps muscles stretched to a comfortable tension is modified by an unnatural position, as when the arm is pushed up by an arm rest, then the muscles take up the slack and shorten; when the shortening is prolonged, they cramp and become painful. If the muscles are *overstretched* from sitting improperly, they fail to keep the ligaments and joints in line, and the sagging of the body results not only in muscle injury but in joint strain, too.

Most chairs have at least one of nine major faults:

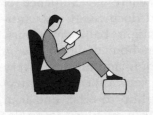

No support for the lower back. Hours of "relaxing" in a chair that fails to support the lumbar region may cause so much muscle fatigue that you become tense, nervous and worn out. A chair back should have some extra padding to fit your lower back. If it hasn't, you can achieve this effect by propping a small cushion against the small of your back. Also, an occasional chair is more likely to be comfortable if it has an opening between the back rest and seat, allowing clearance for body spread.

Back too scooped. To support you properly, a chair should allow your shoulder blades to drop back slightly behind the center of your spine. But a high-back scooped chair like the barrel or Windsor chair rounds your back, rolls your shoulders forward and may cause severe muscle strain. Libraries, conference rooms and restaurants commonly have the scoop-backed chair. What a pity, for these are just the places where one should be able to lean back and relax in comfort!

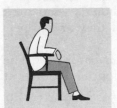

Arm rests too high. These push your shoulders upward and forward. As a result, after any length of time, cramped muscles may cause stiffness and pain across the shoulders and in the back of the neck.

The big upholstered armchairs that look so comfortable are often bad offenders because, when you sink down, the arm rests become too high. A desk or work table that's too high in relation to your chair has the same effect.

Insufficient slope to the back. Any chair with a nearly vertical back forces you to droop forward in a round-shouldered position. The familiar straight dining-room chair, the erect ballroom chair, and the gilt French parlor chair so charming to the eye may be menaces to the human frame if sat in for any length of time.

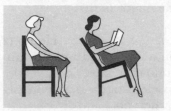

I recall attending a medical convention where an audience of five hundred doctors sat in beautiful little straight ballroom chairs. After half an hour I never saw so much squirming and turning. Every one of those restless people was trying to find a position that would allow him to relax and lean back. If the backs of these chairs had been tilted 15 to 20 degrees behind the vertical, they would have been more comfortable. On easy chairs and sofas, loose back cushions are useful to provide an adjustable incline.

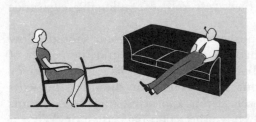

Back too short. Have you ever come out of the movies with a stiff and aching neck? If the back of the movie seat were high enough to support your upper back and neck or if practical neck rests could be devised for movie and theater seats, their comfort would add immeasurably to one's enjoyment. Usually, I advise patients with shoulder and neck pains not to go to the theater or movies until they are 90 percent recovered.

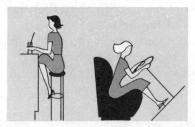

Jackknifing at hips or knees. The ideal sitting position requires at least a 90-degree angle at the waist and also at the knees. If your hips and knees are jackknifed into an angle sharper than that, overstretching of the back muscles follows, together with shortening and cramping of the muscles behind the bent knees, including the calf muscles.

Jackknifing at the hips occurs in any chair which has a seat that sinks way down but has a relatively firm front edge—as, for example, an auto driver's seat when the springs are old and saggy. If you keep driving for very long, your back muscles protest. One

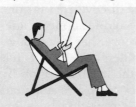

solution is a wedge-shaped cushion that raises the seat at the back and makes it horizontal.

Chairs that give you "shelter legs." During World War II, physicians in London noted an astonishing number of cases of swollen feet. It was found that these people had been sleeping at night in air-raid shelters, in folding deck chairs. Circulation of the blood to and from the lower legs was partially cut off by the pressure which the edge of the chair exerted underneath the thigh, just above the knees, where the main artery and veins cross the bone. The result was pain and swelling. Any chair or sofa with a high, hard front edge may produce this condition.

Chairs with bucket seats. The bucket chair now in vogue has a definite fault. Nature supplies you with bony structures in the middle of each buttock to support the weight of the body when sitting. The bucket seat undoes this work of nature. It puts the weight on the *sides* of the buttocks, so that the center sags, rolling the thighs inward. This distortion, if it lasts, causes discomfort.

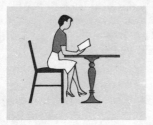

The wrong size for you. Women with short legs should be especially mindful of the chairs they sit in. When feet dangle without touching the floor, the weight of the legs compresses the blood vessels under the thighs and shuts off circulation. The average straight chair measures 17 inches from the front of the seat down to the floor. But some women have legs that measure only 15 or even 14 inches from underneath the knee to the heel. A small footstool can often solve this problem.

In selecting chairs, you should know your measurements and those of other members of the family—the length of legs from knee to floor, and from hip to knee. Thus you can tell right away whether a chair is the right height from the floor and whether its seat is the right depth.

Actually, our ancestors had some chairs more comfortable than most of those we use today. Long ago they discovered that one of the best chairs in the world is the now old-fashioned cane-seated porch rocker with a high back. This rocker has low enough arm rests. It gives support to the upper shoulders and neck. It has a firm, flat back that can be padded to fit the lumbar region by adding a small cushion. It can be tilted back to ensure sufficient "slope." And the motion of rocking favors circulation by alternately relaxing and contracting the muscles and so keeps them from getting stiff.

There's no such thing as one chair to fit every person, nor is there one chair to suit every purpose. But, with an awareness of the general principles involved, you may find it easier to select chairs that will make sitting more comfortable and more restful.

SOMEHOW I WISH, instead of jet planes and atomic artillery, all the world would come to associate us with a gentler invention of ours—the rocking chair. Surely the great capitals and that many-windowed palace dedicated to peace on the East River, New York, might fruitfully ponder the motto carved into the decorative headpiece of many an old rocker: *Sit Ye, Rock and Think.* —Thomas E. Saxe, Jr.

CHAPTER 7

The Laboratories of the Body

LIVER

GALLBLADDER

KIDNEYS

STOMACH

PANCREAS

COLON

FOR THE vast majority of us, the body's great laboratories—stomach, liver, colon, gall-bladder, pancreas and kidneys—will give a life-time of efficient, unfailing service. But these are among the most mistreated organs of our human body. A little knowledge, a little thought and a little care can keep these hidden partners working tirelessly and well in their unseen world.

Treat Your Stomach with Respect

by Richard Carter

In recent years doctors have come to a number of surprising discoveries about the stomach:

Its purpose, which most laymen think they understand, is actually something of a mystery. The stomach is just one stop in an elaborate digestive process by which food is broken down so that it can be absorbed by the body as nutrition. The organ seems to do considerably less digestive work than the intestines, for example.

Present in the stomach is an acid so corrosive that it would blister your palm. Also present is a protective substance so effective that virtually nothing can penetrate to the stomach walls—including the acid.

Perhaps the most illuminating finding is that the normal undiseased stomach is impartial to any edible material which is not extremely hot, cold or excessively spiced, and not eaten under emotional circumstances so pressing that the diner's anxiety disturbs his digestive nerves and muscles.

Emotion makes trouble even in the most carefully coddled stomach. The kind of trouble depends on the nature of the stress. For example: two workmen are sharply chastised by their boss.

The stomach of one may feel as if there is a blowtorch or a volcano in it, while the other's feels as if it has had five rides on a roller coaster. The first man is angry. In this situation his stomach boils combatively, turns fiery red and splashes acid around the innards. The man with the butterflies in his stomach, on the other hand, is more frightened than angry, and his stomach lies still and pale, nauseated and in abject surrender.

The stomach is often unjustly blamed for the derelictions of other organs. In heart trouble the misplaced blame can be catastrophic. People have died because angina pectoris was mistaken for indigestion, or coronary thrombosis for a severe stomach upset. A malfunctioning liver, pancreas, gallbladder or kidney may send out danger signals which only a doctor can distinguish from stomach trouble. In such cases the pain the sufferer feels may actually occur in the region of the stomach—telegraphed there by the nerves—although the trouble is elsewhere. The same difficulty sometimes occurs in cancer, appendicitis, hernia, polio, pneumonia, mumps, spinal tumors and tuberculosis of the bone. In these cases self-diagnosis and self-treatment may be dangerous. The sufferer should head for his doctor.

Naturally, not even the most ardent advocate of mind-over-matter would insist that *all* stomach distress is emotional. A person can be made highly uncomfortable, for example, by extreme overeating. Other digestive upsets often stem from the body's effort to rid itself of some kind of poison, virus or bacteria. Perhaps the best-known example of this is the illness we commonly call "intestinal flu." The diarrhea and vomiting which accompany this ailment are part of a reflex action set off when virus gets into the intestinal walls. The body automatically tries to throw off the infected material. The same is true of food poisoning: the body reacts violently—and often painfully—to rid itself of the infectious matter as quickly as possible. Often it is the intestine that does most of the reacting and these sicknesses should not really be blamed on the stomach at all.

Contrary to popular belief, the stomach is not situated behind the soft façade of the belly but is mainly behind the lower ribs, slightly to the left of center. When empty, it hangs from the gullet, or esophagus, as limply as a deflated balloon and may measure as much as 16 inches from top to bottom (where it opens into the small intestine). When everything is happy and there is food to be digested, it contracts into a shape roughly resembling an outsized kidney bean and may measure only 8 inches from top to bottom and about 4 inches across.

Before the first mouthful of a meal has reached it, the stomach has usually begun to writhe expectantly and secrete juice. These activities are touched off by the nervous system after the brain has been excited by the sight, smell or even the thought of food. Whether or not food is on the way, the stomach contracts every three or four hours in an involuntary cycle, causing the sensation known as hunger pangs.

The most remarkable thing about the stomach is its juice, the

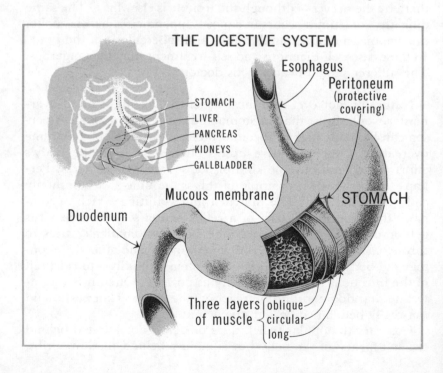

THE DIGESTIVE SYSTEM

Esophagus

Peritoneum (protective covering)

STOMACH
LIVER
PANCREAS
KIDNEYS
GALLBLADDER

Mucous membrane

STOMACH

Duodenum

Three layers of muscle { oblique, circular, long }

best-known constituent of which is powerful hydrochloric acid. When bathed in this fluid and crushed by the stomach's kneading motion, the toughest meat soon loses its individuality and becomes part of a gray mush called chyme. Enzymes contained in the gastric juice help the chemical breakdown.

How does the stomach manage to avoid being digested by its own secretions? The answer seems to be a marvelously resistant mucus which covers the stomach lining. This mucus is the refutation of all theories about "irritating foods." Nothing that we swallow at a meal—even chili, curry, vinegar, kippered herring, for instance—is nearly so irritating as the juice which is in our stomachs to begin with. Experiments have shown that the mucus provides as stout an armor against "irritating foods" as it does against gastric juice.

Despite its complex role, researchers still are not sure just how important the stomach is. Some people, after surgery, manage to get along virtually without one. Under careful medical management, thousands of humans (mostly cancer patients) have lived for years after having the *entire* stomach removed.

Of all "stomach" ailments, perhaps the best known and most cordially detested is the ulcer, a condition which most physicians now associate with emotional stress. An ulcer looks like a larger version of the canker sores that we sometimes get in our mouths. Its diameter is between one quarter and three quarters of an inch, and most cases are accompanied by sharp pain midway between chest and navel.

Some ulcers occur in the stomach itself. Most, however, are found in the duodenum, which is the portion of small intestine that lies directly below the stomach's outlet valve. These are believed to be caused by the stomach's activities.

The ulcer sufferer's stomach is too active, secreting more juice than is needed and contracting more often than is necessary. These contractions make the stomach's outlet valve open too frequently and squirt large amounts of acid at the duodenum. Since the duodenum has no coating of protective mucus, this acid may eventually eat away at the lining of the intestine to produce the ulcer.

There are two modern ways to treat ulcers. One is to prevent overactivity by means of surgery, drugs, X ray or psychotherapy. The other method of preventing stomach juice from burning away the lining of the duodenum—assuming this is the cause of duodenal ulcer—is to give it plenty of food to work on instead. For a long time it was believed that the best foods for ulcer sufferers were mild ones, particularly milk. In a recent experiment, however, a group of ulcer patients given frequent servings of normal food recovered from their ulcers somewhat more rapidly than a group fed frequently on the old-fashioned bland diet.

The sufferer from a duodenal ulcer can take solace from one fact: he almost never gets stomach cancer. At least 70 percent of stomach cancer arises in underactive low-acid stomachs—the opposite of the kind of stomach associated with duodenal ulcer.

In sum, although the stomach is often blamed for anything that goes wrong inside the body, most doctors agree that the stomach is really an exceptionally tough, trustworthy and hard-working organ; that it rarely causes serious trouble, and then only if grossly abused.

Most indigestion is emotional. When you and I are upset—by anger, fear, jealousy, whatnot—food ferments and poisons enter the blood instead of the materials we need for health and sanity. The nagged husband, the bullied wife, has a physiological hangover the next day as definite, as tangible, as though a dose of poison or too much alcohol had been taken the night before.   —George A. Dorsey

Have you heard about the fellow who underwent major stomach surgery? When his midriff was opened up, out flew a flock of butterflies. "Well," exclaimed his doc, stepping back, "I'll be hanged—the guy was right!"   —Cedric Adams in Minneapolis Star

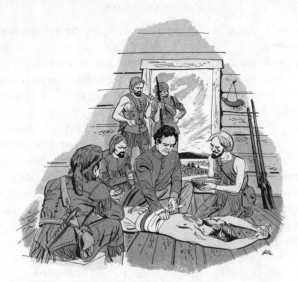

The Window
in St. Martin's Stomach

by Richard Match

One June day in 1822, tipsy fur trappers crowded into the store of John Jacob Astor's American Fur Company on Mackinac Island, Michigan. A gun went off accidentally, and a young French-Canadian, Alexis St. Martin, fell with a huge wound in his side.

Bystanders summoned the only doctor within three hundred miles, at the Army post nearby. Dr. William Beaumont, thirty-seven, a handsome, erect figure in the high-collared blue uniform of the period, knelt at St. Martin's side. In Sir William Osler's memorable phrase, "The man and the opportunity had met." Dr. Beaumont was to achieve medical immortality by observing the inside of the human stomach at work—and making discoveries about the digestive apparatus that became milestones in medical progress.

The charge of duck shot had gouged a hole as big as a man's hand in St. Martin's left side. A portion of the stomach was protruding, and it was punctured. Beaumont did "not believe it possible for the patient to survive 20 minutes," as he wrote later.

St. Martin was a young canoeman, known as a sly, shiftless and alcoholic character. To Beaumont's astonishment, the dark, wiry little fellow clung tenaciously to life. After nearly a year, healthy scar tissue had formed around the opening. But the patient cantankerously refused to submit to an operation to suture its edges together. During all this time St. Martin felt no pain in his stomach, not even nausea.

Instead of dropping back into the abdominal cavity, the rim of St. Martin's stomach puncture adhered to the rim of his external wound, in much the way that a trouser pocket is attached to the outside fabric of the suit. Doctors call such openings a gastric fistula. Eventually an inner coat of St. Martin's stomach folded across the fistulous opening, forming a leakproof valve which could be easily depressed from the outside. There remained, permanently, a round hole large enough to admit the doctor's forefinger directly into the stomach.

Two years passed. St. Martin, now a servant in the doctor's household, was eating "crude food in abundant quantities." While dressing the fistula one day, Beaumont made a momentous observation: "When Alexis lies on his right side, I can look directly into the stomach and almost see the process of digestion."

Beaumont realized that St. Martin's fistula represented a window miraculously opened into the stomach of a healthy, active human being. Here was the means of solving the age-old riddle of how our digestive organs break food down to basic nutritive elements which can be utilized by the body.

That the human stomach secreted a peculiar fluid of its own had been widely acknowledged since the work of the Frenchman Réaumur and the Italian Spallanzani in the preceding century. By swallowing a sponge tied to a string Spallanzani had obtained fluid from his own stomach. He claimed that it possessed the powers of a chemical solvent and named it the "gastric juice." In 1824 an Englishman named Prout added that he had found hydrochloric acid in a freshly killed animal's gastric juice. But many "authorities" scoffed at the idea of living tissues producing a powerful acid capable of dissolving solids.

Pushing the walls of the fistula apart with his thermometer, Beaumont could look into his "human test tube" to a depth of five or six inches. The stomach walls were pale-pink in color, soft and velvety-looking, and filmed with a mucous fluid. Beaumont inserted a few bread crumbs. Promptly the pink hue of the stomach lining brightened, and hundreds of minute droplets began to rise through the mucous film and trickle down the walls. Here was Spallanzani's "gastric juice," but not neutral as the Italian believed; it tasted distinctly of Prout's hydrochloric acid.

Next morning, with the aid of a rubber tube, Beaumont collected some gastric juice in a vial. He dropped a small chunk of boiled beef into the transparent fluid and heated it to the normal temperature of Alexis' stomach. Beaumont's record of this experiment, one of the most decisive ever performed in an American laboratory, states: "In 40 minutes digestion had commenced over the surface of the meat." In two hours "the cellular texture seemed to be entirely destroyed, leaving the muscular fibers loose and unconnected, floating about in fine small shreds." Four hours later "they were nearly all digested, a few fibers only remaining." In ten hours "every part of the meat was completely digested."

No other fluid Beaumont tested reduced the meat's size, shape or weight in the slightest. Beaumont declared, "Gastric juice is the most general solvent of food in nature. Even the hardest bone cannot withstand its action." After a month of soaking in the juice, the solid bone of a hog's rib had been completely dissolved.

Excited over his discovery, Beaumont felt the need for a laboratory and medical library. Securing a transfer eastward, Beaumont packed his wife, his children and St. Martin aboard a Great Lakes steamer. But before the Beaumonts reached Fort Niagara, Alexis vanished, presumably northward.

It is possible to forgive St. Martin for running out on science. The only body chemistry he cared about was that of alcoholic fermentation. And he could see ahead interminable tubes, strings, bags moving in and out of his stomach, along with diets and fasts.

Glumly Dr. Beaumont resumed his Army duties, but he kept the far-flung American Fur agents on watch for St. Martin. Four years later the truant was found living in a village near Montreal. He would come back, yes, but only with his household, now consisting of a wife and two children. His benefactor reluctantly agreed, and shortly the St. Martins debarked at Prairie du Chien, on the upper Mississippi, where Beaumont was now stationed.

In the four years following Alexis' return, Beaumont carried out an amazing variety of experiments. He charted the fluctuations of gastric secretion under all possible conditions. He clocked the digestion times of endless foods, from hash to venison steak, fat and lean, raw and cooked, chewed and whole.

Time and again Beaumont recorded: "Alexis became angry during this experiment," or "He was vexed at being detained from his breakfast." The doctor finally noticed that every time Alexis lost his temper during a meal, digestion was measurably slower. Roast beef eaten in anger lingered in St. Martin's stomach twice as long as it did when Alexis was calm and contented. "Fear and anger," Beaumont wrote, "check the secretion of the gastric juice." He had established for the first time the central role of emotional influences in digestion.

Many of Beaumont's observations could profitably serve as guides to our own eating habits. Fatty foods, he found, are difficult to digest, since they require extra digestive steps. Hot, humid weather depresses gastric secretion—a good argument for light, digestible summer meals. A given amount of gastric juice is capable of combining with only limited quantities of food. When more food is presented than it will dissolve, wrote Beaumont, "indigestion" ensues. The excess food may remain undigested for twenty-four to forty-eight hours, "as insoluble in the stomach as lead. The system," Beaumont concluded, "requires much less than is generally supplied to it." In short, most of us overeat.

In 1831 Mrs. St. Martin announced that she was going home. On the Frenchman's solemn promise to return, Beaumont bought Alexis a large canoe, and the fabulous invalid paddled his wife and children (four by now) down the Mississippi, up the Ohio, and through the Great Lakes and St. Lawrence to Montreal—some two thousand miles.

The unpredictable Alexis reappeared on schedule, and for two more years Beaumont worked ceaselessly to conclude his series of 238 experiments. In 1833 he published his *Experiments and Observations on the Gastric Juice and the Physiology of Digestion*—a book which Harvey Cushing, a century later, called "the most notable and original classic of American medicine."

Enjoying scientific acclaim and planning new experiments, Beaumont drew up a contract in which he agreed to pay Alexis $200 a year to "promote by all means in his power such experiments as the said William Beaumont shall direct. . . ." Alexis signed with his X. Apparently this document gave the doctor a false sense of security. Before leaving for a new Army assignment at St. Louis he let Alexis make a visit to Canada. It was a fatal mistake. He never saw Alexis again. Until he died twenty years later, Beaumont tried to get Alexis back, but in vain.

St. Martin outlived his doctor by more than a quarter of a century. Apparently his trials and tribulations did not affect his rugged physique. He sired seventeen children in all, and at the time of his death in 1880 he was chopping cordwood for a living. He was then nearly eighty years old. For fifty-eight years he had lived comfortably with a hole in his vitals that ought to have killed him in twenty minutes.

FROM start to finish in the digestive process, bafflingly complex organs must work in perfect harmony. It is not surprising that such a system gives occasional trouble. It is a wonder that it works at all. —J. D. Ratcliff

Your Liver Is Your Life

by Paul de Kruif

Ask your doctor to teach you how to take care of your liver.
Follow his advice, and your liver will take care of you. The
chemical genius of this mysterious organ is basic to the strong
beat of your heart, the wide-open channels of your blood vessels,
the soundness of your digestion, sharpness of your brain, strength
of your muscles.

The liver's cells brew a vast and varied chemistry essential to
the smooth functioning of all our organs. Some examples: Our
kidneys couldn't dispose of waste nitrogen if the liver didn't turn it
into urea for excretion. The liver stores vitamins necessary to the
birth of blood in the marrow of our bones. Although sex activity
begins in our gonads, it's the liver that balances their hormones so
that we're neither impotent nor sexually wild. The liver builds
amino acids into the albumin that regulates the balance of salt
and water without which we could not live. And the liver's bile
governs intestinal activity to keep us from being poisoned by the
products of our own digestion.

When we're hit by hemorrhage, we would die if it weren't for
the liver. It not only helps control bleeding, but helps by another
substance to guard us against clotting that might otherwise

fatally block coronary arteries of the heart and blood vessels of the brain. It combats viruses and bacterial poisons and tosses them out of the body. It gets rid of dangerous excesses of medicines, and keeps our tissues safe from chemicals encountered industrially.

This superchemist releases energy from food. From carbohydrates it makes and stores glycogen and splits it into sugar (in the form of glucose)—slowly in life's routine and lightning-fast in emergencies. And it sees to the widespread deposit of fat for reserve food when we're ill or starving.

It's no wonder, in view of its tremendous activity, that the liver is the largest of all our glands, one fortieth of the total weight of the body. Dark-red, dome-shaped, it fits snugly beneath the diaphragm, high up in the right side of the abdomen under the protective bony cage of the ribs.

Here's the liver's mystery: Its complex duties are all performed by just one kind of tiny cell. Present in millions, they are arranged in cords, one cell in thickness, bathed in a never-ending river of blood. Part of this blood, rich in foodstuffs for the liver's chemical kitchen, comes by way of a great vein from the digestive tract; another part, high in oxygen, comes by way of an artery direct from the heart. The liver mixes these two streams of blood just before they merge to flow round the cells, the working units of the master laboratory.

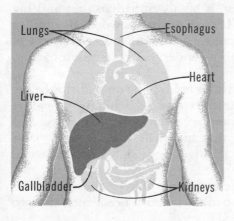

You'd think the incessant labor of the liver's cells would wear them out, kill them. It does just that. But the liver has a unique virtue: potential immortality. Brain cells, heart cells, dying, cannot be replaced. But the liver, amazingly, regenerates itself over and over. Experimenters have removed big pieces of the liver from an animal again and again at intervals, until the total amount taken out exceeded by far the total original weight of the organ. That's the secret of the liver's durability.

Yet the liver sometimes does break down under the mighty load it carries. The final consequence of breakdown is the dread cirrhosis of the liver, believed to afflict two or three of every hundred persons in the U.S.A. and Canada. When—despite their remarkable trick of regenerating—liver cells die too fast, they leave behind them fibrous masses of hard connective tissue.

Luckily, as our liver begins sinking into this desperate state, it signals its plight. Vascular spiders—little blood vessels radiating out in fine branches—appear on the face and shoulders of victims of approaching liver failure. There's deep fatigue, muscles waste, sex urge fails. The liver enlarges, and chemical tests show it's no longer keeping up the level of the vital albumin of the blood. The formerly healthy liver cells, in their one-sided battle against unending chemical insults, fill up with fat and die.

What wrecks liver cells is often *nutritional* failure under their overload of chemical work. Of course, our livers are prone to many ills, including cancer and virus diseases such as serum jaundice and infectious hepatitis. But dominating all these, statistically, is the death of liver cells *due to their own malnutrition*.

The problem is to fight this deadly hidden hunger of the liver cells of human beings, many of whom are far gone with alcoholic cirrhosis. The treatment? Rest, a highly nutritious diet and big doses of liver extract, dried brewer's-yeast powder, B-complex and other vitamins—and, of course, no alcohol. The recovery of many seemingly hopeless cirrhotics under this regimen is amazing.

Nutritional treatment of cirrhosis holds hope not only for heavy drinkers but for us all. While liver disease is highly prevalent among alcoholics—some of whom are notoriously poor eaters and thus threatened with hunger that hits their livers—many of us may teeter on the brink of malnutrition, though we think we're eating adequately.

We're in luck, in view of the frequency of liver disease, that its predominating cause, malnutrition, doesn't need specialists to mend it. The general practitioner can not only treat it but prevent it.

Most doctors feed patients a diet high in calories, average-to-high in proteins, high in carbohydrates and average in fat. Though the diet itself is rich in vitamins, the patients are given supplements. Vitamin C is prescribed in big doses since only a little of it is stored in the body. Crystalline B vitamins and vitamin B_{12}—a powerful fat mover—are administered in large amounts. Patients severely ill are also given crude liver extract, not only for its B complex but because of possible vitamin factors still not defined. And all patients are forbidden to take alcohol.

If the nutritional treatment of advanced cirrhosis is so powerfully curative, why not use it to guard the liver while its cells are still normal? The answer is that if we give our liver the right nutriments to work with, its cells will help to guard themselves. It takes far less to prevent liver failure than to relieve it.

Not long ago I was hospitalized by a severe case of hepatitis, a liver ailment which often turns one's skin a jaundiced yellow. (And I am a girl who never did look well in yellow.) Feeling a bit more chipper one morning, I decided to go down to the hospital newsstand for the morning paper. I spruced myself with a little powder and lipstick and made my way to the elevator. The sole other occupant was a fine-looking intern— tall, dark and handsome—and my heart fluttered as I noticed him looking at me with interest. Modestly, I glanced away. But as the elevator descended and I became more and more aware that he was gazing at me, I wished I'd applied my makeup more carefully. Then he inched closer, and I just knew he was going to speak to me. Pleased, I waited. He leaned forward, looked deep in my eyes and said triumphantly: "Liver?"

—Jane Porter

Your Gallbladder:

TROUBLE HOT SPOT

by J. D. Ratcliff

Every machine has its weak spots. The most complex, most awesome of all machines—the human body—is no exception. One frequent breakdown point is the little, pear-shaped, glistening blue sac in the upper right abdomen, the gallbladder. This organ, the records of many hospitals show, is an even more frequent target for abdominal surgery than the appendix. Estimates indicate that as much as 25 percent of our adult population may have gallbladders that are faulty in one way or another.

What is the gallbladder? What is its function in the body?

The gallbladder is attached to the underside of the liver, to which it is connected by a series of ducts. The duct system also links it with the duodenum, the first looping section of the small intestine. Its main job is to store the bile—a bitter, golden-yellow fluid essential in digesting fats—which is continuously secreted in droplet quantities by the liver.

At mealtime, a hormone released from the small intestine carries a message to the gallbladder. Its muscular walls contract. A valve at the duodenum opens. Bile is delivered into the stream of food in process of digestion. With the help of pancreatic enzymes, it breaks down fats so they can be picked up by the bloodstream and distributed around the body.

No one is quite sure why the harmless-looking little gallbladder is host to so many ills. Some difficulties are apparently caused by hormonal disturbances. In pregnancy, for example, the gall-bladder may not empty properly, and digestive upset may result.

Inflammation is more serious. Under normal circumstances, the gallbladder concentrates bile, extracting water and reducing the yellow digestive juice to approximately one sixth of its original volume. But at times the process is carried too far. Overconcentrated, the bile becomes an irritant. The walls and ducts of the organ become inflamed. This opens the way for bacterial invasion.

Infection originating in the gallbladder may spread to other organs. As inflammation progresses, the walls of the gallbladder and its ducts often become gangrenous. Unless the infection is brought under rapid control they may rupture and empty the contents of the gallbladder into the abdominal cavity. Peritonitis, sometimes fatal, may follow. Surgery—usually removal of the "hot" gallbladder—can be lifesaving in this critical situation.

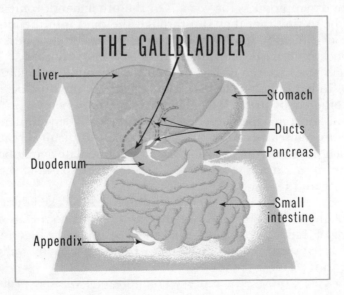

Fortunately, after the gallbladder is removed, the bile can pass directly from the liver through the main duct to the duodenum (if it is clear of obstruction) with no disturbance in function.

Stones are a more frequent cause of gallbladder trouble. Researchers aren't quite sure how or why gallstones are formed. Many hold the reasonable belief that when the bile in the gallbladder becomes too concentrated, its constituents start crystallizing. One doctor sums up this course of events: "Bile turns to sludge, sludge to gravel, gravel to stones."

Gallstones occur at all ages, but are most frequent in the higher age brackets. They appear more often in women than in men. A study of autopsy reports suggests that approximately one person in six in the Western world will have gallstones by the age of fifty. They are less common among the people of Asia and Africa.

Stones may be tiny, and hundreds may be present. Or there may be a single stone, as large as a hen's egg. They are made of three main building materials: calcium, cholesterol, bile pigments.

Generally speaking, large stones cause less difficulty than smaller ones. Being too large to enter a duct, they may lie harmless and symptomless for years. On the other hand, some stones may be so tiny that they slip through the duct into the intestine without difficulty. It is the middle-sized stones, those large enough to block quill-sized ducts, that create the most trouble.

Such blockage can cause some of the most acute pain known to man. In lightninglike flashes, pain radiates to the shoulder, back and other body areas. The colicky attack may be over in a few seconds, or it may persist for an hour or more. The victim may be violently nauseated, sweat profusely and have difficulty breathing. In such situations doctors can take little immediate action beyond administering drugs to relieve pain and reduce spasm of the gallbladder and its ducts.

Blockage often produces other symptoms. A blocked duct may, for example, back bile into the liver, which has no means of disposing of it. Excess bile may then be picked up by the bloodstream and distributed about the body to produce a sickly yellowish coloration. This is jaundice.

For years, quacks have preyed on gallstone victims, promising to break up stones in the body by various nonsurgical means. As of today, however, surgery is the one and only way of ridding the body of these offenders.

Actually there are few ailments for which diagnosis is so positive, or surgery so effective, as for gallstones. A series of perhaps six X rays will be wanted. If stones are obstructing a duct, a decision must be made as to whether or not to operate. Various considerations—severity of pain, frequency of attacks and the patient's age, for example—influence the decision. (Gallbladder surgery can be serious business for people over sixty.)

Fifty years ago the gallbladder operation was frequently unsuccessful because of crude techniques, the danger of infection, the hazards of anesthesia. The death of one patient in sixteen was considered a reasonable score. Today, in proper hands, the operation is one of the safest of the major surgical procedures—except for "hot" gallbladder operations, where infection is present.

The operation takes approximately an hour. Removal of the gallbladder itself—usually the preferred procedure—presents no particular problem to the skilled surgeon. Checking for stones in ducts is slightly more difficult. The surgeon may explore the ducts with a probe. A more satisfactory method is to inject a radioopaque dye into the duct system, then take an X ray while the patient is still on the table.

Sometimes it is necessary to cut out a blocked section of duct and stitch open ends together. Often, however, the block is big enough to make it impossible to draw ends together. There are several solutions. One is to draw up a loop of intestine, make a new opening and attach the duct stub to it. After successful gallbladder surgery, most patients find that they can eat normally without difficulty.

Can anything be done to *prevent* gallbladder difficulties? Some doctors answer with a flat no. Others, noting that gallbladder trouble often accompanies gross overweight, think that diet control and exercise may be helpful.

You may, or may not, be able to prevent gallbladder misery. But you have the consolation that if it does strike, surgery can correct it.

The Kidneys

by J. D. Ratcliff

Kidneys are the body's master chemists. They maintain an exact proportion of water in the blood. They keep us in exact mineral balance—a little too much potassium would stop the heart as effectively as a bullet through it. They control the acid-alkali balance—a swing too far in either direction is lethal. They dispose of waste which, if permitted to accumulate, would be very detrimental to body health.

In a day's time the kidneys sweep clean of wastes over a *ton* of blood (as the body's supply circulates and recirculates). And as a built-in safety feature they have well over twice the capacity needed to maintain health: thus if it is necessary to remove a diseased kidney, the remaining healthy one does double duty with ease.

The fist-size, reddish-brown organs, weighing about a quarter pound each, contain the body's most intricate and fascinating plumbing. Each of our two kidneys—located on either side of the spine at the level of the lowest ribs—has approximately a *million* nephrons, the functional units of the organs. To the naked eye a single nephron resembles a grain of sand, but under a microscope it looks like a big-headed worm with a tortuously twisted, tail-like body. The head is the glomerulus, the tail is the tubule.

The head is covered with a cobwebby net of capillaries which steadily filters blood, permitting the watery part to flow into the pouchlike glomerulus but preventing almost all the blood cells and proteins from entering. More than 98 percent of this fluid is reabsorbed in the tubules. There are approximately 140 *miles* of these in each kidney! In a highly selective process, the tubules take up vital amino acids, proteins, glucose, minerals needed in health, and cast aside wastes and excess water at the rate of one or two quarts a day.

Microscopic droplets from the tubules collect in a tiny reservoir connected to the bladder by a ureter. Every ten to thirty seconds a wavelike contraction of muscles pushes the fluid along to the bladder.

Considering the magnitude of the tasks thrust upon the kidneys, they give astonishingly little trouble, but when they do, it can be serious. The severity of diseases of the kidneys varies according to the nature and cause of the specific disease and the different parts of the kidneys affected. For example, there are

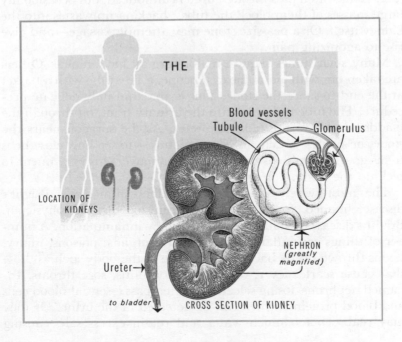

THE KIDNEY

Blood vessels
Tubule
Glomerulus

LOCATION OF KIDNEYS

NEPHRON
(greatly magnified)

Ureter→

to bladder

CROSS SECTION OF KIDNEY

kidney diseases which may not impair function significantly but which cause illness. An example is the invasion of the kidneys by certain bacteria, resulting in infection manifesting itself by fever, backache and other symptoms.

Such kidney infection is by far the most important disease of these organs. If recognized and treated promptly with modern drugs, however, it may not immediately interfere with the work of the kidneys. On the other hand, some of the major kidney troubles result in impairment of kidney function, which if unchecked can cause a serious state of ill health known as uremia. Depending on the severity and type of disease, the kidneys and one's day-to-day health and general functioning will be affected.

Kidney stones, one of the commonest ailments, result when— for reasons still not clear—mineral salts, uric acid and other substances begin to crystallize out and form masses that vary in size from pinhead "gravel" to lumps as large as baseballs. Tiny stones often pass through ureters unnoticed, but occasionally large masses of them block the tubes, backing up wastes into the kidney itself. Or a pea-size stone may attempt passage—and give rise to agonizing pain.

Many such stones require major surgery for removal. Others are taken out with aid of the cystoscope, a tiny tube with a basket at the end to snare the stone. This is an exquisitely delicate procedure. The tube is slipped into the urinary tract, on through the bladder and into the blocked ureter. As the surgeon nears the stone, he pauses to take an X-ray picture—to see how close he is to his goal. When he is on target he maneuvers his instrument to pick up the stone.

The most widely known of all kidney ailments is Bright's disease, named for a nineteenth-century British physician. Bright's disease actually means *any* kidney inflammation. A number of things can inflame these sensitive organs: poisons, injury, toxins thrown off by bacteria elsewhere in the body such as those that cause scarlet fever, diphtheria, tonsillitis, sore throats. Inflamed nephrons, losing selectivity, often pass essential blood cells and blood proteins, which can be detected in the urine. Or they may reabsorb too much water and retain excess salt, causing puffy swelling of arms, legs, eyes. Acute nephritis is an inflammation of the glomeruli which may follow a bacterial infection anywhere in the body as a late complication. Now, thanks to antibiotics, it can be prevented if the bacterial infection is detected and treated early enough.

Until recently, the most lethal of all kidney disorders was kidney shutdown. If kidneys cease to secrete urine, wastes rapidly accumulate in the body. This can result from several types of circulatory failure, when an inadequate supply of blood is delivered to the kidneys. Severe burns or injuries followed by shock may cause the kidneys to stop working. Poisons can so damage nephrons that they cease to function, and severe infections can have much the same effect.

Up to a few years ago—in spite of the gallant struggles of doctors to restore kidney function—a dishearteningly large proportion of the victims of kidney shutdown drifted off into a sleep from which there was no awakening.

The first crude artificial kidney was developed during World War II. Blood sent through cellophane tubing immersed in a "rinsing solution" was cleansed of wastes. Some patients were kept alive thirty days or longer—frequently time enough for damaged kidney tissue to start functioning again—and made complete recoveries. In the last few years artificial kidneys have been improved enormously, and scores of hospital staffs have learned how to use them.

While *partial* kidney shutdown isn't as grave a problem as complete shutdown, it is far more widespread. When kidneys go on a slowdown strike, fluid accumulates in spaces around body cells, and legs, feet and abdomen often become bloated—a condition known as dropsy. Since 1953 there have become available several types of potent diuretics (agents which increase the flow of urine) in pill form. Under the wondrous prod of these medicines, water-logged patients often lose thirty or more pints (pounds) of excess fluid in as little as a week!

One of the most dramatic developments in today's treatment of kidney failure is the surgical transplanting of a kidney from one person to another. For over half a century this was an elusive dream; surgeons who attempted it found that antibodies attacked and destroyed the "foreign" tissue. Then in December, 1954, a twenty-three-year-old ex-Coast Guardsman was brought to the Peter Bent Brigham Hospital in Boston with both kidneys destroyed by disease. By all past reckoning his doom was sealed. His single chance for survival was a transplanted kidney from his identical twin brother. The surgeons removed the left kidney from the healthy brother, installed it in the right side of the sick one. An uneventful recovery followed.

This achievement, of course, was not the answer to any considerable portion of kidney problems, since identical twins are rare. Two years ago the Boston specialist approached the larger problem in a novel manner. Since it is antibodies that destroy transplanted organs, why not try to prevent their formation? Massive, near-lethal doses of radiation, the doctors knew, would temporarily suppress the body's means of producing antibodies. As the body's defense mechanism gradually recovered, wasn't there a chance it would "accept" the transplanted organ?

A patient was available on whom this theorizing could be tested—a young man who, once a husky six-footer, had wasted away to a cadaverous ninety-eight pounds. He had almost totally inactive kidneys. In two sessions, he got near-killing doses of radiation. Then a kidney was transplanted from a fraternal, but not identical, twin. (Fraternal twins are often as chemically different as any random sampling of human beings.) Gradual recovery followed, and now, several years later, history's first patient for such surgery is in apparent good health.

Surgeons elsewhere have used the same approach with the same promising results. The goal at the moment is a safer, possibly a chemical, means of controlling antibody production, to avoid giving massive doses of X ray.

For years kidneys were thought to have but one unglamorous function: to dispose of body wastes. Today's gifted researchers, who have made dazzling progress in understanding kidneys, know better.

What Urinalysis
Tells the Doctor

by J. D. Ratcliff

Modern medicine has at hand an array of tests which reveal to the doctor information about virtually every organ, tissue and fluid in the body. The most widely used test, and one of the most informative, is the humble urinalysis.

Even physicians of ancient times recognized urine as an important diagnostic agent. The color, the glints of light, the sediments were the data upon which they based their diagnosis. Modern urinalysis covers a wide range—from the simple sugar test that diabetics must do themselves daily to the physician's office tests, and on to complex procedures requiring the services of expert chemists.

What are the most common urinalysis tests?

Protein: Normally, kidney filters permit only very small amounts of blood protein to escape into the urine. When there is an excess of protein, it may mean that kidneys are inflamed, infected or degenerated, that a cyst or tumor is present, or that toxins or bacterial infection elsewhere in the body are lowering kidney efficiency. At certain times—after violent exercise, for instance—protein may appear in the urine without having any alarming significance. The expert knows how to interpret such findings with other tests and diagnoses.

Sugar: Sugar in the blood should stay within narrowly defined limits. When it rises too high it is excreted by the kidneys. Sugar in the urine suggestes diabetes, but it can also mean that the patient has been gorging on sweets.

Specific gravity: The weight of urine, in relation to the weight of pure water, gives a good clue to efficiency of kidney function. If urine is too watery, the kidneys may be doing a poor job of concentrating wastes, and disease is suspected.

Acidity: Normally, urine is acid. If it is alkaline in several specimens, something may be wrong. This happens frequently in infections of the bladder or kidneys. In certain stages of pneumonia the urine may also be alkaline and in some nervous diseases the urine is persistently alkaline. Or the acidity test may simply point at the person's dietary habits. A vegetable regime tends to make the urine alkaline; meat increases the acidity.

Bile pigments: Various diseases of the liver or biliary tract (gallbladder and ducts) may cause bile to back up into the blood and then to filter into the urine. Thus, the urinalysis discloses the telltale message that disease is present and further medical attention is necessary.

Microscopic examinations: The study of urine sediments under the microscope can often spot trouble. Pus cells may indicate infection somewhere in the urinary tract. If kidneys are diseased, protein material may accumulate and be excreted in the form of "casts"—impressions of the tiny tubules which make up the kidney. Visible under the microscope, certain types of cast suggest not only kidney disease but possibly other diseases, such as those of the liver. Bacteria also are found occasionally in urine, indicating infection. Diseases affecting the bones may be spotted by the amount of calcium found.

Far more elaborate tests are made on urine for specialized jobs. A cancer along the urinary tract often will shed telltale cells which can be identified under the microscope. End products of hormones show up in the urine, their quantity being a guide to the function of glands, particularly the sex and adrenal glands. Urine tests also indicate pregnancy, since pregnant women shed excess female hormones into the urine in readily detectable amounts.

During pregnancy, urinalysis becomes a vital safeguard of health. The pregnant woman's body is doubly burdened: her kidneys must dispose of not only her own wastes but the wastes of her baby. Monthly checks of urine warn if trouble is brewing, so that the doctor can take steps to forestall it.

A patient may hotly deny that he takes narcotics, but if he is an addict, his urine will reveal it. Urine is similarly valuable in detecting the presence of industrial poisons, like lead and arsenic, in the body.

A urinalysis is part of every physical examination, yielding its information simply and inexpensively. It is essential that the specimen be examined promptly. (Many doctors have facilities in their offices to run immediate tests.) Thus the sample taken to a drugstore or mailed to a laboratory may lose its value unless special preservatives are added.

The time a urine specimen is taken is also important; urine varies in its composition at different times of the day. Physicians frequently specify whether it should be collected before breakfast—as it is usually done in routine hospital examination—or after eating or drinking. After a meal the test may show excessive sugar. Drinking too much water may wash away the clues. Always it is wise to follow the doctor's instructions.

The urinalysis is not a magic divining rod that can spot the exact location of disease. But correlated with other tests and the study of the whole man, it is one of our most informative aids to medical diagnosis. Many people are alive today because of it.

Modesty has ruined more kidneys than bad liquor.   —Dr. S. Morris

The Pancreas and Diabetes

Adapted from "A Million Unknown Diabetics"
by C. Lester Walker
and "A New Day for Diabetics" by Paul de Kruif

The pancreas is a tongue-shaped organ lying behind the stomach whose job it is to manufacture two types of secretion. The pancreas turns one of these, the pancreatic juices, into the intestinal canal, the other into the bloodstream. The second secretion contains insulin: this is where diabetes comes in.

One million two hundred and fifty thousand Americans today have diabetes and are unaware of it. Another million and a half *know* they have diabetes. And there is disturbing evidence that this disease, eighth on the list today as a cause of death in the United States, is on the increase.

In the digestive process, sugars, starches and some fats and proteins are turned into glucose, a special kind of sugar that the body "burns" for fuel. Any unburned glucose is stored, as fat or glycogen, in your liver or your muscles. But neither the burning process nor the storing away can take place without the assistance of that second secretion from the pancreas, insulin. Why? Nobody knows. "Take away insulin," as one doctor puts it, "and you shut tight the draft of the stove."

In the pancreas there are groups of special cells—probably a million of them. These may get out of kilter. You begin to have great thirst, you are troubled with frequent and excessive urination. Fatigue attacks you easily. Perhaps you notice that a small cut is slow to heal. And you are hungry most of the time, but despite all you eat you lose weight. For lack of insulin the body is unable to burn its food and is drawing on its reserve fats for fuel. Actually you are in the process of starving.

If this process runs on unchecked, the diabetic one day collapses into a state of coma, from which nothing will revive him but insulin and fluids. Mashed-up cattle pancreas from the slaughterhouse is still the only source of insulin, but the chemists have refined and purified it so that today simple or "unmodified" insulin comes as a clear watery liquid or as crystals. Injected, it acts at once to lower the diabetic's blood sugar. However, it is effective for only five to six hours, at the end of which, without fail, it must be taken again.

In 1936, the slow-acting insulins were developed, which are compounds of insulin with other materials, such as simple proteins with a trace of zinc. Injected under the skin, such compounds release their insulin slowly and for a long period. Then came intermediate insulins, which work faster and more intensely than the slow-acting compounds, but not over such a long period. They too act less promptly and intensely than plain insulin, but are effective over a much longer time.

In sum, there is now plain—or fast—insulin, which causes the greatest reduction of sugar in from 2 to 4 hours; intermediate insulins, which reach their peak effect in from 8 to 12 hours; and slow-acting insulins which may take 18 to 24 hours to reach their maximum effect and last for another 24 hours or more. Because of this variety most diabetes can now be controlled by a sort of insulin "cocktail"—a mixture of types in one dose—which the diabetic takes but once a day.

One of the dangers of the insulin treatment has been "insulin shock," in which the blood sugar has dropped *too low* after shots of insulin. Patients grew giddy, became confused, even blacked out completely. This effect is so serious that railroadmen and others in hazardous occupations may be taken off the job if found to be insulin-using diabetics.

If the patient gets a little carbohydrate quickly—in the form of sugar, for example, or of candy, crackers, soft drinks, orange juice—the symptoms are likely to disappear within ten minutes. That's why many diabetics carry a few lumps of sugar or several crackers in their pockets or handbags. In severe cases, a doctor may have to inject glucose, or glucagon, another pancreatic hormone which seems to counteract the effects of insulin.

A new drug known as Orinase which can be taken orally has solved for many the problems of repeated injections and the danger of insulin shock. A sulfa drug, Orinase apparently prods the diabetic's pancreas into making its own insulin.

No diabetic less than twenty years old is a candidate for Orinase. In such patients the pancreas rarely has the power to produce insulin, which it must if the drug is to exert its effect. But in the age group between twenty and forty, one out of four may replace insulin by Orinase. And in the age group over forty—to which the great majority of diabetics belong—success with Orinase is about 80 percent.

Many investigators agree that with the pancreas making its own insulin—as it does with Orinase—there is better control of the disease. The hormone is released steadily; there is far less fatigue; patients volunteer that they feel much better; there is no shortness of breath and weakness and no longer the fear of the dreaded low-blood-sugar reactions that plague users of insulin. There is just one caution to be observed: Insulin should be on hand to be used under the doctor's direction in case of sudden need.

New knowledge of diet has also improved the technique of diabetes treatment. Before the discovery of insulin the diabetic's meals were a tasteless nightmare of high-fat, starchless, sugarless foods. "Spinach—cooked three times," old-time diabetics still reminiscently moan. Today the diabetic has to watch what he eats but can include satisfying amounts of carbohydrates, fats and even sugars provided he keeps his weight down. Even alcohol is not entirely taboo, though sweet wines, champagne and beer are forbidden.

At one time a diabetic's life expectancy was only five years— five grim, wasting-away years. Today his chances are excellent of living as long with diabetes, under proper treatment, as he might have expected to live without it. And a diabetic can even take out insurance, upon a physician's statement that the disease is under control.

It is a well-established fact that diabetes prefers fat people. In a group of a thousand diabetics the chances are that 90 percent have at some time in their lives been obese. It is only as the disease advances that they lose weight. But the exact cause-and-effect relationship of overweight and diabetes is something on which the doctors do not yet completely agree.

Diabetes is definitely inheritable. It is what the geneticists call a Mendelian recessive—that is, it follows the same inheritance path as baldness and color blindness and may skip a generation. If both husband and wife have *active* diabetes, the records show that *all* their children will have it if they live long enough.

Before insulin, women with diabetes could seldom become pregnant and, if they did, five out of ten pregnancies were failures. A study of pregnant diabetics disclosed an imbalance in the female sex hormones—hormones necessary for the development of the fetus and for its birth. After the diabetic mothers were given the missing hormones—estrogens and progesterone—90 percent bore healthy babies. Now, with this type of prenatal treatment, the diabetic mother has more than a 25-to-1 chance to bear a live and healthy child.

Before insulin, most deaths from diabetes were due to diabetic coma. Today, diabetic coma causes only 3 percent of the deaths. Atherosclerosis now brings on 66 percent of diabetic deaths. The diabetic is much more susceptible to atherosclerosis than the nondiabetic. This hardening of the arteries may strike anywhere—the heart, the brain, the kidneys. When it works in the hands or feet, circulation is impaired and gangrene often develops. Attacking the retina of the eye, it brings blindness. Proper treatment of the diabetes does not always insure against it. But doctors, observing that diabetics have more progression of atherosclerosis than can be attributed solely to a person's aging, are led to hope that one day we shall see the riddle of atherosclerosis solved by successful research in diabetes.

Meanwhile, what is to be done about the million Americans who have diabetes and are ignorant of the fact? The American Diabetes Association hopes to find them—through publicity and with the aid of general practitioners in many communities. Through its affiliate associations or county or local medical societies, a urine-sugar test often is offered free of charge to anyone.

In its current search for diabetic unknowns, the association emphasizes one cardinal precept: Have a blood-sugar test made (1) if you are over forty and overweight, (2) if any one of your ancestors ever had diabetes.

Your Long-Suffering Colon

by William Harley Glafke, M.D.

The public spends over a hundred million dollars a year for laxatives. More of these drugs are bought than of any other home medicaments.

Possibly custom explains much of this large expenditure. Considering digestive waste as unclean, it is easy to reason (quite wrongly) that if it remains in the colon it will poison us. Nothing seems more logical, then, than to "clear out the system," to "get rid of the poison" that seemingly causes our dizzy feeling, poor appetite or "dopiness." So the poor old colon has been needlessly driven and drugged, until it's a wonder there's anything left of it.

Drug manufacturers have played upon these fears in advertising their cathartic pills, liquids, gums, candies. This state of affairs is dangerous. Every drug used in these "harmless" laxatives acts *because it irritates* and thus causes the digestive tract to push forward its contents faster than normally. Both vegetable cathartics (like cascara and castor oil) and saline cathartics (like Epsom salts, magnesia, Seidlitz powders) as well as such agents as calomel and phenolphthalein irritate the sensitive membrane that lines the intestines.

The thirty-foot-long digestive tract may be divided into three parts. The esophagus (gullet) and stomach receive the food and prepare it for assimilation. The long small intestine absorbs the nutriments from the food. The relatively short large intestine, or colon, extrudes from the body the residues which are left. It is the colon which bears the greatest brunt of irritation when cathartics are used.

The propulsion of intestinal contents is accomplished by a series of contraction waves of the muscle fibers in the bowel wall. When the lining is irritated, these muscular walls squeeze the contents along faster. The intestine is trying to get rid of the hurt. In the small intestine the principal effect of this hurried propulsion is that only part of the nutriment is absorbed through the lining into the blood. The greatest damage occurs in the colon, because there the squeezing motions are normally slower and the cathartic is in contact with the walls for a longer time. The colonic lining becomes inflamed, and since the contents are hurried along there is not time enough for the normal absorption of water from them. There is also a disturbance of the normal interchange of gases between intestinal contents and blood in the bowel wall. This brings abdominal distention, cramplike pains, gurgling and rumbling.

Because of the close association of nerves and digestive tract, in cases of severe irritation our patient has psychic depression and "dopiness"; nausea is common; vomiting may occur. The patient is generally miserable. What does he usually do? Takes more cathartic!

The passage of food through the digestive tract takes a surprising amount of time. To pass through the stomach alone, an average meal requires 4 to 6 hours, and to pass through the whole 30 feet of tube it takes at least 36 to 48 hours. Food eaten Monday (breakfast, lunch and dinner) becomes a liquid in the stomach and then passes through the small intestine during Monday and Monday night. On Tuesday morning the residue has progressed only to the colon, still in liquid state. During Tuesday and Tuesday night this residue is propelled slowly through the colon, being dehydrated as it goes, to be expelled Wednesday morning. Meantime, the food eaten Tuesday has reached the upper colon as a residue, to be expelled Thursday. The normal colon is never empty.

Let's see what happens to this timing when we take a cathartic. We'll assume we take it Monday night on retiring. On Tuesday morning when it acts, not only is Tuesday's movement brought about, but also Wednesday's. When Wednesday comes, the bowel hasn't had time to catch up and no movement may be forthcoming. Reasoning on the old idea that our bowels should move every day, we take another pill. What we should do is to let the bowel alone, and avoid driving it a day ahead of itself. If the evacuation does not occur tomorrow, it will the next day.

Terms such as "autointoxication," "toxic absorption," "colonic stagnation" are bugaboos. The colon's lining is a protective membrane standing between the bloodstream and the products inside the colon. It absorbs practically nothing but water. Fecal material within a normal colon can be thought of as *outside* the body; that is, in a cavity devised for its care until a convenient time for extrusion occurs.

However, repeated irritation breaks down the barrierlike action of the colon membrane and it becomes swollen and thickened. The surface cells lose their continuity with one another. Through this unhealthy lining, products of putrefaction and fermentation can pass into the blood and cause bodily disorders. Our treatment must be not to sweep out the "poisons" in the colon with further cathartics which keep the membrane unhealthy, but to build up the normal barrierlike action of the lining by healing measures.

It has long been known that the greater the bulk of residue, the more active are the bowel muscles. The average diet consists of "smooth" foods, which are absorbed in the small intestine almost completely, and "roughage" foods which leave residues, such as seeds, skins of fruits and vegetables. Most people get enough residue so that they have one passage each day. Others get enough to have more than one, but so long as the colon is not overstimulated by this diet, no harm results. Still other people have one evacuation every two days. So long as it is normal, no harm is done.

Some people, on the other hand, have evacuations that are loose if they eat the average diet; their colons are irritable. They should cut down on roughage foods and take more smooth foods. Still another group of people eat plenty of roughage and still have evacuations that are really constipated. These are the "lazy-colon" tribe and we help them by giving a "bulk producer"—agar, derivatives of psyllium seed, the gum of kabaya or bassorin plant, and the like—products which absorb water and swell up to become bulky in the intestinal tract. Their smooth, nonirritating bulk increases the residue and stimulates colonic muscular action. They are not drugs but nonirritant mechanical helps.

There has been much discussion in medical circles about the use of mineral oil in constipation. Many doctors believe that mineral oil absorbs the so-called fat-soluble vitamins (Vitamins A and D) and therefore should not be used regularly. Also, it seems to make some people flatulent. Aside from these factors, mineral oil appears to be harmless. It is not an irritant like most cathartics; it is a lubricant. It can be used either in its natural form or in the various emulsions which make it more palatable.

For temporary help in regulation of the bowel, the low enema, using one to two pints of plain water, may be used to start expulsive action. Any "stoppage" is in the last few inches of colon and the use of a mechanical help such as the enema is much more logical than starting with a cathartic at the upper end of the digestive tube thirty feet away. Colonic irrigations using many quarts or gallons of water are not recommended, as they disturb the next day's evacuation.

Simple suppositories such as the glycerin type may also be useful in starting expulsive impulses. In training a colon to take up its normal rhythm, either a suppository or an enema may be used daily. All this, of course, should be with your doctor's advice. It is even possible, without mechanical measures, to further the development of a regular evacuation by setting a definite time of day as one's "appointment" and keeping to this schedule.

The unreasoning use of cathartics leads to serious trouble in cases of appendicitis, the beginning pain of which is often felt in the pit of the stomach, not necessarily in the lower right side where the appendix lies. The pain is blamed by many patients on indigestion—and a laxative is taken. Such self-treatment is responsible for a large number of deaths, because nature's effort to put up a "fire wall" about the inflamed area is defeated. The intestinal coils are forced to writhe and squirm upon themselves, the adherent loops are torn apart and the fire can spread throughout the abdomen to cause deadly peritonitis.

There is still another count in the indictment of cathartics. If any inflammation occurs in the digestive tube, it not only sends waves of muscular action downward at a faster rate but also sends waves upward, the wrong way—the progress of food is slowed or stopped and we suffer a lack of appetite, belching or nausea. In such cases it is necessary to quiet the irritated colon and soothe it back to normal. This means smooth foods for a few weeks, a smooth bulk such as agar to give a gentle push to the colon without hurting it, and the avoidance of roughage foods entirely until the bowel has a chance to recover.

Don't fear the "terrible consequences" of constipation—most of them never happen. Merely use common sense in regulating your digestion. Learn whether your colon has any special quirks, whether it is touchy or lazy, whether it needs little bulk or a great deal. Treat it kindly. Normally it is a protective organ which will serve you well, if given proper material to work with.

CHAPTER 8

The Body's Chemical Wizardry

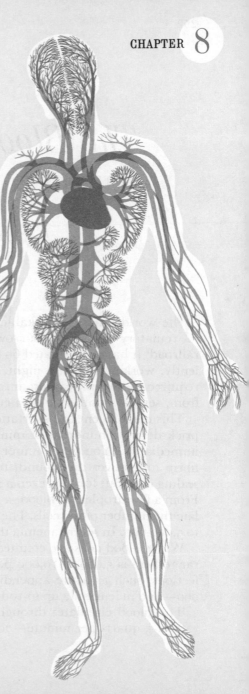

THE BLOODSTREAM and its extraordinary cargo of delicate substances circulated from the body's glands and major organs guides the basic pattern of human responses in many ways.

New breakthroughs in science disclose the intricate interplay of these chemicals and indicate what we ourselves can do to assist them in their task.

The Bloodstream:
CHEMISTRY IN ACTION

by J. D. Ratcliff

The world's most remarkable transportation system is the circulatory system of your own body. Longer than any U.S. railroad, it has an estimated 60,000 to 100,000 miles of route. Silently, working day and night, it provides the exact blood flow required by any tissue or organ, carrying food to, and wastes away from, several hundred *trillion* customers—the body cells.

This magnificent transportation system is self-repairing. A pinprick destroys hundreds of minute capillaries. New ones sprout immediately. You get a minor cut: instantly a cottony web of fibrin forms over the wound, trapping red cells and building a sealing clot. But for this, even a minor wound might mean death. From a few droplets of blood, a laboratory technician can calculate the number of red cells. The count should be about 4,500,000 to 5,000,000. In severe anemia the count may be under 1,000,000.

White blood cells are counted in similar fashion. The healthy range here is 5,000 to 10,000 per cubic millimeter. In severe infections, such as acute appendicitis, the count may rise to 20,000—and in leukemia up to 100 times normal.

The blood circulates through the system at the approximate rate of 5 quarts per minute—7000 to 9000 quarts every twenty-four hours. Arteries are more than simple piping. They are pulsing muscular tubes. Blood enters them from the heart in surging gushes. Arteries even this flow by relaxing with each beat, contracting between beats. Thus blood reaches the tiniest branches of the circulatory system as a smooth-flowing stream.

On death, arteries empty themselves. Finding them empty, ancient anatomists thought they were air passages, and so the word artery derives from the Latin for windpipe. Not until 1628 did William Harvey, the great English physician, announce his discovery of circulation of the blood.

Circulation has two responsibilities. Arterial blood transports a mixed cargo to the cells: amino acids for tissue repair, sugar for energy, minerals and vitamins, hormones, oxygen. On the return trip through the veins, blood carts off carbon dioxide from combustion that has taken place in the cells. It also removes excess water and debris from protein metabolism.

Follow the fate of a bite of steak eaten at dinner. In the stomach and small intestine, acid and enzymes break down the steak protein into some twenty amino acids. The wall of the small intestine is lined with villi, minute hairlike protuberances which look, under the microscope, like the nap of a carpet. There are an estimated five million of them, each containing tiny blood vessels whose walls are porous enough to admit molecules of amino acids.

Thus the remnants of your steak are taken aboard the bloodstream. The first stop is the liver, the blood's master regulatory organ. It is the liver's job to see that blood contains at all times the exact amount of sugar needed by muscles and the precise quantities of amino acids required for tissue building and repair. If you have eaten too much steak, the blood entering the liver will contain too many aminos. Some will be stored, some destroyed.

From this point onward the blood acts like a conveyor belt. In time it will reach every cell in the body, unloading a portion of its cargo wherever needed—cargo which will build muscle in a growing child, or produce a new film of skin over a burned finger.

The sugar in your coffee and the mashed potatoes follow much the same course. In the small intestine both are converted into glucose. This, too, is carried to the liver. If there is an excess, the liver converts it into glycogen and stores it. When needed as fuel for muscles, it is reconverted into glucose and dribbled out. During exercise the liver will draw on the twelve-to-twenty-four-hour reserve it keeps on hand at all times.

Fats represent another stockpile of fuel. Broken down in the intestine into fatty acids, they are picked up by the lymphatic system, which feeds them into the blood as needed. In times of emergency these fat deposits can be drawn upon, supplying the body's energy requirements for weeks after the liver's sugar storage has been exhausted.

The array of proteins which the blood carries is particularly remarkable. Each protein appears to have a special transport function—just as railroad refrigerator, coal or grain cars have special functions. One is designed to carry iodine needed by the thyroid gland; another carries phosphorus for the teeth; a third, calcium for bones.

At all times there is approximately a quart of oxygen in circulation. Hemoglobin, the iron-containing protein which gives blood its red color, is the carrier of this life-sustaining gas. In the presence of excess oxygen, hemoglobin gives up carbon dioxide and, like a sponge, soaks up oxygen. This takes place in the lungs. In cells along the circulatory system the reverse takes place. Hemoglobin gives up oxygen and takes aboard carbon dioxide.

The most important and fascinating part of the circulatory system is the great network of capillaries, the microscopic junction points between arteries and veins. It is in these tiny vessels, so small that red blood cells must pass through single-file, that blood fulfills its ultimate destiny—the nourishing of cells and the absorption of cellular wastes. Just how this is accomplished is not yet clear, but the general outline is known. Each cell in our body lives in a bath of salty fluid which must be constantly replenished. To this end, capillary walls are relatively porous, so that oxygen from the blood can pass through the walls in one direction, and carbon dioxide wastes from the body cells in the other. There is also a seepage of fluid from the capillaries into the intercellular spaces, bathing the cells in liquid nourishment.

Blood in the veins, as we have seen, carries a variety of

wastes—mainly carbon dioxide, water and the nitrogenous by-products of protein metabolism. The circulatory system has two chief dumps for these unwanted materials: lungs and kidneys.

To determine the speed of the blood flow through the body, scientists have exercised considerable ingenuity. One method is to inject a bitter-tasting chemical in, say, an ankle or arm vein; then with a stop watch check the elapsed time before it is tasted by the tongue. Injected radioactive substances, checked with a Geiger counter, have also been used to determine rate of flow. Most such studies agree that the blood moves through the body at about six inches a second.

The unbelievably complex task of blood-traffic control is handled by the vasomotor center in the base of the brain. Nerve impulses go out from this point, tightening or loosening the muscular walls of arteries—in effect opening and closing sluiceways.

There are other lesser control centers for blood distribution. After meals, the major attention of the circulatory system must be directed to digestion. Blood is routed to the abdominal region and the brain may be put on short rations. Then we become drowsy. Swimming after meals can be dangerous for a similar reason—there isn't enough blood for digestive organs *and* muscles. Since the blood pays first heed to digestion, muscles are starved and are likely to cramp if used strenuously.

The blood itself is quite as remarkable as the circulatory system. Look at the red cells. The approximately six quarts of blood in the adult body contain many trillions of these minute discs. Formed mainly in bone marrow, they are born and destroyed at a stupendous rate: seventy-two million a *minute*. As they pass through the liver, aged red cells—their life span is 120 days—are plucked out by microscopic fingers of cells shaped like starfish. They are destroyed, but the ever-frugal body salvages 85 percent of their vital iron. This is carried back to bone marrow by the blood for the manufacture of new hemoglobin. Without this miraculous iron recovery most of us would face the pale death of anemia, since iron is scarce in the average diet.

Besides red cells, blood contains a variety of infection-fighting white cells, some of which engulf and eat invading bacteria. It also contains an array of clotting materials whose subtle chemistry has yet to be fully understood.

Another fascinating blood component is the assortment of chemicals which determine blood "types." How many of these chemicals there are no one knows. New ones are discovered all the time and it may be that the blood of each individual differs from the blood of all others—and that in time detailed blood typing will become as reliable as fingerprinting in establishing identity.

For surgery, the doctor will want to know the broad blood type, essential information for transfusion. One way is to add a drop of the patient's blood to a solution to form a cell suspension. Then a drop of the suspension is mixed with serum of a known blood category and watched for the clumping characteristics which reveal the type of the unknown sample.

It is also essential for the surgeon to know clotting time— hemorrhage is a deadly possibility when clotting lags. Samples of blood are placed in test tubes the size of pencil leads. At intervals the technician tilts the tubes; when blood no longer flows, it has clotted. Normal time: two to eight minutes.

The sedimentation test measures the time it takes red cells to settle out of a sample of blood. This is useful in some chronic illnesses; the faster the red cells settle, the graver the illness. Tests for the protein and protein end products present in blood serum are important in determining kidney function; bile pigments present are a measure of liver performance. There are tests for measuring the amounts of sodium, potassium and other electrolytes, of critical importance in the fluid balance of the body. The slightest imbalance, uncorrected, can be fatal.

All in all, your blood is a remarkable fluid, and the transport system which carries it a marvel. The throb you feel when you press fingers to wrist is the faint murmuring of one of the wonders of the universe.

A GREAT SURGEON once said to his students, "A man will bleed to death from a severed carotid artery in three minutes. You can tie this artery in two minutes *if you are not in a hurry.*"
—Don Herold

Lymph,

THE MYSTERIOUS FLUID

by Henry Morton Robinson

Over the entire human body, permeating the skin and the tissues beneath, stretches a remarkable network of tiny, transparent vessels, somewhat like knotted lace in appearance. This is the little-known lymphatic system. Through its microscopic conduits flows a mysterious, straw-colored fluid—the lymph—which in its leisurely course performs marvels of biochemistry for the maintenance of your health.

You've probably witnessed one small miracle of the lymph without knowing it. A cut finger was neglected for a day. Then a droplet of pale yellow fluid oozed from the cut. This was the lymph, loaded with specialized cells which help the white corpuscles kill off disease organisms.

When infection penetrates deeper than a cut, the invading organisms are caught up in the lymphatic system and carried to the nearest lymph node. Here another attempt is made to destroy them. These lymph nodes, varying in size from a mustard seed to a large lima bean, produce lymphocytes, a type of white corpuscle which is an important disease-fighting unit of the blood. Lymph nodes are located abundantly throughout the body with the largest clustered in the neck, groin, armpits and intestines.

These mechanical filters are designed to trap not only bacteria but any cell debris or other foreign matter as well. One physiologist aptly calls them "dust bins of the body."

But this vitally important protective function is only a small part of the lymphatics' job. Life itself depends on this body fluid which closely resembles blood in chemical composition and yet emphatically is not blood. The lymph derives from the blood system and passes back into it eventually. But in the interim, employing its own private network, it performs a miraculous physiological duty. That duty is to salvage vital proteins—the very building blocks of which our body is made—which would be lost were they not thriftily gathered up by the lymphatic system. Greatly simplified, here's what happens:

Under pressure from the heart, fluids seep through the porous walls of the capillaries—the tiniest blood vessels—carrying nutriment to tissues and absorbing waste products. These fluids consist of molecules of protein, salts and water. The salts and water can and do pass back into the veins. But the proteins cannot directly re-enter the venous system. Here a potentially awkward situation develops. If these proteins accumulate, the superfluous concentration may damage surrounding tissues. They must be distributed to other parts of the body, where they are sorely needed.

With blotterlike action, the lymphatics soak up the protein-laden filtrate. Through its own circulatory system, quite separate from the veins and arteries, the lymph now proceeds toward the center of the body. In the intestines the lymph vessels take up an emulsion of fats from foods that have been transformed by the digestive juices.

Now the lymph, laden with both fats and proteins, is ready to return to the bloodstream. Tiny flaplike valves on the interior walls of the lymph ducts prevent any backward movement of the fluid. The lymph can flow in one direction only—toward the heart.

But unlike the bloodstream, which depends on the pumping action of the heart, the lymph has no driving force behind it. Its progress depends solely on the body's muscular and breathing movements. For example, lymph ducts twine themselves around the muscles of the arms and legs: when these muscles contract and expand they exert pressure on the lymph vessels. In the intestines a powerful force is required to squeeze upward the heavy emulsion of fats that has been taken on. Now occurs a marvel that ranks high among physiological wonders. The lymph vessel winds itself around the mightiest of arteries—the aorta—and utilizes the powerful pulsations of that huge blood vessel to propel the lymph.

Usually the lymph current moves at a rather sluggish pace. But it can be whipped up, with definite advantages to health and body tone, by exercise, deep breathing and massage.

At a point just above the gateway to the heart, the main lymph stream pours into a major vein. Thus the choicest products of digestion have been gathered up and delivered safely to the bloodstream in a roundabout and biologically ingenious manner.

But all along the line, the straw-colored fluid has passed through the myriad wayside filtering stations, the lymph nodes. These glands are subjected to many severe trials. For example, an infection of the hand may cause painful swelling of the lymph glands in the armpit; an infection of the foot or leg may produce an inflammation of the glands in the groin. This is nature struggling to annihilate the invading disease organisms. Unless the battle is won, the bacteria will pass on to the bloodstream, causing blood poisoning.

Sometimes the trapped bacteria infect the lymph nodes, causing acute inflammation and abscess formation; then it may become necessary to remove the infected glands. The lymph nodes filter out cancer cells; but then the glands themselves may become the site of new malignant growths. Thus in the treatment of cancer, attention must be paid to the lymph glands that drain the area of the primary growth.

The lymphatic system is also subject to diseases of its own. In elephantiasis, for example, a threadlike parasite renders the lymphatic tissue incapable of draining off the fluids that collect in the tissue spaces. The result: swollen, waterlogged lower limbs and coarsened skin.

But the miracle of the lymph in the normal body suggests a question: What would happen if the vital fluid were prevented from returning to the blood? Scientists found a definite answer in the case of a young woman who had been stabbed in the neck. The wound severed the main pathway of the lymph stream on its way back to the heart. The patient suffered serious loss of weight and was losing ground so rapidly that death seemed inevitable. Then the lymph lines were repaired surgically so that again the lymph flowed back into the bloodstream. Within a few weeks the patient regained her weight and left the hospital in good health.

Silently, invisibly, the lymph river winds through our cells and organs, bathing them in a vital alkaline fluid. It is one of the most remarkable of the adaptive mechanisms that enable the human body to maintain its interior balance and economy. It is an instrument of survival, versatile and awe-inspiring as the blood from which it springs and which, by the strangest of physiological processes, it nourishes and sustains.

Kiss and Tell

We have radio to thank for the information that love is "a matter of vitamin B-1, phosphorus and starch metabolism." During a WOR broadcast, Dr. Carlton Fredericks was asked to explain the relationship between nutrition and kissing, and he told it—in full!

"When a fellow kisses a girl," said Dr. Fredericks, "the adrenosympathetic system calls on the liver for glycogen for energy. This in turn forces the release of insulin, vitamin B-1, and phosphorus to burn the sugar. In his brain, if he is doing any thinking, which is problematical, there is an exchange of starch, phosphorus and thiamine between the thalamic and the cortical brain. As the pulse and respiration rates rise, there is increased exchange of oxygen on the intracellular level, which would mean increased consumption of thiamine and phosphorus."   —Marie Torre

THE BODY'S MASTER CHEMICALS

Three mysterious substances, in minute quantities, control the chemistry of the human body. Some of the most important facts about them have been unearthed only within recent years. These substances are the hormones, those powerful chemicals secreted in the body by the endocrine glands; the enzymes, which turn one chemical substance into another; and the vitamins. These magic chemicals maintain an extraordinary balance among forces so powerful that any of them could be destructive if unchecked.

—Bruce Bliven, Jr.

The Endocrine Glands:
CENTERS OF CONTROL

by J. D. Ratcliff

Hormones circulating in your bloodstream are much like miniature hydrogen bombs—powerful almost beyond belief. During her thirty childbearing years a woman's ovaries secrete an amount of the hormone estrogen approximately equal in weight to a postage stamp. At the time of puberty an amount equivalent to the tiniest corner of the stamp is sufficient to bring about an amazing metamorphosis—the resculpturing of a girl's body into that of a woman.

The thyroid gland in your neck produces no more than a teaspoonful of hormone in a year. But if the teaspoon is only partially filled, a newborn baby can develop into a cretin—a malformed idiot.

The adrenal glands produce only a teaspoonful of hormone in a *lifetime*. But let their hairline balance be upset and we are prey to a host of crippling and disabling diseases. Or let them go on strike for any reason and life unreels at a dizzy clip: in months, a vigorous young male can become a tottering old man.

Our amazing endocrine glands take some part in virtually everything we do. Lift an eyelid—it was hormones that made sure sugar was in the blood to provide muscle power. Cut a finger and hormones will be there to help control inflammation and wall off infection.

Hormones are common denominators of animal life. Some of the movie starlet's sex hormones are identical with those of a whale; some of a prize fighter's pituitary products match those of a mouse.

Scientists have come up with a host of wonder-working hormones which cure eye diseases that once led to blindness, snatch back lives from illnesses once regarded as fatal, wash pain from inflamed arthritic joints. On an experimental basis hormones have been used successfully both to combat the shock that so often kills badly debilitated people on operating tables and to help give elderly invalids a new lease on life. Many researchers are convinced that hormones will play key parts in resolving much of medicine's unfinished business: cancer, hardening of the arteries, heart and kidney diseases.

So let us take a closer look at the remarkable endocrine system. Some glands—salivary, digestive-juice, sweat—pour their secretions to the outside. The endocrines empty theirs into the bloodstream and are therefore known as ductless glands. There are eight of them, which together weigh only about two ounces. This tiny amount of tissue acts as a kind of council of ministers for the body, directing myriad activities. So harmoniously do these glands work together that if one is sluggish, another gives it a prod, or assumes part of its function.

Four of the endocrine glands may be quickly dismissed. The

function of the pancreas, whose million little "island" cells secrete insulin (which promotes the utilization of sugar), is already widely known. The parathyroids, four little wheat grains attached to the thyroid, seem to have but one function—that of governing the amount of calcium, phosphorus and other electrolytes circulating in the blood—and rarely give trouble. The pineal, whose function is just beginning to be understood, is a tiny, cone-shaped gland attached to the underside of the brain—thought to be the remnant of a third eye man inherited from some primordial ancestor. The thymus in the upper chest is similarly mysterious, although it appears to play some role in the maturing process.

This leaves the big four: the pituitary, thyroid, adrenals and sex glands. They are the body's master chemists, producing hormones of enormous complexity. The pituitary is perhaps the most remarkable component of the human body. Because of its influence on other glands it has been compared to the conductor of a great symphony—the symphony of life. About the size of a large pea, it resides in a bony cavern on the underside of the brain, approximately in the center of the head. Something like 50,000 nerve fibers enter this fragment of tissue, while its enormously rich blood supply carries its chemical messengers—hormones—to the rest of the body. Some of these hormones act as stimulants on specific targets.

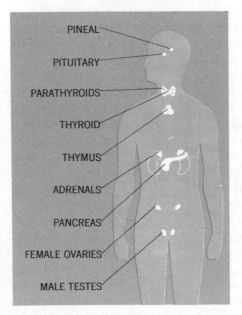

Silhouette of human body showing locations of endocrine glands

PINEAL

PITUITARY

PARATHYROIDS

THYROID

THYMUS

ADRENALS

PANCREAS

FEMALE OVARIES

MALE TESTES

Thus one jogs the thyroid into activity, while others activate the adrenals, pancreas and sex glands. One helps to govern salt balance in the body. Another acts as a brake on the kidneys: with this brake removed, as much as three gallons of urine a day may be secreted.

One of the most fascinating of pituitary chemicals is the growth hormone: the circus midget has too little, the giant too much. Under the influence of this powerful stuff, experimental rats have grown to twice normal size. It has been similarly used to prod slow-growing children.

The pituitary plays a major role in the birth process. After delivery of a baby it releases a minute squirt of hormone which causes contraction of the mother's womb—one of nature's safety measures against hemorrhage. And a few days after birth it releases one of the most extraordinary chemicals ever discovered— prolactin, which stimulates breasts to produce milk.

Most endocrinologists rank the adrenals next in importance to the pituitary. Like little tricorn hats, these yellowish-brown glands sit atop the kidneys. The blood supply that comes to them is an indication of their importance: each minute they receive six times their own weight!

Because of their role in preparing us for emergencies, they have been called the "fight-or-run" glands. For example, a man, badly injured himself, rushes into a burning plane and saves others, then collapses. It was the adrenals that provided energy for the act.

In time of stress, their hormone output may shoot up to ten times normal levels—increasing heart and respiration rates, hoisting the level of energizing blood sugar. Not sure how a possible encounter may come out, the adrenals also quicken the clotting time of blood—to reduce loss if bloodshed ensues.

There are more than forty hormones or hormonelike chemicals produced directly or indirectly by the adrenal glands. One influences mineral levels in the blood; others perform other, similar, tasks. The adrenals also produce sex hormones. But possibly the most important hormones produced by the adrenals are those of the cortisone family. Synthetic hormones of this group have been used successfully against some one hundred diseases.

The thyroid, a butterfly-shaped gland that straddles the windpipe, acts something like a car's accelerator; it speeds up or slows down bodily activity. Whether we live in a sluggish, sleepy, half-alive world, or in a racing, energy-charged world depends on thyroid hormone—secreted normally at a rate of 1/2800 of an ounce a day.

With advancing age the thyroid frequently tapers off activity. That's why grandmother moves closer to the fire—her body isn't producing enough heat. Or, a young woman may be unable to have children—all bodily activity has slowed because of a sluggish thyroid. In these cases hormone pills can quicken the tempo of life.

At the other extreme the thyroid may be too active, burning food into energy far too fast. Result: wolfish appetite, pounding heart, high blood pressure, tremor, sweating and heat intolerance. Surgery, radioactive iodine or drugs can exert a calming influence.

Of the sex glands, look first at the almond-shaped ovaries which lie on either side of a woman's lower abdomen. They produce two hormones. Under the stimulus of one—estrogen—ovaries each month produce a single egg cell. Once the egg has been released, a second hormone—progesterone—causes the womb to lie quietly and make a safe nest for the new life in the event of fertilization.

Lately researchers have come up with some surprising findings about female hormones. For example, there are indications that doses of these hormones may sometimes help ward off hardening of the arteries in both men and women. They are also showing signs of usefulness in the animal world. Normally sheep bear but one lamb a year—in the spring. Under female-hormone stimulus they have been made to bear an additional lamb in the autumn, thereby doubling meat production.

The ancients knew the vital role played by the testes, the male sex glands. Removal changed the snorting bull into the docile ox, the aggressive rooster into the passive capon, the virile male into the safest of harem watchmen. The testes produce the hormone testosterone, which has now been found to have considerable importance in the body economy outside the reproductive cycle. It appears, for example, to play a large part in the utilization of all-important protein. Minute amounts improve the appetite and general well-being of oldsters. The same hormone also seems to hasten fracture healing. In women, testosterone has proved an effective treatment for uterine bleeding.

Almost certainly hormones hold the solution for many of today's disease riddles. And most researchers believe that they will also help solve one of the most pressing problems of tomorrow— the problem of an aging population. Even if they do not lengthen life, they will provide a *better* life—through keeping older people in youthful chemical balance.

A MAN weighing 140 pounds contains enough fat for 7 cakes of soap, carbon for 9000 pencils, phosphorus to make 2200 match heads, magnesium for one dose of salts, iron to make one medium-sized nail, sufficient lime to whitewash a chicken coop, enough sulphur to rid one dog of fleas and water to fill a 10-gallon barrel.   —Dr. F. E. Lawson

THERE is no such thing as an especially de luxe set of glands filling one to bursting with energy. They are no more a source of energy than the heart or lungs. A person with gilt-edged glands may be exhausted by emotional strains. Something more than hormones is driving the person who is a Human Dynamo. It is interest.   —Marie Beynon Ray

Enzymes:

NATURE'S "CONVERTERS"

by J. D. Ratcliff

Enzymes are large protein molecules, present in all living things from bacteria to whales to marigolds. They are nature's chemists. All activity of living things depends on them—the greening of leaves in the spring, the bolt from an electric eel, the wagging of a dog's tail, the illumination of a firefly.

From the instant of conception, enzymes play the supreme role in all life processes. Without them the fragile male sperm could never gain entrance to the enormously larger and tougher female egg to complete the act of fertilization. As it is, the sperm is equipped with a minute amount of enzyme to dissolve a tiny crevice in the egg membrane, thereby gaining admittance.

Virtually all the foods we eat (alcohol is a notable exception) are totally indigestible until enzymes work on them and break down complex foods into simpler substances which can be absorbed into the bloodstream. But for enzymes, we could gorge ourselves with food—and starve. Or the food we eat could be lethal as cyanide. (Digesting a lamb chop, for example, could liberate enough ammonia to kill, were it not for enzymes which instantly synthesize ammonia into harmless end products.)

In a twinkling, enzymes perform chemical transformations that are difficult or impossible to perform in the laboratory. To digest a piece of steak in the laboratory—to break it down into its component amino acids—it is necessary to boil the steak for nearly a day in concentrated acid. At body temperature, enzymes accomplish the same thing in a few hours!

No one knows for sure how enzymes achieve their chemical wizardry. But each enzyme is specific in its action—it usually acts on only one substance. Thus, the enzymes which are known to be able to break up a pat of butter are powerless to break up sugar, and the sugar enzymes are unable to split proteins.

But enzymes do not merely break substances down, they also create new matter. From the bloodstream they take amino acids, say, that originated from cow muscle (steak), and use them as building blocks to produce human muscle—quite a different substance. They change sugar into glycogen, which the liver can store to supply energy needs as they arise.

Chew a piece of bread for a few minutes. You will note that it gradually becomes sweet. This is enzyme action. The body can't utilize starch, but it can absorb certain sugars. So an enzyme in saliva has converted some of the starch into sugar, a process later completed by enzymes of the digestive tract.

Pour a little hydrogen peroxide on a small wound. It foams up. An enzyme in the skin is breaking down the chemical into water and free oxygen, which makes the foam. In a single second one molecule of this enzyme can split 80,000 molecules of peroxide. In the intestine, a molecule of the enzyme invertase can break down a million times its own weight of sugar.

How many different enzymes are there in the human body? More than 650 are known and researchers guess that many more will be discovered. There are trillions of cells in the body. But even the smallest is estimated to contain at least 100,000 enzyme particles. If a cell is regarded as a factory, the enzymes are the machinery that makes the factory work.

Some of the enzymes are oxidants—fuel burners. They take a minute fragment of food and start it on a series of chemical reactions that produces one of the most extraordinary substances on earth: adenosine triphosphate, or ATP for short. In effect, ATP is a minute storage battery which releases stored energy to make muscle fibers contract. Every time your heart beats, every time your eyelids blink, every time you take a breath, it is ATP that provides energy for the action.

Much the same type of thing takes place in nerves. Enzymes

produce a remarkable stuff called acetylcholine—minute squirts of which make possible transmission of messages across nerve junctions. However, once it has done its job acetylcholine must be instantly destroyed—otherwise the heart would stop. Here again, an enzyme comes to the rescue—in a few thousandths of a second.

Many enzymes are now being put to work by physicians. Researchers extract them from plants, molds, bacteria, human blood. Among the more helpful is an enzyme called hyaluronidase, which doctors bring to the aid of infants who have been severely dehydrated by diarrhea or by burns. Such patients must get fluid in their circulatory systems or die. But with gravely ill infants it is often difficult or impossible for physicians to find veins for transfusion. The enzyme solves the problem. Administered by injection, it dissolves the binding stuff of muscle and makes tissue so permeable that fluids can be dripped via a transfusion needle directly into muscle and be absorbed into the circulation.

One enzyme—streptokinase (SK for short) promises to be effective in dissolving blood clots lodging in heart arteries. Another dissolves clots in leg blood vessels, which cause thrombophlebitis.

Today, many researchers are convinced that a number of diseases trace to missing or faulty enzymes. They theorize that there is a specific gene—an inheritance factor in the chromosome—to govern the production of each enzyme in the body. When the gene is missing or defective, so is the enzyme.

Diabetes, researchers think, may be due in part to the lack of an enzyme governing the production of insulin in the pancreas. And there is mounting evidence that leukemia and other cancers trace to faulty enzyme behavior. To date, an estimated forty-four diseases have been related to enzyme disturbances.

Such observations lead in an obvious direction. If enzymes are deficient or lacking, it should eventually be possible to make up the lack with synthetic enzymes. Or, if one group of enzymes is *too* active, it should be possible to offset their activity with chemical controls.

With the solid accomplishments already at hand, and with exciting goals ahead, enzymology represents research's wave of the future.

Vitamins –

KEYS TO WELL-BEING

by Paul de Kruif

A brilliant new science of nutrition, grown out of the discovery of synthetic vitamins, is demonstrating that old age need no longer be regarded as a sad dragging out of existence. There is today chemical hope that for many it can be a period of active, productive life.

We now know that the time to try to push back senility is before we're old in years. Old age begins to sneak up on us even in our twenties. Nutrition scientists have uncovered a fantastic fact: Though it's true that we are what we eat, what we eat—while seemingly adequate—may mean the *premature* aging of many of us. But by using chemical knowledge now available this premature aging can be reversed. Keys to this reversal are the synthetic vitamins. Here are a few examples:

An industrialist, though well-fed, felt old and *was* old ahead of his time, suffering the pain of what seemed permanently disabling neuritis. Injections of a B vitamin, thiamine, abolished his agony and brought back his vigor. A middle-aged woman was about to be institutionalized for senile dementia. A few massive shots of another B vitamin, niacin, rapidly restored her sanity. A medical-school professor knew what to eat and ate it; yet his rheumy, inflamed eyes threatened him with blindness. Still another B vitamin, riboflavin, brought his sight back.

These patients maintained their recovery by the addition of vitamins to highly nutritious diets. But why were extra vitamins necessary? The synthetic vitamins are identical to those naturally present in our food. Why do we need to add more?

Spectacular cures like these give the answer. Even in the best diets vitamins may exist only in borderline amounts; and some people, because of their inborn chemistry, require far more vitamins than others. As we grow older, the need of most of us for vitamins rises; we can't absorb or use them so well. So, a diet ample for one person may be deficient for another.

Hidden hunger for vitamins, however, is rarely for only one of these chemicals. In an epic twenty-year investigation, Dr. Tom D. Spies and his associates screened 5700 chronically sick people in the Birmingham, Alabama, area. Of these, 893 were so feeble that most of them hadn't worked for years. They did not have tuberculosis, heart disease or any standard, chronic sickness; these were ruled out by complete clinical and laboratory diagnoses. Their complaints masqueraded under symptoms of digestive, nervous and mental ailments. They were down-and-out physically and in morale. From age thirty on they all were old.

What they had in common was nutritional failure, due to the lack of several vitamins. This was revealed by the fading of one symptom after another in response to a specific vitamin.

Then the Birmingham medical researchers went out for total recovery of all their 893 nutritionally disabled patients. They fed them diets rich in proteins, natural vitamins and minerals, supercharged by big doses of synthetic vitamins. They added dried brewer's-yeast powder and liver extracts to furnish chemicals still unknown. It was a rugged test for the new science—the seemingly impossible task of rehabilitating these feeble people.

But the nutritionists won. All the patients went back to full-time work, as miners, shipbuilders, steelworkers, housekeepers, farmers. Among them were 41 young men, prematurely aged invalids, now vigorous enough to be accepted for unlimited service in the armed forces. The majority of these people had been brought to the nutrition clinic after they'd been given up by doctors as hopeless. Their salvation has encouraged many practicing physicians;

their new vigor testifies that premature aging can be reversed. Nearly twenty years ago the Spies group began following the long-term insidious effect of substandard nutrition on the health of 1000 children in the Birmingham area. They found the diets of these youngsters had this in common: they were high in carbohydrates (like bread) and fats, and low in proteins (like meat, eggs). Dr. Spies tried an inexpensive *and palatable* supplement.

To the daily diets of a group of these blighted children, under close supervision, he added six ounces of instant nonfat dry milk, dissolved in ten ounces of water—equaling two quarts of skim milk. The response was spectacular. The children's growth increased measurably. Their strength improved. Those who had been backward in school work became better.

To study this supplement further, Dr. Spies worked out a test diet representing food commonly consumed by many people in the area. It was made up of lard, sugar, white corn meal and white flour and enriched with certain vitamins. He then fed this ration to a group of healthy young white rats—their nutritional needs are strikingly close to those of human beings.

At the start of the experiment their nutrition was good, as shown by the husky little rat in Figure 1. But the result of forty days on the test diet is indicated by the horrible little rodent in Figure 2. They had stopped growing; they wept bloody tears; their skins were inflamed. Then to the test diet of the runts was added the dry-milk supplement given to the stunted children. Figure 3 shows the state of the animals forty days later, tripled in weight, models of robust rathood.

These curative triumphs evoke an inevitable question: Why shouldn't we all supplement our daily diets with large amounts of vitamins? Pediatricians and physicians regularly prescribe vitamins to make babies and children far healthier than youngsters of a generation ago. Why is the same supercharge thought to be needless in adolescence and later life?

Mainly because of the belief in the virtues of the well-balanced diet. Many people—among them some physicians—smile at the effect of high vitamin intake as a matter of imagination. Look, they say, at the old codgers who are balls of fire at eighty, and have never taken a single synthetic vitamin! They forget that such people are the fortunate ones whose internal chemistry is such that they can obtain the full benefits of a well-balanced diet.

Imagination? Then why do farmers now regularly supercharge the old-fashioned rations of their poultry, pigs and cattle with vitamins, minerals and hormones? They do it because this has enormously boosted the health, growth and vigor of their domestic animals. Is this upsurge, which has revolutionized American agriculture, due to the imagination of our cows, pigs and chickens?

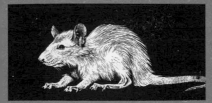
Fig. 1. Healthy male rat six weeks old

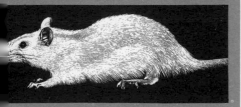
Fig. 2. Same rat after 40 days on test diet

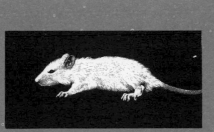
Fig. 3. Same rat 40 days later on corrected diet

Another obstacle retards the routine use of vitamins by human beings. It is objected that an adequate vitamin supercharge is expensive. But think back to the 893 prematurely aged, and the thousands since that first experiment, who have gone back to work as the result of vitamins added to nutritious diets. The cost of these chemicals for each person rejuvenated in the Birmingham experiment was *less than the price of a pack of cigarettes a day.*

"The expensive way to use vitamins," said Dr. Spies, "is to avoid them, develop nutritional failure, lose your job." The way to keep yourself a productive, independent citizen is to have your doctor check you carefully to rule out other serious disease and then to prescribe these potent chemicals that will help stretch out your span of productive vitality.

Another helpful development is a remarkable form of milk, which is a major source of old-age-fighting protein. Whole milk, an excellent food, is widely avoided in corrective diets because of its high content of fat. Skim milk, though rich in protein, may be rejected as less tasty than whole milk. Dr. Spies, reporting his reversal of hundreds of prematurely aged children, told of his success with a form of fat-free, dry milk solids, soluble in water and rich in proteins, B vitamins and calcium.

Dr. Spies taught that man cannot live by pills alone, and the supercharging of well-balanced diets will not, of course, ward off all diseases. But it will help the body fight them better, and snap back more quickly, because it brings a new and more lasting integrity to our tissue.

Dr. Spies explained that the real heroes are the cells of his patients' bodies. He said the big and little pains are alarms from damaged tissues. They do not mean the tissues are finished. Give the starved cells the nutriments they need and they'll recover. More and more physicians, following Dr. Spies' recommendation, now make part of their treatment of all their patients a regimen of therapeutic vitamins.

THAT old saw about a human being containing only 98 cents' worth of chemical components may have to be revised. Now that we know about the energy value of chemicals, the Du Pont Company says those in an average human body could produce 85 billion dollars' worth of energy.

—UPI

CHAPTER 9

The Changing Cycles of Life

Never still, seldom dormant, the clustered cells of the human organism move in their predestined patterns to prepare the body for life's changing demands. An understanding of this process of change—and the delights as well as the hazards it involves—can smooth the transition from one stage to another and renew the hope that "the best is yet to be."

Childhood—

WONDERFUL AND ALARMING

by Herbert S. Benjamin, M.D.

There is nothing quite like the shock a medical student experiences when he examines a child patient for the first time. He has spent long hours in adult wards making physical examinations, learning to diagnose disease. Then he goes over to the children's wards.

In the children's wards the medical student sees many amazing things. He sees infants who are very ill because they got a few ounces too much of this or that in their diet. He sees a baby with a chest full of pus who gets perfectly well in a couple of days. (In an adult this would surely have been fatal.)

A young child who has fallen headfirst from a window onto a metal roof two stories below is happy with his toys the next day. The worst kinds of pneumonia may last only a few days, and there are rarely complications. The entire half of a brain is removed surgically: a paralyzed mentally deficient child picks up in intelligence and begins to use his muscles.

A child recovers without complications so quickly from pneumonia, or from pus in the chest space, because his flexible organism can withstand attacks better than the rigid system of an adult. A child's skull is soft and elastic and can withstand falls much better than an adult's hard skull.

How can the removal of half a baby brain, instead of making things worse, increase intelligence and bring back power in paralyzed muscles? The diseased half was interfering with the function of the whole brain and nervous system. After it was removed, the remaining healthy half had enough extra young, undeveloped cells to take over the functions of the lost half. Only in children are such wonders possible.

The greatest natural athletes in the world are children. Parents know how trying it is to keep up with their endless physical activity. Tommy, aged eleven, plays ball in the hot summer sun from morning until dusk, and begs to be allowed to play more games after dark. Janet, aged nine, jumps rope for hours, and comes home reluctantly when called to meals.

After exercise, children's blood pressure, pulse and respiration rate return to normal in a fraction of the time it would take a healthy adult's. The warming-up period which athletes require before a contest is not necessary for children, who are always physiologically ready for great physical stress.

Because the warmth-regulating center in a child's brain is not completely developed yet, certain great changes in temperature hardly faze children, who adapt to freezing cold with comparatively little discomfort.

A family is tragically stranded in the mountains in subfreezing temperatures. The parents perish, but the children survive unharmed, and recuperate in a relatively short period of time. During a heat spell in the midsummer months, large numbers of adults are treated for sunstroke or heat prostration. Children seem to be immune.

After injuries, children's wounds heal faster. Recuperation from shock is quicker. Fevers drop faster. Response to medication is more prompt.

Broken bones knit in less than half the time it takes for adult bones, without residual defects. A fractured leg, for instance, can be strapped for weeks in the best possible position to heal, with the child lying straight on his back and his foot extended to a frame spanned directly above. (An adult couldn't tolerate such a posture more than twenty minutes.)

Loss of large amounts of blood from injuries sometimes causes a severe condition called "secondary anemia." A child's flexible blood-building apparatus replaces the lost blood in a few days; for an adult it might take a dangerously long time.

Having a tooth pulled is a painful, bloody event in an adult's life. He may not get over it for many days, while his jaw aches and chewing is uncomfortable. A child has his tooth pulled, the bleeding stops quickly, he eats a normal meal thirty minutes later and forgets the whole thing in an hour.

The elastic growing lenses of younger eyes allow children to observe moving objects, like television or outdoor spectacles, indefinitely—an occupation which tires adult eyes. The resilience of their hearing apparatus allows them to listen longer, too. And an opera star would envy the voice power and sturdy lungs of a child, who can talk, sing or cry with all its might all day long.

Children's skin is softer—bathed in more abundant sebum from their skin glands—their muscles and ligaments more elastic, their mental reactions quicker, their fantasies richer, their emotional spontaneity greater than an adult's. And as the child reaches puberty, around fourteen years of age, his natural health and physiological efficiency reach their peak.

But woe to the infant, baby or child, if something goes wrong with his nourishment. His kidneys are not able to work so well yet and can't keep fluids concentrated in the blood. So if an infant does not get just the right proportions of salts and starches and fluids in his diet, or if he loses extra water from diarrhea, his cells will dry out, and he will get a fever and be terribly sick. Also, an enormous amount of what he takes in is used only for purposes of growing, and a child has to grow to live.

In fact, almost everything in a child's life revolves around the two simple words "growth" and "development." A disease in an adult is a disease, but in a child it is a "disease in a growing organism." His whole life force is devoted to *becoming* something, to getting formed, to reaching that goal of being grown up, without stopping on the way.

The child's muscle reflexes are different because certain parts of the nerve fibers haven't developed insulating sheaths. And that staring expression of uncritical interest and wonder on the baby's face—Johnny is busy developing mentally, too. He is collecting impressions of the world and forming his points of view.

Psychiatrists say that a child turns into a "criminal type" or an adjusted member of society from the very beginning, out of the first experiences he has of this world, not suddenly in later life. They stress the enormous importance of the first experiences at the mother's breast, where the child takes in not only milk but also warmth and love and security. They say if the child is frustrated frequently at the mother's breast, he could become a frustrated person his whole life. Personality and character develop in the early years just as firmly as arms and legs.

Some children get over diseases of retarded development quickly, when the nurses and attendants are patient and affectionate. On the other hand, some children perish in the hospital when there is no love waiting for them at home.

CHANGES IN FORM AND PROPORTION (PARALLEL LINES FOR EASY COMPARISON)

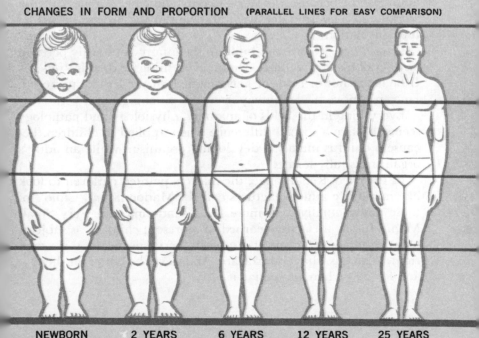

NEWBORN   2 YEARS   6 YEARS   12 YEARS   25 YEARS

Every child develops differently, at his own rate; and when a child seems retarded in certain ways it does not necessarily mean that there is something organically wrong. He may be just taking his time growing up.

One of the most interesting and helpful explanations of the differences between children and adults lies in the brain and spinal cord. Baby has almost as much "gray matter," or brain cells, as the adult; but the "white matter," or connecting pathways between cells, is very poorly developed in comparison. It is as if, in a radio, all the tubes and amplifiers and transformers and current were there, but the wires had not been connected yet. The radio won't work until the wires make the right connections.

Actually, it is a question of the insulating sheaths around the wires. These insulating sheaths around the long nerve fibers connecting up the gray matter develop slowly in the infant and child; and as they develop, the child becomes capable of performing more and more physical activities and mental functions.

The slow development of these nerve sheaths explains much about the child's behavior. He twists and fidgets more than an adult partly because the nerves controlling his muscles are not working in a coördinated way, all being in the process of getting their insulation.

Before these sheaths are built up the infant can hardly perform any act of his own willing. Almost everything he does is "reflex." If he is too hot or cold, or gets pinched on the leg, he just cries. He can't move his legs away from the pinching hand yet.

Everything in the fields of anatomy, physiology and pathology seems to have a special difference when applied to children, because a child is mainly a developing organism, while an adult's organism is fully formed.

In the early Renaissance, the masters painted children to look like miniature adults. Pictures called "Madonna and Child" of those days actually look more like "Madonna and Very Small Man." Later, the artists learned to represent children as subjects quite different from adults, subjects very special in their own right. Which is what children are. And it will be better for them— and for us—when we realize it.

Why Adolescents Act That Way

by J. D. Ratcliff

Within the human body chemical magic wands constantly perform wonders that rival the magic of fairy tales. Consider the transformation that takes place at puberty, when a happy-go-lucky little boy is turned into a troubled, rebellious semiadult—a stranger both to himself and to his parents. Consider the magic which resculptures a reedy, angular little tomboy into a curvaceous, reserved young woman.

The hurdle separating childhood from adulthood is perhaps the greatest barrier human beings are called on to surmount. In the chemical ferment of puberty an entirely new human being is born, and the process is a time of trial for all families.

There is, of course, a grand design in this transformation: the child body is being prepared for its ultimate task of reproduction, to ensure continuance of the race. Scarcely an organ or tissue is untouched by the dramatic events taking place within the body.

Heart and lungs may begin growing at rates even triple those of prepuberty years. The thyroid in the neck begins enlarging to adult proportions, and the mysterious thymus in the chest begins shrinking—in time it will virtually disappear. Muscles harden, and fat is deposited in new patterns. During childhood, bone ends are capped with soft cartilage to facilitate growth. But during and shortly after puberty, calcium begins to infiltrate the cartilage. Bone ends harden; growth slows and finally stops. Even the texture of the skin changes. Fat glands become more active, oil secretions increase and pores enlarge. When bacteria gain entrance to the skin, the result may be acne, that age-old curse of puberty.

Puberty is triggered by the pea-size pituitary gland on the underside of the brain. What prompts it to move into action remains a mystery. But the results are instantly apparent when it begins producing tiny amounts of gonadotropic hormone—which stimulates ovaries in girls, testes in boys. During childhood these glands have remained quiescent. But under the pituitary stimulus they begin producing hormones of their own.

In the adolescent girl newly activated ovaries produce estrogen in fantastically small amounts—a daily output equal to 1/1000 of a grain of sugar! But that is enough of this potent stuff to propel the girl-child into womanhood. She begins shooting up at a rate of as much as three inches a year, leaving laggard boys behind—a fact that further contributes to the antipathy between the sexes at this age. (Propelling a girl half a head taller around a dance floor represents exquisite torture for the boy—and the girl suffers equally.)

Pelvic bones begin to grow, widening hips and providing a bony cradle for babies-to-be. Breast tissue proliferates—slowly at first, but ever faster under the hormone influence. Tissue in the birth canal thickens and toughens to be ready to withstand the rigors of childbirth. The womb, too, enlarges from the plum size of childhood to the pear size of adulthood.

It takes perhaps two years to transform the female body in preparation for potential motherhood. Now important events begin in the ovaries themselves. These glands contain at birth the lifetime supply of undeveloped egg cells, estimated at 420,000— an astonishing number, since only 400 to 500 will be expelled during a woman's fruitful years.

In some mysterious fashion one of the two ovaries selects a

single egg cell for development. When fully developed, the tiny cell approaches the surface of the ovary—contained in a marble-size blister. Membranes of the blister stretch and finally rupture. The liberated egg starts its journey to the womb.

In the week or so preceding release of the egg the womb itself gets hormonal attention. Its walls thicken and a new network of blood vessels appears, to provide nourishment for a possible baby-to-be. Unneeded unless pregnancy occurs, this new tissue breaks down, and the young girl has her first menstrual period. The grand design has been completed. She has reached adulthood and is ready for childbearing.

When the boy's turn comes for pubertal development, no less momentous events take place in his body. Under the urging of pituitary hormone, testicular tissue begins proliferating, maturing. When fully developed it will serve a dual purpose: production of the male hormone, testosterone, which is emptied into the bloodstream, and production of the sperm cells necessary to fertilize the egg.

Effects of the hormone are instantly visible. Hair patterns of the body change, and a beard begins to sprout. Body growth often goes at a dizzy clip—perhaps six inches in a year, plus twenty-five pounds of added weight. The boy shoots past the towering girl, to the relief of both. Hands and feet grow at an inordinate rate—to produce an awkward, coltish effect.

Pitch of voice is determined by the mass, length and elasticity of vocal cords. In women they remain relatively short; hence women have higher voices. But at puberty the cords begin to elongate in boys. Until they are brought under muscular control, speaking is an embarrassing and uncertain thing—rumbling bass one moment, falsetto squeak the next.

Male hormone also triggers the development of the prostate, which helps provide the fluid that propels and nourishes sperm cells. This gland grows from the size of a bean to about that of a chestnut. However unready he may be socially, the boy is now able, physically, to father children.

If the physical changes of this period have been enormous,

the emotional changes have been no less so. This is a period of profound readjustment. Emotionally, two people are living within the same body, and each is fighting for supremacy. One wants to retain the privileges of childhood; the other tries to exercise all the prerogatives of adulthood without having adult understanding or responsibility.

The once friendly, tractable boy becomes the arrogant show-off. He challenges all authority. Teachers become unfair tyrants to be treated with disdain. Parents, once adored, become barely tolerable dunces. Given the tools of the adult world to work with, yet having only the reactions of childhood to guide him, the youngster does countless foolish things. He is often a menace in an automobile. He dives into streams from perilous heights. He experiments with sex.

The pattern is standardized, yet each generation is surprised at seeing it repeated. The father who gobbled live goldfish thirty years ago is baffled by a son who finds hot rods more enticing than algebra; the mother who did the Charleston in above-the-knee skirts has difficulty understanding a daughter sent into ecstasies by a rock-'n'-roller.

The quite normal revolt that occurs as the child moves into the adult world takes odd twists. Knowing that parents insist on personal cleanliness, the boy prides himself on being dirty. He is obsessed with self and will spend hours gazing into the mirror, examining each minor blemish. He may express his rebellion in bizarre haircuts—flattops, ducktails and so on.

So great becomes the ferment in his mind that he pays little attention to what he sees or hears. Parents and teachers complain that boys are fuzzy-minded, inattentive, lazy. This is only partly true. It is well known that worry produces fatigue. The pubescent boy worries most of the time and is tired most of the time—not lazy. Under the stress of his internal physical and emotional activity, he *does* become fuzzy-minded.

Girls face problems equally great as they bid good-by to childhood and grope their way into an alien world. Often, they are self-conscious about their new bodies. They may attempt to hide their breasts under tight straps, react with shame to monthly periods. They become secretive, withdrawn into a strange world of their own creation. Parents, once trusted, become unsympathetic taskmasters. Any criticism is likely to bring a reaction of rage or tears or sullen hurt. As with boys, there is complete preoccupation with self—the slightest physical imperfection becomes a major tragedy.

Loyalties shift. Boys of the same age, because they are less mature, become repulsive to the developing girl. Older boys are far more desirable. But the child-woman usually decides that it is safer to adore them from a distance. Hero worship is another phenomenon. When squealing girls besiege the latest pelvis-wriggling singer they are following normal behavior patterns.

If this is a trying period for new adults in the making, it is equally trying for parents, teachers and others. About the best we can do is face the situation with patience and understanding. There is always the comforting thought that it will soon be over.

There is usually a temporary rise in IQ at the time of puberty. This occurs earlier in girls than in boys. But in another year or so the boys catch up with the girls, and from then on it is neck and neck.

—Donald and Eleanor Laird

It was the teen-aged daughter's first dance, and she desperately wanted a strapless frock. Her mother felt she wasn't old enough to wear anything so sophisticated. There was a heated family discussion, and it was the father who finally settled the problem. "Well," he proposed, "let her try on one. If it stays up—she's old enough to wear it." —Margaret Helms

Acne:

YOUTH'S MYSTERIOUS ENEMY

by Paul de Kruif

Though acne tends to fade from the skin after adolescence, its aftermath is often cruel. Striking when boys and girls regard their face as their fortune, acne leads to social embarrassment, saps ambition, causes timidity in the search for a mate. After it has burned out it may leave permanent scars not only on the skin but on the personality—setting behavior patterns of feeling unwanted and alone. For millions thus threatened, this need no longer be. Modern science can douse the flame of nine out of ten acne eruptions.

Acne is no mere complexion problem but a complex chemical mystery far more than just skin-deep. It's an internal chemical upheaval at a critical time of life, a disturbance so widespread that few escape some evidence of it.

The sex hormones, hugely increasing in the blood at puberty as they turn boys and girls into men and women, usually are the basic cause of this trouble of the skin. This temporary excess of hormones triggers overproduction of oil by the little lubricating glands attached to the hair follicles in the pores, especially those of the face, chest and back.

The excess oil, mixed with skin-cell debris, dries on the surface of the skin, plugging up the pores, forming the blackheads which are the first subtle sign of acne's subsequent red flame. Underneath the blackheads the oil keeps pouring into the plugged-up hair follicles; body chemicals, unable to escape, irritate the distended follicle walls; normally harmless skin microbes, trapped inside, cause infection.

This gives rise to the eruptions of bumps, papules and pimples. In young people whose oil glands are especially susceptible, it leads to serious, disfiguring all-out acne.

The first step in treating acne is for the sufferer to learn how to wash his face. The customary lick and a promise isn't nearly enough. Hot water and soap should be worked into a lather and rubbed in thoroughly with a turkish washcloth several times a day, followed by a drying lotion. This systematic washing softens blackheads, dries up excess oil and causes a mild peeling that unplugs the pores.

The patient's next duty seems still simpler, until you remember how hard it is to stop the fascinating yet dangerous indoor sport of squeezing and needling blackheads, bumps or pimples before a mirror. Because of the peril of wrecking already damaged hair follicles, this minor surgery is best left to the doctor.

Even when treatment has had its effect, however, there may be relapses. The mysterious flare-ups are sometimes caused by iodine, seafood, shellfish and the bromides in cough medicines and sedatives. Chocolate may trigger new eruptions. The same *may* happen after excess eating of sweets or fats, of peanuts or sharp cheese.

The affliction may be perpetuated by an upset chemistry, beyond the hormonal, of the entire human being. Persistent acne often clears up after treatment of infected sinuses, tonsils or teeth. A regimen of plenty of sleep, outdoor exercise and a well-balanced diet may often speed the action of skin care. It seems as if a sick skin can be healed only by a healthy body.

And now comes new hope against what, until the past few years, have been the most stubborn and vicious culprits perpetuating severe acne. These are the ordinarily harmless microbes that live invisibly and placidly in the skin of every human being. These microbes—especially the staphylococcus—seem to resent imprisonment in the plugged skin pores that are the beginning of acne. Then they get nasty, preying upon the hair follicles that have been damaged by distension with excess oil, or allergically irritated by certain foods, or wrecked by their owner's squeezing and picking. These formerly gentle microbes are responsible for acne's purulent inflammation.

They do not yield to local antiseptics; in severe acne there are too many pussy pimples for doctors to treat them with locally injected penicillin. But now to the aid of the physicians have come the new wide-spectrum antibiotics. They are the most powerful of all medical weapons against severe purulent acne.

These drugs are taken internally; the secret of their success is the keeping up of an effective antibiotic concentration in the blood. This demands that patients keep up their daily intake, in the exact dose prescribed by the doctor.

Though there is no "magic-bullet" cure for acne, the splendid hope to control this blight of youth is shown by the success of physicians associated with the Vanderbilt Clinic at the College of Physicians and Surgeons, Columbia University. They used many weapons. Their patients were 384 disfigured unfortunate chronic sufferers.

The medical attack started with small, safe doses of the synthetic female hormone, stilbestrol. In both boys and girls, it is a disturbed balance of their natural hormones that starts acne mischief. Stilbestrol, restoring hormone balance, began to clear eruptions in many.

Then the disease was dealt another wallop. Antibiotics were administered. The doctors selected the antibiotic to which the microbes in each case were found to be most sensitive. Now, in many more patients among the 384 treated, the eruption was controlled.

They went on from this to the treatment of the whole young man or woman. Patients were put on low-fat, low-carbohydrate, high-protein diets, plus vitamins and liver. Since acne in some cases may be aggravated by worry, the doctors corrected emotional upsets. They taught all victims thorough care of the skin.

Summing up the result of their multibarreled treatment of these stubborn cases, the Columbia doctors describe their success as "overwhelming—pleasing to a degree beyond expectation." They report that 94 percent of their patients were improved or cleared up completely. Even when acne has left skin scars, much disfigurement can be wiped away by skin-planing operations.

Now doctors, making use of what was learned at New York University and Columbia, should be able to clear up or at least control most cases. They can change youthful despair to hope and confidence—if the young acne victims, encouraged by their parents, will only consult them and follow their advice.

Menstruation:

NEW HELP FOR NEEDLESS MISERY

Adapted from "Premenstrual Tension: The Needless Misery" *by Robert B. Greenblatt, M.D., with Richard L. Frey and* "The Truth about Menstruation" *by Maxine Davis*

The frenzied thump of Elsie's iron sends its warning down the shirt factory's production line. Today Elsie's fingers are all thumbs, her rhythm is gone, the flow of work is slowed all along her row. The whole team of girls is suffering because Elsie is having one of her "bad days."

In a California high school Belle flubs every problem in

algebra, her favorite subject. At lunch she slaps her best friend. Later she runs away from home—the third time this has happened in the few months since she turned sixteen, and each time just before her menstrual period.

In a New York State prison for women, a convicted killer warns the matron, "It's time to lock me up for a couple of days." A Kansas housewife, trembling with the jitters that caused her to crash a tray full of breakfast dishes, piles into her car and drives off to meet a bus—head-on. And when Dr. Abraham Stone was a frequent marriage consultant as director of the Margaret Sanger Research Bureau in New York, he listened often to a familiar story—that for ten days every month an irritable, weepy, "touch-me-not" attitude rises like a wall between wife and husband. "I don't understand it," a woman would say. "I only know I can't help it."

She can't help it. But she can be helped. She is the victim, not of a malady, but of the myth that nothing can be done about it.

Premenstrual tension is a mystery that has puzzled men of medicine for centuries. Why, as a woman's period nears, does a feeling of pressure build up inside her? Why do many women suffer no more than uneasy discomfort, while in others the pressure pounds higher and higher until they feel ready to explode? And why does it slacken when the menstrual flow begins?

The average age when menstruation begins is 13.8 years, but it may begin any time between 11 and 17. Blondes tend to be earlier than brunettes. According to the books, menstruation occurs every twenty-eight days, but the interval is not the same in every woman. Each has a different chronometer, set by some mysterious combination of forces in our bodies. Susie may menstruate every three weeks, Joan every six weeks and Sally every twenty-eight days, but this does not mean there is something wrong with any of them. Each is normal according to her own timing. Scientists have long agreed that "the only regular thing about menstruation is its irregularity."

A period may last from three to seven days, though five is the average. It won't be the same every month, year in and year out, for many things cause irregularity. Diseases—from tuber-culosis to the flu or just a cold in the head—affect it, as do glandu-lar disorders. Change of altitude or climate causes periods to be early or late, long or short. Certain psychological hazards may hasten or retard them. Fear of pregnancy or wanting a baby very much may cause menstruation to occur quite late, or may pro-duce every symptom of early pregnancy.

Then, too, most women are extremely irregular at the begin-ning and close of their reproductive life. It is not unusual for a child to menstruate once and then wait several months before her next experience, or for a woman nearing fifty to have two or more months elapse between periods.

It is important to get rid of old superstitions concerning menstruation, such as the necessity for rest and the danger of taking baths or exercising during the period. This is nonsense. It is wise to remember that menstruation is a normal function.

Most women have some general symptoms before or at the beginning of their periods. Their breasts may be somewhat en-larged and sensitive. They may have slight aches. They may suffer a sense of tension and feel depressed. In such cases there is nothing to do but remember that tomorrow everything will look brighter.

There may be a very slight staining in the middle of the in-terval between periods. This is a common experience. It occurs at the time of ovulation. Typically, it is accompanied by a little pain for two or three hours on one side or the other. It will recur, perhaps, for two or three months; then a woman will not notice it again for seven or eight months or for several years. It is natural and normal. And it is useful in ascertaining the period of fertility if the woman is anxious to have a baby, for she may become pregnant at the time of ovulation.

Premenstrual tension is the most common of all female nervous disorders. A week to ten days prior to menstruation, a sizable number of females—schoolgirls, businesswomen, housewives—get jittery, become inefficient, irritable, depressed. Some have headache, backache, sore breasts. It hits 50 percent of the women of childbearing age, doctors say.

Four times as many unpremeditated crimes of violence are committed by females in premenstrual days as on other days, studies show. In 500 serious auto crashes involving women drivers, a significantly high proportion was found related to the menstrual cycle.

Factory studies made by Dr. Harvey E. Billig of Los Angeles, in West Coast aircraft and other factories, indicate that premenstrual tension costs $150 a year per female employe, in absence and reduced efficiency—some two and a half billion dollars a year in production loss alone.

This problem has been a challenge to the medical profession. Attempting to solve it, doctors have studied everything from hormones to weight. This last is perhaps the most marked physical symptom. Beginning about a week before menstruation, something causes a woman's body to store up extra fluids. It is usual for her to gain as much as 2 pounds, but severe sufferers gain 5, 6, even 8 or 10 pounds. No wonder they complain of feeling "heavy."

With the onset of menstruation, fluids are released, tension subsides. Drs. S. Charles Freed of San Francisco and J. P. Greenhill of Chicago asked themselves, why not give premenstrual sufferers a powerful diuretic (agent to increase urine flow) to pull out the water? They tested ammonium chloride and found that it gave many women relief. However, there were those it did not help, for fluid is only one of the culprits.

In Richmond, Virginia, Dr. William Bickers was testing a proposed remedy for painful menstruation. He found it didn't help much during menstruation, but it *was* highly effective in the premenstrual period, releasing excess fluids and relieving tension. The formula included an antihistamine that brought added comfort by countering allergic reaction and acting as a quieting agent. This and other preparations, equally effective when fluid retention is the chief villain, are now available on a doctor's prescription.

Meanwhile, Dr. Joseph H. Morton, of New York Medical College, observed that the faintness and fatigue, the jitters and the craving for sweets were much like the symptoms of a diabetic who has taken too much insulin. Could the cause be the same? Blood tests said yes. They showed, for these days only, a sharp, vitality-sapping drop in blood sugar.

Combining ingredients, Dr. Morton created a formula aimed not at just one symptom but at many. He included ammonium chloride to dehydrate; a relaxing agent to lessen tension; caffeine as a stimulant to combat mental sluggishness and depression; Vitamin B complex for its tonic effect, and multiple feedings, high in protein, to battle the blood-sugar deficiency. He recommended following this regimen, together with restricted salt intake, for ten days before the expected menstrual period.

Dr. Morton gave this new formula its first large-scale test in a study at Westfield State Farm, a woman's reformatory near New York City. Tension-ridden inmates, 249 of them, volunteered. They were divided into equal groups. One group ate the regular prison fare; the other got additional between-meal snacks of milk and cheese three times a day. Half of each group received the real pill; the others got a fake with no medical content.

The improvement in the prisoners' attitude and behavior was marked. During the three months' study there was no major infraction of prison rules, no need for solitary confinement. Final results showed an improvement in each group much as expected:

> Fake pill, regular diet—15 percent
> Fake pill, special diet—39 percent
> Real pill, regular diet—61 percent
> Real pill, special diet—79 percent

Even the fake pill brought some measure of relief—proof that with some women much of the trouble is emotional and can be alleviated psychologically. The male members of a family, understanding this, could ease many a crisis.

Meanwhile, new medical studies are afoot—in hospitals, in clinics, and especially in industry, where better premenstrual health will carry a multimillion-dollar bonus.

Absenteeism, social friction and erratic production have already been significantly reduced in some factories by supervised premenstrual treatment. Premenstrual tension is still an individual problem, and only the doctor can decide which of a dozen weapons at his command he will use. But, thanks to his new knowledge, many women no longer suffer during those distressing days.

The worst thing that can be said about menstruation is that it interferes so regularly with a woman's life. She can be sensible about this, ignoring all the old wives' tales—and never repeating a single one of them to her daughters.

What to Do about Change of Life

Adapted from "The Facts about Menopause"
by Ruth and Edward Brecher,
"New Help for Women's Change of Life" *by Paul de Kruif*
and "Changing Life Sensibly" *by Lois Mattox Miller*

"The most effective medicine that a physician can give a woman entering the menopause," says a wise physician we know, "is the simplest—an explanation. He can explain to her that the menopause does *not* mark the end of personal attractiveness or of sexual enjoyment. He can explain that the menopause is a time of readjustment that is usually the introduction to a rich period of satisfying work, play and affectionate relationships."

Unfortunately, such explanations often come too late. Even the most skilled doctor finds it hard, during a consultation or two, to sweep out all the mental cobwebs and superstitions that a woman of forty-five to fifty has accumulated. "The time to educate women about the menopause," our physician friend says, "is before the seeds of error are planted. I'd like every girl to learn the facts when she learns about menstruation, and to get a 're-fresher course' from time to time thereafter."

What are the facts? At puberty, a girl's pituitary gland, located near the base of the brain, begins to manufacture and release into the bloodstream a hormone known as gonadotropin. This substance stimulates the ovaries to produce a sex hormone called estrogen. There follows over a period of twenty-eight days or so the familiar monthly cycle. A follicle—an egg-containing sac—in one of the ovaries ripens and an ovum emerges from it. Then the empty follicle manufactures yet another hormone, progesterone, which prepares the lining of the uterus for pregnancy. If no pregnancy occurs, this temporary lining is sloughed off, and menstruation follows. Ordinarily a woman experiences this cycle some 350 to 450 times over a period of thirty to forty years.

Eventually, however, the ovaries produce less estrogen, and in time none; no follicle ripens; no progesterone is secreted. The ovaries, as before puberty, become relatively inactive.

With the quieting of the ovaries, other endocrine glands step up their activity. The adrenal glands, perched atop the kidneys, increase their manufacture of estrogen; the thyroid gland in the neck becomes more active; other glands, too, alter their parts in the "symphony," so that after a while the body establishes a new hormone balance. Thus a woman enters the third major era in her life, a little older, a little wiser, no longer able to have babies—but otherwise not so different in her fifties from what she was in her forties.

Some women have considerable physical discomfort during the changeover. The commonest symptom is the "hot flash"—a sudden rush of blood to the head and upper body. Many women find this embarrassing as well as uncomfortable. Other symptoms are less well defined—headaches, backaches, fatigue or just a sense of feeling miserable all over.

The physical and emotional aspects of the "hard time" in menopause are curiously intermingled. The emotional aspect consists of anxiety, depression and fear. A woman may worry that her relationship with her husband will be jeopardized. Some worry about their appearance. Many worry about the future. "Am I going to feel like this all the rest of my life?" is a common question women ask their doctors. Such anxieties usually have no basis in fact; they are the result of the glandular changes occurring in the body.

A considerable number of women—estimated at 15 to 20 percent—have no symptoms at all; they just gradually stop menstruating. The majority have a few hot flashes, feel blue from time to time, but experience nothing they can't take in stride.

For those who experience distressing symptoms, medical science now has two remedies to offer—hormones and reassurance. "Hormones are excellent," we were told by a gynecologist, "but reassurance is even better."

Women who are having hot flashes or other menopausal symptoms need to be assured that these discomforts won't last forever. Here the sympathetic physician often makes a telling point. It is true, he says, that for some women menopausal symptoms may be spread over a period of a year or more. But this does not mean a year of uninterrupted distress. There will be weeks and even months along the way when they will feel as healthy and vigorous as ever.

Then there is the general fact of aging and appearance. But aging begins, of course, on the day one is born; the menopause does not hasten the appearance of age, nor does it cause women to put on fat. During this period, as always, fat comes chiefly from eating too much.

There is now no need to endure the more severe forms of melancholy sickness that blight the happiness of some women at their change of life. Some years ago hormones had to be given by cumbersome injections; there were doubts as to their safety; they were too costly. But now at last they can transfigure the stormy afternoon of life, in many cases, into a time of serenity and vigor.

There are two forms of the main female hormone, natural and synthetic; both are classified as "estrogens." Both can now be taken as simple tablets; when administered under a doctor's supervision they are as safe as they are powerful; and they're within the reach of any woman who can pay from three to eight cents a day.

When the symptoms are severe in women undergoing change of life, they feel nervous, jumpy, trembly; sometimes they want to scream. Even mildly disagreeable news overexcites them; they're irritable at the noise of children playing. Formerly calm women sometimes become argumentative; some become intensely jealous of faithful husbands. They are likely to suffer gnawing headaches and vague abdominal pains.

Worst of all is the depression, the melancholy that haunts many women in this condition, so that they lose interest in life, cry for no reason at all, lie awake nights with anxiety that something dreadful is going to happen, begin to believe that the world and even their dear ones are against them.

What's at the bottom of this upset that causes unhappiness to millions? Long ago it was suspected that failing ovaries were the culprits—but that couldn't be proved till chemists actually isolated the female hormone. Twenty-five years ago when Drs. Edward A. Doisy and Edgar Allen, of St. Louis, took the ovaries out of rats and mice, they found that all sex activity vanished and the womb withered. But when the experimenters injected the rodents with fluid from the ovarian egg sacs of normal animals, they saw a great surge of growth in the withered organs and a renewal of sex activity. This was the first hint of the existence of a female sex hormone.

Then from the urine of pregnant women, Dr. Doisy trapped the female hormone, crystal pure. Its power over the sex organs and sex activity of females of every species of animal was truly fantastic. For suffering women a hopeful premonition was that the hormone was chemically identical in whatever animal found—had the same strange power whether it came from doves or turtles. It controls the monthly growth of the lining of the human womb, is essential to childbearing and menstruation and causes the development of women's bodily contours. It's what makes women womanly.

Would the female sex hormone extend its power beyond this purely physical action so as to mend the jangled emotional and mental life of certain women? Dr. August A. Werner of St. Louis was a pioneer in searching for the answer. Boldly he started with women whose ovaries had been removed. He gave hormone injections to 16 such prematurely aged people (some in their twenties or early thirties). The results, published in *The Journal of the American Medical Association*, were astounding. The patients' nervousness, "hot flashes" and headaches vanished. Their depression and crying spells disappeared. Their energy zoomed. Their married life again became natural and normal.

Dr. Werner now spread his experiment to 96 women not deprived of their ovaries, but nervously sick and physically fatigued during natural change of life. Again, shots of hormones sent them surging back to nervous steadiness, mental calm, return of vigor.

Clinical investigation by Dr. L. F. Hawkinson, of Brainerd, Minnesota, confirmed this hope. Estrogen, injected into 1000 women incapacitated by the change of life, relieved 691 of most of their mental and physical misery and definitely improved 149 others.

Rarely has a medical discovery found such unanimous acceptance. Hundreds of investigators here and abroad confirmed the claim that the female hormone was a chemical substitute for worn-out ovaries.

Then why didn't physicians give the hormone to all women with severe change-of-life symptoms? The big obstacle was the necessity of giving it by injection. The ills of the change of life may last from months to six years and even longer, and to control them the injections would have to be given once or twice weekly. They're expensive, and also time-consuming for doctors, nurses and the sufferers themselves. And even in the best of hands the needle isn't painless.

The search continued. In 1939 English chemists synthesized an epoch-making drug, stilbestrol, which controlled the hot flashes and nervous troubles of many women, could be taken by mouth and could be bought by prescription at a few cents a day. But stilbestrol had one drawback—it produced nausea in a certain number of women.

Other organic chemists brought out a synthetic replica of the natural hormone—ethinyl estradiol. This turned out to be the most powerful female hormone known, but like stilbestrol it nauseated some of the patients.

In the early 1940s, Canadian hormone hunters concentrated a mixture of natural female hormones from the urine of pregnant mares. The astonishing dominion of this estrogenic mixture over the nervous and mental agony of severe change of life was first reported by Dr. J. R. Goodall of McGill University. One of his patients, formerly a lovable character, had become in a few months so irritable that her home became "a sea of storms of misunderstandings and intolerance." Within a week after she started taking the mixed estrogens, by mouth, the reversal of her character began. The speed of her return to her old calm and cheerful self was extraordinary.

Many scientific reports have confirmed the efficacy of this mixture. It is not only well tolerated by the vast majority of the many thousands of women upon whom it has been tested, but seems to control midlife distress better than any other estrogen that can be taken by mouth. Thousands of women report that they not only lose their jumpy nerves, headaches and melancholy while they're taking it, but also experience a peculiar lift, a surge of vigor which doctors call a "feeling of well-being."

As Dr. Doisy pointed out, with every woman of forty or so a prospective patient, an experiment of tremendous magnitude is in progress. Indeed, in sheer numbers of suffering people involved it is probably the greatest medical experiment in history, extend-ing to ages long before, and long after, the period of the change of life. For endocrinologists and gynecologists are discovering other powers of these amazing female hormones.

The estrogens conquer the failure of young girls to develop sexually; Dr. E. C. Hamblen of Durham, North Carolina, has re-ported that nowhere in medicine is there a more dramatic thera-peutic effect than this one. In older women, lack of the female hormone pulls calcium out of the bones so that they break easily. Doctors at the Massachusetts General Hospital have found that administration of estrogens speeds up the healing of such frac-tures. Estrogens also heal the vaginitis (inflammation of the vagina) that tortures many older women.

Furthermore, estrogens can relieve the suffering of certain stricken men. They lighten the terrible pain of cancer of the prostate gland, shrink the prostate cancer and prolong life—although they cannot cure the tumor.

But now that women can take the female hormone so con-veniently by mouth, the extreme simplicity of the treatment requires certain warnings. First and foremost—*Never take female hormones without supervision by a doctor!*

Gynecologists and endocrinologists who have had the most experience with the estrogens emphasize that the female hor-mones must never be prescribed until the physician is satisfied that the patient has no cancerous or nonmalignant growths. This necessitates careful examination of the breasts and pelvis. While the female hormones do not cause cancer, there is clinical evidence that they may cause unsuspected tumors to grow with dangerous rapidity. So the safe course, for doctor and patient both, is the cancer-detection examination preceding any attempts at estrogenic therapy.

Dosage must be controlled carefully under the doctor's obser-vation, and women vary greatly in the amount required. When the estrogens are taken in large doses by women who have passed their menopause, bleeding like that of menstruation may be resumed. If this persists, curettage (scraping of the uterus) is necessary; and curettage, performed repeatedly, is bad.

While estrogens are not cure-alls for the domestic conflicts of women in midlife, they may bring harmony to many troubled homes. Whether estrogen therapy is needed at all is something that must be decided in each case by the doctor.

Doctors have observed that business and professional women, absorbed in a variety of interests, are least given to self-pity during the change in life. Housewives and unoccupied women have too much idle time in which to worry about themselves. For this reason doctors strongly favor careers for women in middle life. Any activity outside the home will help during the dangerous lull in life when children have grown, the family has ceased to depend so largely upon her and she is left with little to think about except herself.

If a woman finds that she is one of those for whom the menopause comes and goes with little discomfort, she will be wise to heed the doctor's advice: Learn to laugh at the old wives' tales about cancer, insanity and the other ills supposed to come with the change of life. If you have a career, keep at it; if you haven't, multiply your activities and keep your mind off yourself. Don't dramatize your ailments, or act like an invalid. Most women who claim that their husbands "lost interest" because of the menopause have largely themselves to blame.

Above all, don't talk about your change of life, or listen to women who are eager to tell you about theirs. For generations this has ranked with operations as a prime topic of conversation for women among themselves. Discreet silence will do much to lay the ghost of an "affliction" which through education and medical progress has lost its aura of tragedy and suffering.

MIDDLE AGE: When you begin to exchange your emotions for symptoms.
—Irvin S. Cobb

Prostate Trouble

by Paul de Kruif

◦✎◦

Sunk deep in the male pelvic cavity is a small horse-chestnut-shaped gland—the prostate—which menaces with misery and disability three out of every ten men past fifty. The prostate is a vital organ because it plays a major role in reproduction, secreting a fluid which carries and nourishes the sperm, giving it vigor and motility. But the prostate is as dangerous as it is vital, because its position at the outlet of the bladder causes it, when enlarged, to block urination, thus setting up a train of consequences that may jeopardize health and life itself.

Commonest of prostate disorders is prostatitis, a chronic inflammation occurring when the gland becomes infected, usually by streptococcus, colon bacillus, gonococcus or other disease organisms. The earliest sign of prostatitis, which may occur at any age, is frequent urination, especially at night, accompanied by pain, burning and difficulty in emptying the bladder. The patient may suffer from an aching back, and feels below par generally. Temporary sterility is a not uncommon result of prostatic inflammation; when the condition is cleared up, the sperm regains its fertilizing power.

The modern physician has at his disposal highly effective means of treating this male malady. He can prescribe magic-working sulfa drugs with virtual certainty of a good result. Massage of the prostate, by a skilled physician, is valuable. So too is diathermy, either in the form of short wave, or hot baths and a special type of enema—all of which dilate the blood vessels locally, increasing circulation. Any measure that promotes general good health is of assistance in clearing up prostatitis. Body tone and circulation should be maintained by a program of moderate exercise such as walking or golf. Constipation should be avoided. Plenty of water and a balanced diet under the care of a physician complete the preventive measures that should be taken. Sane sex hygiene, plus early and thoroughgoing care of the inflamed prostate, will do much to stave off later, more serious, complications.

As men advance in years (between fifty and seventy) the prostate may become permanently enlarged and increasingly troublesome. Urination becomes a crisis, recurring with distressing frequency as the sufferer makes painful and futile attempts to empty his bladder completely. Serious, even fatal damage to the kidneys, followed by systemic poisoning (uremia), may result unless the prostate obstruction is removed. At this critical point, surgery steps in with alternative techniques for relieving the prostatic victim.

Since the beginning of the century skilled surgeons have grappled with this martyrdom afflicting men only, constantly improving operative methods by which enlarged prostate masses may be removed. In 1903 Dr. Hugh Young devised a technique of making a small incision in the crotch, and was thus able to reach and remove obstructing portions of the prostate.

The perfecting of the electrical scalpel—an instrument of sheer wizardry—in the early 1930s, revolutionized the outlook for prostatic sufferers by making it no longer necessary in most cases for surgeons to lay open the body. In the modern transurethral operation a slender rod, tipped with a minute electric light and a hair-thin loop of wire, is adroitly inserted into the male urinary canal. Through the eyepiece, the surgeon sees (as through an illuminated periscope) the obstructing prostate. Now a double-barreled miracle takes place. First, high-frequency current passing along the loop of wire cuts away offending tissue; the surgeon sees an eerie spectacle as blood vessels spurt in flamelike hemorrhages. The second part of the miracle occurs when the magic electric current seals up the vessels and stops the flow of blood.

This cutting-and-coagulating process (done painlessly under low-spinal anesthesia) continues until the perilous obstruction is removed and the urine can flow free once more. The patient is usually able to leave the hospital within ten days and in a short time is restored to normal life. Statistics? Plenty of them, all attesting to the dramatic results of the transurethral operation. At many hospitals this is the operation of choice for benign prostate trouble. In one series of 1000 cases the mortality rate reached the phenomenal low of less than one percent—approximately the same mortality as that of appendicitis!

Urologists specially trained in prostate surgery are bringing fresh strength and renewed vigor to thousands of men at a time when they are carrying the peak load of life's responsibility. With modern improvements in technique, both the transurethral method and open surgery are about equally safe and relatively free from danger. It is merely a question of the surgeon's discretion in fitting the operation to the individual case.

To augment the blessings of prostatic surgery, operators use antibiotics to conquer the hazards of infection which were formerly a principal cause of death. Antibiotics given after the operation have so reduced this deadly danger that 300 consecutive transurethral operations have been performed in a single clinic without a fatality.

There seems to be no end to the diabolic activities of the diseased prostate. Not only does it dam up the urine, damage the kidneys, jangle the sexual life of the victim, but when infected, poisons seep from the prostate, via the blood, to the joints, tendons, muscles, bones—even to the eye. In seeking the cause of many a mysterious disease condition among men past middle life, physicians should consider the possibility of prostate infection. On the other hand, abscessed teeth or tonsils may spread their infection, by way of the bloodstream or lymphatic glands, to the prostate itself, causing it to become inflamed.

In about 10 percent of the cases of prostate enlargement, cancer is the cause. Fortunately, cancer usually starts in that part of the gland which can be felt by the physician during rectal examination, thus leading to early diagnosis. Some cases of prostatic cancer can be cured by surgery, and beneficial results in its treatment have been obtained by the use of the female hormone. For men over fifty, rectal examination should be a routine part of every physical checkup—done by a doctor whose finger is expertly sensitized in the detection of early prostatic disorders.

Protected by the latest advances of surgical and chemical science, prostate sufferers need no longer lead bedraggled lives. While his experience and judgment are at their peak, no man should condemn himself to carry the burden of prostate trouble, nor need he, when medical science now promises a lengthening of life's prime.

To make oneself eligible for this desirable extension of vigor and vitality, every man over fifty should regularly submit himself to a most rigorous physical examination at the hands of his own physician. This checkup will consist not only of a rectal examination but also will include a complete diagnostic survey of kidney, bladder and sexual functions. Doctors everywhere are urging this, and it is nothing less than folly to neglect it in your own case.

Don't make the mistake of confusing emotional immaturity with true youthfulness. It takes a mature person to be really young. Men and women who refuse to grow up emotionally are usually the first ones to grow old; and the reason why, in later years, some people relapse into second childhood is that they never really emerged from their first. Masquerading as much younger than you are is a sure sign that you've not grown up emotionally.   —George Lawton

Sex Life
after Middle Age

by Margaret Culkin Banning

The young man taking his seat on the airplane noted carelessly that the motherly-looking woman by the window was deep in thought, and that the old fellow across the aisle—he was at least sixty—looked half asleep. Well, said the young man to himself, when you get to be old, at least you don't have all this woman trouble *I* have.

He did not know that the woman was on her way to buy a trousseau for her wedding and was planning it with delight. He had no idea that the man across the aisle was dreaming with excitement of the coming reunion with his middle-aged wife, whom he had not seen for two lonesome weeks. If the young man had been told these things he probably would have said in derisive astonishment, "The old fools!"

But they were happier than he was. They had learned how to manage the problems of sex life which were bewildering and torturing him. They knew far more about the generosities and skills of love. They were aware of their own capacities, able to give happiness and to get it in return. They were far from being "old fools"; their desires and plans were both normal and sensible.

Today, as life expectancy has grown longer, the scientific

study of the later years has become increasingly intensive. All kinds of ways to occupy the minds and abilities of those past middle age are being explored in an effort to prevent unhappiness. But too often the problem that interests people most deeply, their own human relations and the continuance of their sex life, is left to conjecture, wishful thinking or worry. Are the post-childbearing years also a postsexual period? Many people are unsure.

In this area of human behavior, ignorance and shame can do as great harm in maturity as in adolescence. It is constantly revealed to doctors that many women believe sex life is wrong, unhappy or shameful after the menopause; that many men believe their powers will fail before they attain normal life expectancy.

These two complete misconceptions have resulted in jealousy, cruelty and infidelity, and have wrecked many happy marriages. There is no reason why they should continue to do so, for a great deal of authoritative information is available that should destroy such worries and fears.

There is no sin, no wrong, no outrage in long-continued sex life in marriage. Says Dr. Leland Foster Wood, secretary for the Committee on Marriage and the Home of the Federal Council of Churches: "For both husbands and wives who fully understand the meaning of marriage and the interrelationships between the physical, emotional and spiritual factors, the sex relationship after the menopause can still be a rich and rewarding expression of love."

The Catholic religion concurs. A statement that is attributed to A. Ballerini, professor at the Catholic Gregorian University in Rome, says explicitly: "Married people are at liberty to make use of their marital rights even when the wife can no longer conceive because of age."

In *The Changing Years*, Madeline Gray writes: "For those of the Jewish faith, sex communion between husband and wife from the celebration of marriage until death is a ritual and a trust."

Woman's sex desire after the menopause is generally about the same as before, and in some cases actually increases. The late Dr. Frederic Loomis, in his book *Consultation Room*, stated, "There is a definite upward surge in the sexual lives of many women at 40, or 45 or even 50—a recrudescence of the flame that has perhaps been dimmed by work or worry." With the fear of pregnancy removed, many women enjoy sex life more than at any other time during their marrige. Their families are complete, and they can offer their husbands love without the thought of the increased responsibility it can bring.

As for the man, his fears of losing his sex capacities are usually needless. Dr. Miriam Lincoln writes, "Nature has endowed the male with an almost lifetime possession of physical ability and emotional interest." Dr. Edmund Bergler, an authority in the field of impotence, says, "Sexual activity stabilizes itself in the late thirties or early forties on a moderate level and remains more or less unchanged until the late sixties or early seventies, provided organic disease does not occur."

Nor do operations such as hysterectomies or removal of the prostate gland result in loss of either sex interest or enjoyment, medical authorities point out.

Men especially need these statements and reassurances. For with men the fear of growing old is, as a rule, inextricably and subtly tied up with reluctance to abandon, or to be thought incapable of, sexual activity. This last is a matter of the deepest masculine pride.

True sexual happiness is not to be found, however, merely because religious and medical authorities say it is possible. This happiness is an intangible and mysterious thing; it is based on physical unity but it must draw the physical aspect into mental and spiritual areas if it is to take root and grow. Too often a sense of unsuitability surrounds middle-aged love, particularly among women. That this is so is largely the fault of misunderstanding among older people themselves.

For physical love at its best has long been associated with youth and physical beauty. Young people have always believed that properly it belongs to them; poets and novelists have fostered the idea, and the claim has been generally conceded by older people. If the young man on the plane had called those elderly passengers old fools, he could only have been led to believe this by the adults around him.

You've often heard a member of the older generation call another an old fool when a man of sixty married again or a grandmother took a new husband. In such mockery, however, there is usually a note of jealousy. "At her age . . ." they will say derisively—but a sharp ear can hear the envy.

Many older people *are*, in fact, fools in their attempts to retain the benefits and pleasures of continuing sex life. Since, secretly, they believe that these belong exclusively to youth, they try to falsify their own ages. They become absurd in appearance and in conduct. They deliberately fall out of their own generation and try to find room in a younger one. But they deceive nobody for long and only exhaust themselves trying to compete with the energies of youth. There are far better ways to achieve what they basically want, and mature men and women are beginning to find them out. F. Hugh Herbert says in his play *The Vintage Years:* "Aren't there lots of things that mellow and get better with the years? To the years ahead for us—the vintage years!"

Dr. Bergler has said: "There is no time limit on sex." This is what everyone should be taught, and as early in life as possible. On this foundation each person can fearlessly and honestly build his or her own sex life. The activity will vary with the passing of time, but it need never degenerate. For as sex accompanies later life, it becomes wiser, more informed, less selfish and less crude. It may be physically less beautiful at sixty but it can be even lovelier emotionally. It relates itself to philosophy as well as to poetry and therefore is less dependent on appearance and more dependent on character.

"Sex," wrote D. H. Lawrence, "means the whole relationship between men and women. The relationship is a lifelong change and a lifelong traveling. At periods sex desire itself departs completely. Yet the flow of the relationship goes on all the same, undying, and lasts a lifetime."

Can Science Prolong Our Useful Years?

by Albert Q. Maisel

⊷

Through the ages, men have dreamed of finding a Fountain of Youth: some potion or treatment that would postpone aging and prolong our useful, vigorous years.

Today, instead of just dreaming about it, scientists are actively working toward this goal. Where once they scoffed, they now speak seriously of stretching the *average* human life span to one hundred years or more. In at least six major research centers and in more than three hundred laboratories supported by grants from government (totaling over sixteen million dollars), from private foundations, universities and industry, they are searching for means of slowing down or halting the process of aging.

Until a few years ago, many scientists believed that all living things had a fixed, "natural" life span controlled by a built-in biological clock. If we were lucky, heredity endowed us with a long clock spring and, barring accidents, destined us for a comparatively long life. If we were less lucky, our time simply ran out quickly.

This theory was rudely shaken by a series of brilliant experiments conceived by Dr. Clive Maine McCay, professor of nutrition at Cornell University. He started by dividing a large batch of newly weaned white rats into two groups. To one group he fed a standard ration heavily fortified with sugar and lard. He let them eat to their hearts' content. They lived a normal life span for rats of their type—2 to 2½ years. The oldest died on the 965th day.

Dr. McCay's second group of rats received the same basic diet but with no extra calories—no lard and no sugar. Their growth was retarded, but otherwise they developed normally. And when they were finally allowed to eat their fill—after 300, 600 or, in some instances, 900 days—they resumed growing and went on to maturity. Almost all this group were still youthfully active at 1000 days, long after all the "control" rats had died. The oldest survived for 1400 days.

Over the years other researchers confirmed McCay's results, and the importance of his work became clear beyond doubt. He had proved that heredity fixes no specific limit on an animal's life span. A change of nutritional pattern could extend youth and healthy middle age in rats up to 100 percent.

Other researchers have shown that even a moderate restriction of food intake can produce both a tremendous reduction in disease and increased longevity in experimental animals. They fed the same diet to two groups of rats, but permitted those in Group A to gorge themselves at will. Almost all the Group A rats developed tumors or heart or kidney lesions before they reached an age of 850 days. The rats of Group B, on the other hand, were allowed to consume only a little more than half as much as their free-feeding litter mates. At the age of 850 days, far less than one half of the Bs had developed disease lesions, and their average life span exceeded that of the fat rats by 200 days in the males and 350 days in the females.

Scientists have long known that radiation shortens the life span of all living things. It works its havoc by ionizing cell molecules to produce highly reactive *stripped* molecules—so-called free radicals—which set up damaging chain reactions in living tissues. To block this effect, researchers have tried, with some success, to treat victims of radiation exposure with antioxidizing substances, which combine rapidly with free radicals.

In 1958 Dr. Denham Harman, then working at the Atomic Energy Commission's Donner Laboratory at the University of California, was struck by the fact that free radicals are also released by normal metabolic processes. Here, he thought, might be one of the basic causes of aging. To test his theory, he used mice of strains noted for short life spans. On a standard diet, his control animals lived for an average of only 7.6 months. But mice that were fed the same diet *plus* an antioxidant survived for an average of 10.5 months.

Was this just happenstance? To answer this question, Dr. Harman recently performed (at the University of Nebraska College of Medicine) a series of experiments with two other strains of mice, and with different antioxidants. In both, the aging process was substantially arrested. In one strain, life was prolonged by 15 percent; in the other, by 26.

More than twenty-five years ago, V. B. Wigglesworth, now professor of biology at Cambridge University, England, discovered that in insects a strange "juvenile" hormone released by a tiny gland held off aging until full growth was achieved. Then the gland shut off, and the insect began to molt. Just before it emerged as an adult, the gland turned on again, triggering the growth of sex organs and eggs.

Since only insects possess this Peter Pan gland, the juvenile hormone was long considered merely a scientific curiosity. But in 1959, Professor Carroll M. Williams, of Harvard University, extracted a previously unknown substance from the tissues of newborn rats and injected it into insects ready to molt. Surprisingly, it produced age-postponing effects exactly like those of the insect hormone.

Then followed a series of unexpected discoveries. The same age-postponing substance was detected in the bone, liver, muscle and adrenal-gland tissues of calves. Then it was found in the human placenta and finally in human thymus glands.

Much work must yet be done before researchers learn whether—and how—this substance actually delays aging in higher animals. But a number of experiments indicate that its presence in the young may play a major role in the healing of wounds. Its diminution or absence in the aged may account for reduced ability to replace dead cells and injured tissues.

At the aging-research center in Baltimore extremely delicate surgical techniques are used to link young and aged cockroaches together as artificial Siamese twins. Ordinarily, a young cockroach that loses a leg can quickly grow a complete replacement. Old cockroaches, after their final molt, lose this ability. But in this study whenever a leg from an older member of the Siamese pairs was removed, a new leg promptly grew to replace it. The younger twin's juvenile hormone had restored the old bug's regenerative powers.

At Cornell, Dr. McCay has similarly joined rats. In such unions, the aged member of the pair soon takes on a youthful appearance. More important, it lives far beyond its usual life expectancy, sometimes for more than 400 additional days. These discoveries open up the fascinating possibility that injections of a "juvenile hormone" may one day delay human aging and senescence.

Before such hopes can be realized, however, much more must be learned about the aging process in humans and how it begins. Up to now, most information has been derived from studies of aged patients in hospitals or other institutions. Recently, age researchers have turned to long-term projects that start with the middle-aged and the young.

At the Health Research Center in Boston, a team of consultant specialists are studying 900 war veterans, each of whom qualified for the study by extensive tests showing perfect health. Periodically, each veteran will receive thorough re-examination for the rest of his life. Thus, any physical or mental slowing down will be revealed in its earliest stages. Aging and age-related illnesses can be studied in the light of detailed knowledge of each veteran's living pattern—his eating, smoking and drinking habits, his work and his leisure activities.

A similar long-term project at the center for aging research in Baltimore has had under study for several years some 300 men of all ages from eighteen up. And the University of Michigan has undertaken an even more ambitious project—a study of the entire population of Tecumseh, Michigan. Some 8600 persons have already received their initial examinations, and the researchers hope to follow them through periodic tests for decades to come.

Already studies of this kind have yielded valuable data. We now know that hearing and visual acuity begin to deteriorate in many individuals in the early twenties. In these years, blood pressure may begin to rise, the volume of blood pumped by the heart may decrease, kidney function and muscle strength may begin to decline.

Such findings have convinced research workers that many ills of our later years are not simply the result of aging, but are the late effects of long-hidden metabolic disorders. These workers contend, therefore, that science should hunt for means of halting metabolic imbalances in the young and middle-aged.

Research based on this view has already produced significant advances in the fight against atherosclerosis, the most common cause of death among people in their middle and later years. This form of hardening of the arteries was once thought to be the *result* of aging. Then autopsy studies revealed changes in the arteries of certain persons in their early twenties. Such evidence that atherosclerosis is an early-starting metabolic disorder stimulated a hunt for its underlying causes and vast research into the role of cholesterol in heart disease. Today, although the question is not yet settled, many physicians routinely prescribe cholesterol-controlling drugs or diets not merely for their advanced atherosclerotic patients but as a protective measure for almost anyone with a higher-than-normal cholesterol level.

Fulfillment of the hope of stretching the span of active, healthful life to a full century lies a long way off. It is not likely to be accomplished by any single triumph of research, but rather by the gradual accumulation of small and partial victories. Meanwhile, there is much that we as individuals can do to increase our life expectancy and that of our children. Here are four measures suggested by leading age researchers:

Avoid overeating. A recent study of the mortality records of several million insurance policyholders showed that men who were 20 pounds overweight died, on the average, 1½ years earlier than those of normal weight; 35 pounds of excess weight lowered life expectancy by at least 4 years. On the other hand, overweight men who reduced to the norm for their age and build were found to have almost as favorable life expectancy as those who never allowed themselves to put on surplus fat.

Avoid unnecessary exposure to radiation. The life-shortening effects of even small or intermittent doses of radiation have been demonstrated on many species of animals. No exact data are yet available for man. But, because the danger is there, both the American Medical Association and the American College of Radiology warn against needless or excessive exposure. That does not mean forgoing diagnostic X rays; it does mean avoiding radiation treatments for nonmalignant conditions, and avoiding X rays or fluoroscopies performed by careless technicians.

Keep physically active. Leading heart specialists have long advocated regular exercise for all people, young or old, healthy or infirm. The wisdom of their advice has recently been confirmed by a monumental study, conducted in the United States and in the mountains of Austria, by a research team under Dr. Wilhelm Raab, of the University of Vermont. Athletes, mountaineers, lumberjacks and others given to habitual, vigorous exercise were found to have "young" hearts even when they were in their fifties, with low pulse rates, high muscle efficiency and quick recovery after intensive exertion. On the other hand, the hearts of sedentary office workers, businessmen and medical students—even those in their twenties—had the typical functional characteristics of age and incipient heart disease. Most significant, however, was a third finding: six to twelve weeks of regular exercise restored a more youthful heart function to many of the formerly sedentary.

Keep mentally active. No functions atrophy more rapidly under disuse than those of the mind. But studies of the mentally active have shown that the ability for new learning persists far into our later years. Even when it drops off, the judgment and reasoning power developed by the mentally active compensate for age deterioration. As Professor Ross McFarland of the Harvard University School of Public Health puts it, "The brain, like other organs of the body, shows continuous improvement over the life span *if appropriately exercised*."

How to Keep Young Mentally

by Mary B. Mullett

When Alexander Graham Bell, the famous scientist and inventor, was seventy-five years old, an intimate acquaintance said, "The most remarkable thing about Dr. Bell is that he is younger in mind than most men half his age. Mentally, he seems to have discovered a Fountain of Youth which keeps him perennially alert and vigorous."

I repeated to a very able and highly educated man Dr. Bell's ideas on how to study and to learn. This man said with emphasis, "If anyone would follow that plan consistently, he would learn more than he would get through a college education. It is the best rule for everybody, at any age and in any walk of life, that I have ever heard."

"The education of the mind," said Dr. Bell, "is, after all, not a mere question of remembering facts which someone else gives us. The mind should conduct its own education to a better extent. And it cannot do this unless it thinks for itself. A mind that does not reason is comparatively useless.

"I have given the subject of self-education a great deal of thought and have evolved what you might call a 'Rule of Three' in regard to it. The rule is simply this: 'Observe! Remember! Compare!'. . .

"The very first essential of any real education is to observe concrete facts. Unless you do this, you have no material out of which to manufacture knowledge. Remember what you have observed. Compare the facts you have observed; and you will find yourself thinking out conclusions. These conclusions are real knowledge; and they are your own.

"That was what made John Burroughs a great naturalist, J. P. Morgan a great financier, Napoleon a great general. It is the foundation of all education. And the wonderful thing about it is that gaining an education in this way is not a penance, but a delight.

"As an illustration: Is not a detective story a record of observing, remembering and comparing facts—and of then drawing conclusions? Practically all of us enjoy reading these books because, while we read, we ourselves are observing, remembering, comparing and trying to draw the correct conclusion.

"We can pursue knowledge in just the same way, and can have even more pleasure doing it. Moreover, in pursuing knowledge we may capture something that will contribute to the welfare of the world.

"In any case, we enrich ourselves; we open new windows through which to behold interesting things. Did you ever look up a word in the dictionary without gaining more than the one definition you were seeking? I never do. I have the same sort of experience when I start out with a fact or an idea.

"We cannot perform the simplest act without bringing some principle of science into play. And there is nothing of more enthralling interest than to study these simple acts and to try to learn something from them.

"In dealing with children, the main essential is not to tell them things, but to encourage them to find out things for themselves. Ask them questions, but leave them to find out the answer. If they arrive at the wrong answer, do not tell them they are mistaken; and do not give them the right answer. Ask them other questions, which will show them their mistake, and so make them push their inquiry further.

"For example: Suppose you wanted to teach a child about moisture and condensation. You could state to him that there are minute particles of water vapor in the air exhaled from the lungs, and that this water vapor will be condensed under certain conditions. In other words, you give him a general conclusion which other people have arrived at and ask him to memorize it.

"Now suppose you tell him nothing, but simply ask him to breathe into a glass tumbler. He sees the moisture on the glass. Ask him where it came from. Have him breathe against the outside of the tumbler. Have him try the experiment with a glass that is hot and with one that is ice-cold. Have him try it with other surfaces. And don't do his thinking for him. Make him observe what takes place, stimulating him to remember the different results he observes and, by comparing them, to arrive at conclusions.

"I believe that self-education is a lifelong affair. It comes, naturally and inevitably, through using the mind and following this Rule of Three."

W<small>HEN</small> Oliver Wendell Holmes was still on the Supreme Court bench, he and Justice Brandeis took walks every afternoon. On one of these occasions Holmes, then 92, paused to gaze in frank admiration at a beautiful young girl who passed them. He even turned to look at her as she continued down the street. Then, turning to Brandeis, he sighed: "Ah! What wouldn't I give to be 70 again!"   —Drew Pearson and Robert S. Allen

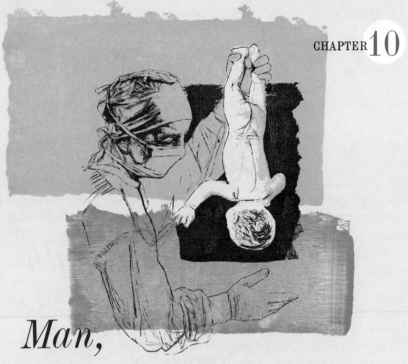

CHAPTER 10

Man, Woman and Fertility

THE profound physical differences of the human male and female are so great that it might be best to imagine the two as of different species. Yet the miracle of fertility in all its stages, despite the difficulties of conception, the plague of miscarriage, the tyranny of civilized living over natural birth and infancy, form a dramatic history in the lives of most couples.

Here is that history—an account of the forces within male and female and all the main events that may confront the human couple in the quest of parenthood.

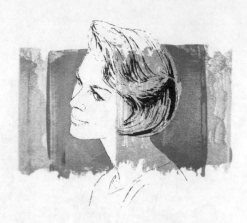

The Secret Strength
of Women

by Caroline Bird

W ITH ALL the talk about putting *man* into space, scientists suggest it actually would be more logical if the first human
space travelers had been women. This is not only because of
woman's smaller size, and the superior thermostat which enables
her to stand extremes of heat and cold better than the male; the
belief is growing in scientific circles that women have a special
talent for survival, a secret weapon against physical and emotional wear and tear.

"Women are the stronger sex," said the late Dr. David Adlers-
berg, a researcher into metabolic aspects of heart disease at New
York's Mount Sinai Hospital. "All their adaptive mechanisms
are better. They stand the stress of surgery better than men.
They have a better resistance to most diseases."

White women in the U.S. and Canada today have a longevity

advantage over men of about six years, and the gap is growing. Though women are sick more often, they resist more successfully than men every major killer except diabetes. Of the 64 killers doctors most commonly put on death certificates—including accidents, birth defects, diseases, as well as murder and suicide—57 kill more men than women.

What is the explanation?

Many think that modern life is particularly hard on men compared with women. But this theory does not hold up when put to the test. Father Francis C. Madigan, a Jesuit, and sociologist Rupert B. Vance of the University of North Carolina studied the life span of some 37,000 teaching monks and nuns. For 50 years both groups had lived the same exemplary lives, equally free from self-indulgence and nervous strain. In 1957, the researchers reported that the sisters had increased their lead over the monks from 0.1 year in 1900 to 5.8 years—just about the gain made by the women of the outside world. Apparently the stresses of modern life have little to do with longevity differences. The sociologists could only hand the mystery back to the biologists.

The first reaction of a biologist is to credit the extra X chromosome, or gene-packed carrier of heredity, that is dealt to females at conception. Thus, at the very start men are exposed to hemophilia, color blindness, hereditary muscular dystrophy and hundreds of other "sex-linked" defects. Research is turning up unexpected sex-linked defects all the time. One is agammaglobulinemia, or lack of gamma globulin, a substance in the blood necessary to the production of antibodies to fight disease germs. Before antibiotics, boy babies born with agammaglobulinemia died before anyone could find out what was wrong.

But the most fruitful and fascinating clue to the role of sex in durability has been the fact that woman's advantage over man is never greater than during her childbearing years. Now that women seldom die in childbirth, we're losing twice as many men as women in the 25-to-44 age group. Some doctors believe that coronary-artery disease accounts for much of the disadvantage; it strikes down five or six men for every woman during these childbearing years. But after 45, women's coronary rate increases—as it also does for young women whose ovaries have been removed or who have stopped menstruating early. Apparently the ability to bear children has something to do with coronary arteries.

The prime suspects are the sex hormones testosterone (male) and the estrogens (female), which have chemically similar molecules. Each sex has both male and female sex hormones, but in differing amounts. Estrogen generally calms; and when a woman's ovaries are functioning they send it to all parts of the body. Testosterone stimulates. Because it raises metabolism, pulse and respiration, doctors think that men may literally burn themselves out sooner than women.

When heart researchers began investigating cholesterol they noticed that men—and older women—have the "bad" blood-fat ratios associated with heart attack. Early in the 1950s, researchers began changing the proportion of blood fats toward the "good" female pattern by giving men and older women doses of estrogen. When testosterone was given, it made the blood pattern "bad."

At Michael Reese Hospital in Chicago, Dr. Ruth Pick gave chickens a diet which has the same effect on their blood as the standard high-fat American bill of fare. When she cut the chickens open, she found that the roosters' coronary arteries were scarred like the arteries of human coronary victims, while those of the hens remained smooth. When Dr. Pick mixed estrogen in the roosters' feed, their arteries stayed smooth, and damaged arteries cleared. "A woman's natural estrogen protects her against the solid fat she serves her husband," Dr. Pick concluded.

Many men here and in England who have had coronary attacks have been taking estrogen, and they show a substantially improved survival rate. About half of them, however, experience side effects. They may feel draggy and depressed; some don't have to shave as often; others are delighted to find hair growing on their bald spots. Although some have fathered children, the loss of the sex drive or fear of such a loss has haunted almost all of them. Researchers are now trying to isolate the protection of estrogen from its feminizing effects.

The effect of estrogen on blood fats may be only one of the hormone's secrets. Dr. Edward Henderson, a research endocrinologist, believes that women when pregnant shake off most infections more easily. He suspects that the increased supply of estrogen stimulates phagocyte cells to step up their scavenging of germs and other foreign troublemakers in the blood.

Dr. Henderson has also observed that pregnancy can temporarily "cure" a woman's arthritis. Other physicians have noticed the same phenomenon. Even though early investigators couldn't cure arthritis with doses of estrogen, they decided that the extra quantity of natural hormones a woman produces in pregnancy must have a beneficial effect. This led to the development of ACTH and hydrocortisone hormone drugs, which ease the suffering of rheumatism and arthritis victims.

Dr. Robert H. Furman of the Oklahoma Medical Research Foundation now suspects that the liver, which processes hormones, may shed further light on women's secret strength. Dr. Furman's interest was aroused by finding that the liver of a man who has had a heart attack so changes the estrogen in his system that a chemist can tell, through urinalysis, that the patient has had a coronary. Dr. Furman has counted several dozen liver processes which differ in men and women. He intends to find out why.

If estrogen is woman's strength, the secret may be in femininity itself. "Men are highly specialized, delicate creatures," suggests Dr. Louis N. Katz of Michael Reese Hospital. "They are like the spermatozoa—a moment's stimulation and their biological job is done. Women may live longer simply because they are the bearers of life."

NATURE meant woman to be her masterpiece.—Lessing

What Doctors Can Do
to Promote Fertility

by Grace Naismith

An interview with Dr. Edward T. Tyler, associate clinical professor of medicine, obstetrics and gynecology at the University of California at Los Angeles School of Medicine, and also president of the Pacific Coast Fertility Society.

Q *Dr. Tyler, is it true that there are more couples unable to bear children than there used to be?*

A Yes. According to statistics, one of every ten married couples is faced with the problem of a barren marriage. Of course, more men—as well as more women—are willing to seek medical aid today. This increases the statistical record.

Q *You said "more men" are seeking medical aid. Isn't it thought that sterility is the woman's fault?*

A Some people still make this mistaken generalization, but between 40 and 50 percent of all sterile marriages may be attributable primarily to the husband. Neither the husband nor the wife is to be "blamed" for a condition which prevents them from conceiving a child. Often these conditions can be corrected.

Q *But don't most people think of sterility as being quite hopeless?*

A Strictly speaking, sterility is, as one doctor defined it, "the *permanent* state of infertility." Today more and more *infertile* couples are being helped to be fertile.

Q *How large a percentage?*

A About 40 percent. And more could be helped if husbands would coöperate with medical examination and treatment. Many specialists and clinics, such as the Margaret Sanger Research Bureau in New York City, will take cases only when both husband and wife come for treatment.

Q *Why don't all husbands coöperate?*

A Perhaps because of the male ego. Many men don't know the difference between "virility" and fertility. But we have found that most infertile male patients are entirely normal with regard to all "he-man" traits.

Q *What causes infertility?*

A There are as many causes as there are vulnerable spots in the reproductive process. Conception requires that a sperm cell from the male and an egg (ovum) from the female meet in the Fallopian tubes. If fertilized, the egg is propelled into the uterus, where it is implanted, nourished and grows until ready for delivery nine months later. Infertility can occur if any link in the chain is broken in this reproductive process. And the entire chain is far more complex than this brief description indicates.

In the fertile woman there must be normally functioning ovaries. She must ovulate (produce an egg). The uterus must be normal and the Fallopian tubes must be clear so that the sperm and egg can meet. In the fertile man there must be production of millions of healthy, active sperm. And in both the man and the woman the hormone-producing glands must be normal.

Q *What tests are made to find out if anything is not normal?*

A For the female, basic tests include, in addition to complete physical examination, a test of the Fallopian tubes for blockage, an X ray of the pelvic organs, a check on thyroid function and a study of tissue samples taken from the lining of the uterus. For the male, tests include complete physical examination, a check on blood iodine, and semen evaluation.

Q *Who can help the childless couple overcome their infertility?*
A Any well-trained physician—the family doctor, a gynecologist, a urologist, an internist or an obstetrician.

Q *How long should a couple try to have a baby before seeking help?*
A No longer than a year. Studies show that, if contraception is not practiced, pregnancy occurs within that time in 90 percent of couples of childbearing age.

Q *Can anything be done for an infertile couple whose tests show that husband and wife are "normal"?*
A Yes. "Normal" is a category which includes between 30 and 40 percent of all infertile couples. For these we try more tests, some of which are new and experimental. One of the most recent and exciting research discoveries leads us to believe that there is some type of "reproductive incompatibility" among certain couples which prevents conception. The male sperm and the female ovum simply do not get along. We might say they are "allergic" to each other.

Q *Then this might account for the childless woman who remarries after divorce or after her husband's death and immediately conceives?*
A Yes. Reproductive incompatibility is difficult to explain. Let me attempt it this way:

Two physicians in the Netherlands, Drs. Philip Rumke and George Hellinga, both associated with the Red Cross Blood Laboratories in Amsterdam, made extensive studies of the blood of some 2000 infertile and fertile persons. In a number of the infertile patients they found that the blood contained substances "hostile" to sperm. These substances are similar to the blood chemicals called antibodies which protect us against certain diseases. It is conjectured that antibodies—described by Webster as any substance that opposes the action of another substance—can make ineffective or neutralize the ability of sperm to fertilize or even to move.

Q *Isn't there another kind of hostility between male and female reproductive secretions—this one related to the acidity of the female's secretions?*
A Yes. The male seminal fluid is alkaline. The fluids in the female vagina are acid—this probably being nature's way of

helping to keep harmful bacteria from causing infection in the vagina. At the same time, acidity is harmful to sperm, and if the semen lacks enough alkaline to neutralize the female's acid fluids, the sperm can be immobilized. Fertility specialists sometimes need to "equalize" the alkaline-acid environment in the vagina to avoid the destruction of the sperm.

Q *Suppose the sperm are weak to begin with?*

A Unfortunately, there are only limited types of treatment available for the husband. Proper diet, rest, a clearing up of certain infected areas—such as bad tonsils—often improve fertility conditions. In some cases, hormones are helpful.

Q *What about the psychological aspects of infertility?*

A Some physicians believe that emotional problems cause infertility in a great number of patients. Dr. Karl Menninger, of the Menninger Clinic, Topeka, Kansas, says that numerous cases have been reported where "reorganization of the psychic life" was followed by pregnancy in marriages barren for ten to twenty years. Reassurance and understanding alone can have a great deal to do with "relaxing" a couple so that pregnancy occurs.

Q *Is it true that many childless couples adopt a child, "relax" and then have one of their own?*

A That is a common belief, but several studies have proved "it ain't necessarily so." Some adoption agencies are now seeking additional statistical information on this adoption fertility theory.

Q *What are the tests for ovulation?*

A First, one must understand that ovulation—the release of the ovum from the ovary—occurs but once during the menstrual cycle. We are not sure how long the sperm are capable of fertilizing the egg or how long the egg is capable of being fertilized.

It is obvious that to the couple wanting a child, the date of ovulation must be pinpointed as closely as possible. There are various methods. One is by a daily check of body temperature. Ovulation is thought to occur at a point when temperature lowers and then rises slightly.

Other tests include vaginal smears, measuring the cervical secretions, and the fern test, which is useful in showing under a microscope a series of patterns indicating the ovulation period.

More recently, a paper-color test based on the detection of glucose in cervical secretions has been developed, but it is not very accurate. We are constantly on the lookout for new ovulation tests—particularly those which women may use themselves—to ascertain the twelve-to-twenty-four-hour fertile period.

Q *What if a woman does not ovulate?*

A Ovulation fails to occur in only about 5 percent of infertile women. One experimental treatment for this condition involves a new pill—an antiestrogen which stimulates the ovaries to produce an egg. *But* this antiestrogen—which is not a hormone, incidentally—must be discontinued immediately after ovulation or it may act as a contraceptive.

Q *Then what helps one couple to have a child may help another to have fewer children?*

A Definitely. One such treatment is the oral contraceptive pill. Many persons, in spite of all the publicity about it, are unaware that the pill was originally developed for *infertile* women. When used as a contraceptive measure, then discontinued, the oral pill may increase the fertility potential. This pill is made of a synthetic hormone closely related to progesterone, which is the hormone formed after ovulation and responsible, among other things, for conditioning the lining of the uterus so that it can adequately receive and nourish the embryo.

The new synthetic progesterone-like hormones, taken by mouth, are effective in inducing and maintaining pregnancy. However, they are extremely potent and must be administered only in carefully diagnosed instances.

Q *Can surgery help?*

A Though surgery is not always successful, surgeons are doing breathlessly minute operations in an effort to bring about conception. It has been possible, for example, to operate on a hopelessly blocked Fallopian tube and transfer a threadlike bit of the intestinal "gut" to serve as a passageway for the ovum from ovary to uterus.

All the work I have mentioned shows how new directions may help to conquer infertility. And, believe me, the satisfaction of helping to bring children into a childless home is great indeed.

Nutrition
and Pregnancy

by Bruce Bliven

News of the greatest importance to every expectant mother is now coming out of the scientific laboratories. It has been discovered that the average mother, during the period of pregnancy, gets a faulty diet, especially in the following particulars: too much carbohydrate and not enough protein; not enough of the vitamins, especially vitamins A and C and members of the B complex; too much fluid.

Having a baby is a severe strain on the mother's nutritional resources of vitamins, calcium, phosphorus, iron and other minerals. By giving all expectant mothers in the United States a special diet, at an additional cost of less than a dollar a day, it would be possible *each year* to:

• Save the lives of many of the 33,000 premature babies who die; of a large part of the approximately 112,000 babies who now die shortly after birth; and of many of the 69,000 stillborn.

• Greatly reduce the number of deaths of mothers during pregnancy and childbirth.

• Prevent a large number of the hundreds of thousands of cases of spontaneous abortion.

• Rescue many thousands of children born with lowered vitality or with malformations which mean lifelong unhappiness.

This new knowledge has been developed in numerous laboratories, notably by Dr. J. H. Ebbs at the University of Toronto, by a group of workers at the Harvard School of Public Health and by Dr. Winslow Tompkins and his associates at Pennsylvania Hospital in Philadelphia.

The work at Pennsylvania Hospital began in the 1930s. Among the patients were several pregnant women who were having fatigue, morning sickness, high blood pressure, swelling of the feet and ankles, excess gain in weight, nervousness and faulty functioning of the kidneys—all symptoms of the condition called toxemia. Suspecting that improper diet might be the cause, the doctors began prescribing special diets. The results were so extraordinary that a scientific study was launched.

The records of 593 mothers receiving special diet instructions have been compared with those of 772 who did not. In the latter group there were 38 percent more babies born dead, 15 percent more deaths in the first few weeks, 70 percent more premature babies and a much larger amount of toxemia.

In studies made by the Harvard School of Public Health, 80 percent of the babies born in poor condition had mothers whose diet had been conspicuously bad. Among 216 cases, with only one exception, the mother had had an inadequate diet in every case of a premature or stillborn baby, or one that died within a few days. And experiments with laboratory animals have shown decisively that inadequate diets are responsible for clubfeet, cleft palates, bone deformities and many cases of blindness at birth.

Years ago doctors used to say to an expectant mother, "Take very little meat, and drink all the fruit juice and water you can." But today we know that plenty of protein is enormously important. We have also discovered that liquids in excessive amounts help to cause swelling.

Here is the minimum daily diet for the pregnant woman as worked out at Pennsylvania Hospital:

Not more than one serving of fresh fruit.
Not more than one glass of fruit juice.
Two cups of cooked vegetables.

One cup of salad made with leafy or other highly colored vegetables, with any dressing desired.

Three squares of butter, or two tablespoons of oil—not both.

Two servings of whole-grain cereal, hot or cold.

At least one egg.

Six ounces of lean meat, fish or fowl. Liver and the other organ meats are especially recommended.

Not more than three slices of whole-wheat bread (*never* white).

Three glasses of milk.

Flavored gelatin or junket, custard or fruit whip.

Severely restricted are potatoes, spaghetti, rice, corn, lima beans and dried beans. Not more than 1½ tablespoonfuls of any one of these may be taken. The patient is told not to eat pastries, ice cream, nuts or candy, because they take away the appetite for the protective foods listed above and produce a harmful gain in weight. Of liquids of all kinds the patient is limited to 8 glasses in twenty-four hours. Salt and salty foods are to be avoided.

Experts at the Pennsylvania Hospital consider a multiple-vitamin preparation (containing vitamin A, thiamin, riboflavin, niacin, ascorbic acid and probably a small quantity of vitamin D) essential for most patients. The dose should be worked out by the physician.

Patients are advised to eat six small meals a day instead of three large ones. The food seems to digest better when the stomach is not overloaded. Patients on this diet have very little morning sickness, even in the first months, and are almost completely free from fatigue, nausea and other disturbances.

The diet mentioned above is a minimum below which no expectant mother can go with safety. Those who can afford it might increase the daily protein intake somewhat: two or three eggs could be taken instead of one, and an additional 25 percent of meat. One and one half ounces of cheese (except cream cheese) is a desirable addition.

One of the most remarkable results of the experiments at the Pennsylvania Hospital has been to cut down the proportion of babies which are very large or very small. A fat baby frequently

causes a difficult delivery. Thus a proper diet means a less difficult labor for the mother, a more prompt return to her full
normal vigor, and a child born with a decidedly better equipment with which to face the world.

The
Rh Factor
in Pregnancy

by J. D. Ratcliff

A baby born in Birmingham, England, in the early 1940s was
jaundiced and dangerously anemic at birth. Death was so
near, the doctors made a dramatic decision. They would drain
off *all* the baby's blood and replace it with new. Within five
minutes of birth the transfusion was begun. A healthy pink came
to the baby's skin. Its troubled breathing settled into steady,
regular respiration.

The reasons behind the dramatic story were frightening to
women around the world. Here was one more case involving the
mysterious newly discovered blood factor, Rh, which sometimes
causes a mother's blood to declare war on the blood of her unborn infant.

Many highly colored and confusing stories have been told
about Rh: that mothers who lacked it could never hope to bear
live babies; that transfusion for them often meant sudden death.
It is time to sweep away the confusion. For Rh is nothing to be

feared, although it is something you should know about. Knowledge of Rh is helping physicians to solve baffling medical
mysteries—mysteries that up to now have caused the deaths of
too many infants.

The story of Rh goes back to the work of the late Dr. Karl
Landsteiner, a giant of medical research. One of his triumphs
was the discovery of the major blood groupings—types A, B, AB
and O—which made safe transfusions possible. With a sharp-
eyed young assistant, Dr. Alexander Wiener, Dr. Landsteiner
was working in his Rockefeller Institute laboratory in 1937,
studying the blood of a rabbit that had just been transfused with
a small amount of rhesus-monkey blood. They noted an entirely
new chemical stuff hidden in the red cells, and named it Rh after
the rhesus monkey. Landsteiner recorded his observations, then
went about his main job. Rh was a sidetrack.

But to Dr. Wiener the sidetrack was fascinating. Would human
blood have this Rh stuff? He found it in the blood of 85 out of
every 100 white Americans! An even larger percentage of
Negroes had it, and 99 percent of all Chinese.

The discovery caused a small amount of interest among research men. But nothing very practical promised to come from it.
Wiener, however, kept thinking about the transfusion accidents
that sometimes occurred. A patient's blood would be typed and
matched with blood of a donor. But instead of getting better after
the transfusion, the patient would have a fearful reaction. There
would be chills, fever, anemia. And sometimes the patient would
go into shock and die. Could these symptoms be the result of
mixing blood containing Rh factors with blood which did not
possess them?

Wiener's theorizing, tested by experimentation, proved correct. Mix Rh-positive with Rh-negative blood and under certain
conditions open warfare ensued. There was fearful destruction of
red cells, in some cases 80 percent or more. Their debris clogged
tiny kidney tubules. The result was a general toxemia, then
death.

Meanwhile, another research man—Dr. Philip Levine of the

Ortho Research Foundation at Linden, New Jersey—was on the track of a disease which had baffled medical men for years: erythroblastosis. It struck at unborn or at newborn babies. In its most severe form it would kill in the first months of pregnancy. Or a baby would be born apparently healthy, then in a short time become jaundiced and die. Since the jaundice was a mark of red-blood-cell destruction, physicians had one weapon against this sickness—transfusion. In rare instances it worked wonders. But oftener it brought violent reaction and death.

Some thought this ugly disease was a malignant process. Others thought it was an inherited sickness of the blood. Levine made a new guess. Wasn't it reasonable to suppose that Rh-negative mothers might have babies with Rh-positive blood inherited from fathers? Then, *under certain conditions*, wouldn't the mother's blood actually declare war on the blood of her own baby—thinning, diluting it until it could hardly be called blood at all?

Levine checked the blood of mothers who had borne dead babies. He checked the blood of the fathers. Over and over again the story was repeated: mothers Rh-negative, fathers Rh-positive. And the story was tragic. One woman had two miscarriages, then a normal child, then a stillbirth. She was transfused with her husband's blood and died.

Dr. Levine found a striking case in a pair of twins. One infant, with Rh-negative blood inherited from its mother, was vigorous, healthy. The other, with Rh-positive blood inherited from the father, had erythroblastosis.

The picture added up grimly but convincingly. But there was a flaw in it. *What was the certain condition that brought it about?* By the law of averages 9 percent of all white marriages are between Rh-negative women and Rh-positive men. Yet erythroblastosis occurs only once in every 40 potential cases, or about once in every 400 births.

Levine remembered a discovery he had made in 1939. An unborn infant has a heart action and circulatory system of its own. But Levine had found that a woman may have a tendency to develop a defective placenta which permits an exchange of red blood cells or other cells between herself and her unborn child. What if such a woman was Rh-negative and her child Rh-positive? That was the clue.

The red blood cells that went from an Rh-positive infant to an Rh-negative mother created something in the mother's blood that turned on and destroyed its own. Or, more commonly, it turned on the blood of the next child the mother carried.

The sequence is very much like the way our common vaccines act. They jolt the blood into building protective factors called antibodies against germs. Getting minute doses of the Rh chemical from the red cells of her baby's blood, the mother builds antibodies which attack red cells containing Rh—the unborn infant's blood.

When her first baby is born, Levine reasoned, the blood of an Rh-negative mother probably would not contain enough antibodies to do material damage. In the course of later pregnancies, however, more antibodies would be created, until there might be enough to cause trouble.

One explanation for the rarity of erythroblastosis, therefore, is that most women today do not have many pregnancies. Another explanation is that Rh is a *dominant* trait. If both parents are negative or both are positive, or if the mother is positive and the father negative, there will be no trouble. So things boil down to this: There is trouble *only* if the mother is negative, the father positive.

One point of caution should be injected here. If the Rh-negative woman received a whole-blood transfusion as a child, the chances are five to one that she received Rh-positive blood. So her blood even before pregnancy contains antibodies ready to declare war on any Rh-positive infant she might conceive.

Doctors now know what precautions to take. An Rh-negative woman married to an Rh-positive man can usually expect two babies without difficulty. If a third child is desired, her physician can watch her blood for a telltale rise in the antibodies which spell Rh trouble. If they stay within safe limits he can permit a normal delivery. If they rise sharply after the sixth month he may decide to bring the baby prematurely. He will have a stock of

Rh-negative blood on hand for immediate transfusion into the infant, and the child should live.

This knowledge of Rh has already saved thousands of lives. Armed-forces surgeons watch for reactions when whole-blood transfusions are made. If the reactions are ominous, they have stocks of Rh-negative blood on hand to correct the trouble. Plasma is always safe because it contains no red cells, hence no Rh factors.

Today, nearly all large, well-equipped hospitals routinely test prospective mothers for Rh. Wherever possible a woman should demand this test with pregnancy. If she is Rh-positive there is nothing to fear. If she is negative her husband should also be tested, and if he is positive the correct precautions can be taken.

✳✳✳

Le Mot Juste

At a dinner party in New York, a South American visitor was telling about his country and himself. He concluded, "And I have a most charming and sympathetic wife but, alas, no children." Then, as his companions seemed to expect further enlightenment, he continued haltingly, "You see, my wife is unbearable."

This was greeted with puzzled glances, so he sought to clear the matter up: "I mean, my wife is inconceivable." Seeing that this, too, was not understood, and floundering deeper and deeper in the intricacies of English, he finally explained triumphantly: "That is, my wife, she is impregnable!"

✳✳✳

I was expecting a baby and wanted to find a practical nurse to help me when I came home from the hospital. I called a woman who had been recommended and told her that the baby was due in about three months.

"My dear," she said in shocked tones, "I'm afraid you're a little late. All the young women consult me at least ten or eleven months before delivery, and we plan this together."   —Mrs. James P. Mondi

Even modern medical science has not been able to duplicate mother's milk, or to explain how the female breast creates this vital food.

For humankind in the Western world, this source of life has become a symbol of sex, completely separated from its natural function. In recent years, because of the myth that breast feeding spoils the female figure and because hospitals for many years discouraged the practice, a campaign to educate modern women in the ways of nature has been going on. Though the breast as a sex symbol is more entrenched than ever in twentieth-century culture, the breast as nature's provision for infant survival and emotional health may be "coming back."

Its Mysteries

by J. D. Ratcliff

The female breast, celebrated throughout history by poets, painters and sculptors as a symbol of femininity, is to the medical researcher a continuous source of wonder. On it all higher forms of life depend. The milk it provides is a near-perfect food to bridge the gap between prenatal life and independent life on earth. A measure of its importance is given by its name. The word "mamma," among the first words uttered by the young, is the Latin word for breast—and not so by coincidence.

The highly complex mechanism of the breast is still imperfectly understood. Even in the newborn it is capable of function. (Stimulated by hormones from the mother, breasts of both male and female infants ooze a few droplets of "witch's milk.") Then the breast lies dormant until at puberty a remarkable chain of events begins, to prepare the girl's body for eventual motherhood.

To understand better what happens, look at the structure of the breast. Each breast contains from 15 to 20 milk-producing systems. Each system is much like an inverted, rootless tree, with trunk emerging at the nipple. Just under the nipple, each of the 15 to 20 trunks widens to make milk cisterns. The branches of the tree are ducts for the transport and storage of milk, and in the leaves are the cells where milk is produced.

Until puberty the milk tree is but a stunted version of its later splendor. Then, as ovaries begin to function, they produce two hormones. One of them, estrogen, prods the development and growth of the duct system. The other, progesterone, stimulates the growth and proliferation of the milk-producing cells. By their action these hormones sculpture the breast to adult proportions.

Visible signs of this internal activity go on for several years. The budding breast is at first a small projecting cone. Then, as glandular tissue proliferates, a protective fat cover is laid over it. Gradually the nipple enlarges to fit an infant mouth, and a pigmented zone (the areola) is laid down around it. The areola is richly equipped with sebaceous (fat) glands to prevent drying and cracking when a baby nurses.

Pregnancy sets off another chain of events timed with hairline precision. For the tasks that lie ahead, the breast starts enlarging as early as the second month. The areola begins to darken; this in itself is an indicator of pregnancy.

For two to four days after the mother is delivered of a baby, her breasts secrete a yellowish, viscous, nonnutritive liquid called colostrum. This is mildly laxative and clears mucus and other waste from the infant's digestive tract. There is also evidence that colostrum contains antibodies that protect the baby against disease in its first days on earth.

For the first few days the newborn infant loses weight; it must have nourishment or die. It is at this juncture that the mother's pituitary gland begins secreting prolactin, the all-important "mother love" hormone which starts the milk-production process. Prolactin has a number of remarkable effects. It is thought to repress the sex urge and often suppresses menstruation. So long as prolactin is produced and nursing continues, the probability of conception is decreased. This is nature's method of seeing that pregnancies don't develop too close together.

The milk that breasts produce is miraculous: chemists have never been able to duplicate it. It is exactly tailored to meet the needs of the infant, whatever the species. Thus, walrus milk contains 12 times the fat of human milk—to provide the fat layer that will protect the young from frigid waters. A calf nearly doubles its birth weight in 60 days, compared with 120 days for human infants. To meet the demands made by this rapid growth, a cow's milk contains twice the protein, four times the calcium, five times the phosphorus of human milk.

The exact means by which the breast produces milk remains one of the mysteries of science. There is but one raw material it could draw on—blood—and the conversion of blood into milk is a stupendous chemical achievement. Estimates indicate that 400 ounces of blood must circulate through breasts to make a single ounce of milk! The components of blood are totally unlike those of milk: sugary glucose in blood, for example, is only distantly related to lactose in milk. The amino acids in blood are far removed from the complex proteins in milk. And the same is true of fatty acids in blood and fats in milk.

Breasts have the remarkable ability of stepping up activity to meet the needs of a growing infant. The few ounces of milk a day produced initially are sufficient for a seven-pound baby. But as the infant grows, the breasts keep producing milk equal to his food requirements—finally producing a quart or more a day.

Nature has contrived to make nursing a highly pleasurable experience for all animals, and for most women. But for this, many animals might abandon their young. A gentle sensual pleasure may result from stimulation of the nipple by the sucking of the infant and from the rhythmic contractions of the uterus caused by hormonal action during nursing. These contractions help to shrink the enlarged womb to normal pear-size. When a child is weaned, the breast is informed by some chemical magic that further milk production is not needed. Milk is permitted to stagnate, and the lactating breast dries up.

In light of the complex workings of the female breast, it is not surprising that the organ should cause occasional trouble. The main danger is cancer—indeed, the breast is the commonest site of cancer in the female. But if women would take the simplest precautions to detect the cancer in its earliest stage, it need not be fatal for most. Teaching women to examine their own breasts offers the best hope of controlling breast disease.

It is curious that primitive people seem to have come closer than civilized societies to a true appreciation of the function of this wondrous organ. To them, the freely displayed breast is not a sex symbol. It is not a cause for ogling—but rather a mark of womanliness to be accepted matter-of-factly, the provider of food on which all mammalian life depends.

A MEDICAL-school class was asked to name five reasons why mother's milk is better for babies than cow's milk. One student wrote:
1. It's faster.
2. It's cleaner.
3. It's safer; the cat can't get it.
4. Easier to handle when traveling.
5. Comes in more attractive containers.

Bosom Worship

by Goodrich C. Schauffler, M.D.

In the course of my work as a gynecologist, I have become increasingly aware of a sort of hysteria which is affecting women in general, and which has become particularly serious in its grasp upon teen-agers and younger married women. This is an exaggerated interest in the female bosom. The trend, stimulated by the press, the movies, TV and radio, is so strong that it is fast becoming a serious problem in a specialized medical practice.

It is not so much that this bosom-consciousness sometimes leads to serious sex complications. What worries most physicians is that the breasts are becoming overemphasized symbols of sex, and that their splendid biological purpose is rapidly falling into the discard. The fact that about 65 percent of our babies today are bottle-fed proves that breast nursing is becoming a lost art. This is so in spite of the almost universal medical opinion that the healthiest babies are breast-fed babies.

Once the symbol of motherhood, the breast has come to be regarded by many young girls as the prime indicator of their sex potential. From the business of attracting a boy friend in grade school to getting dates or even a husband in later life, bosom-consciousness is becoming too deeply intrenched in teen-agers' thinking. In "the good old days" there was such a thing as modesty, which seems less common today. From five to six, our cute little would-be ballet dancers and drum majorettes begin to worry about these matters and by twelve or thirteen have achieved an impressive mass awareness of bosom appeal. To see striplings devoting themselves to bust-development programs may seem to have a humorous aspect; it might, indeed, be funny if so many young girls and women were not so serious about it.

I have seen children of ten and eleven in my office so concerned about breast development that they are wearing miniature falsies. Little girls with real or fancied breast irregularities have actually become psychiatric cases, one of my patients even attempting suicide. Such serious cases are rare, of course, but they are sufficiently frequent to indicate that an abnormal emphasis is being placed upon these matters at an abnormal age.

The increasingly common advertisements for drugs offering hope to frustrated women and the endless variety of foam-rubber substitutes on the market indicate the extent of bosom worship in our culture. Any physician can tell you that two out of three of our women already adequately equipped by nature are supplementing their chest contours by the use of falsies. And far too many adopt such misguided procedures as plastic surgery, paraffin injections and other unnatural means of tampering with their figures.

A deplorable phase of this whole matter is in the activities of the press, movies, radio and TV. Jokes and innuendoes are made about the breasts with frightening regularity. One magazine recently made a survey of its risqué humor. Those items having the bosom theme exceeded all other types; nudity was a close second. A temperate or sensible use of such material is acceptable and amusing, but such exaggeration and reiteration—a continuous idiotic striptease—is unwholesome and, not infrequently, harmful.

That woman was made for motherhood more essentially than for the satisfaction of her own or the male's sexual desires has become an almost forgotten aphorism. The increased antagonism to breast nursing by young mothers is part of this lopsided modern emphasis on the nonreproductive sexual role of women. The reason usually given for the decline in breast feeding is that young mothers are too lazy or too unwilling to bind themselves to their babies' needs, lest the social program be interfered with. But I am afraid that the current esthetic objection to breast feeding—defensible or not—has a great deal to do with the matter.

Many women obviously fear that breast nursing will destroy the shapeliness, and therefore the esthetic appeal, of the bosom. This, of course, is not true. Far from being a harmful influence, normal nursing can be shown to contribute often and substantially to breast contours. Frequently our flat-chested young patients, distressed by their boyish figures, have added a full size to the bra after nursing a first baby.

Nursing one or two lusty infants is better for the health and elastic quality of the breast than the unnatural process of tying up the breasts and drying the natural secretions with unnatural hormone pills. Some research gives evidence that failure to use the breast for its biological purpose may predispose to breast cancer. This theory is as yet unproved, but it is straight scientific knowledge that the functional neglect of the breast creates a condition favorable to breast disorders. There is need for a normal demand upon the complicated functional structure of the milk apparatus.

Many mothers hide their real reasons for not nursing their babies by saying they cannot, or that the baby refuses the breast. Actually, a newborn baby has a healthy normal interest in its mother's breast. One of the first things it tries to do is to shove soft and available things into its hungry little mug.

Unsuccessful breast feeding is a typical modern urban problem in the United States and Canada. In most other countries it is a simple, successful process. In modern Sweden some 90 percent of the mothers breast-feed. Mother and baby expect the mother to nurse, and there is milk. Whereupon both mother and baby enjoy this natural, intimate relationship.

Breast feeding as a means to making the baby psychologically "secure" gets a lot of high-falutin' discussion today. I know only that good nursing makes good-natured babies. But perhaps not enough is said about the good effect upon the *mother*.

Nursing releases functional hormones to the entire body as

well as to the uterus and breast. Biologically, this is part of the female cycle. The late Dr. C. Anderson Aldrich emphasized this in an article in *The Journal of the American Medical Association.* "Breast feeding," he said, "is a physiological maturation process for mothers." The reproductive role of the woman is complete only after conception, childbirth and normal lactation have taken place.

Why do so many women refuse to nurse their babies and so cheat themselves of one of the most beautiful physical experiences in life? Because nobody tells them these facts. The magazines and the television shows are too busy glorifying the breast as an externalized sex appendage designed only to attract men.

For the health of the baby, for the health of the mother, for the pleasure of both, the beneficial aspects of breast feeding should be emphasized to the prospective mother. Doctors and hospitals should be less anxious to thwart the desire of many mothers who really want to breast-feed their babies. Writes Dr. Niles Newton, of the Jefferson Hospital, Philadelphia, "If institutions and physicians would stop promoting feeding methods that cause lactation failure, stop education for artificial feeding and stop forcing early weaning on mothers who enjoy breast feeding, there would be many more contented mothers and babies."

As for husbands, there is many a man still left in this world who is proud of his nursing wife. He looks upon her, with their baby at her breast, as the most beautiful madonna in the world. The role of motherhood is spiritual; no man denies it. In spite of all the cheap and unwholesome sex fetish about the bosom, no woman should fear the loss of her husband's love or desire as a result of breast nursing.

The curves and lines and warmth and beauty of the female body are God's gift, and they are all the more beautiful when they are understood—and employed—in the role intended for them: motherhood.

❦

Breast-Fed Is Best Fed

by Eleanor Lake

Breast feeding, once as outmoded as the bustle, is fortunately on its way back. Today, many hospitals are trying to help mothers to breast-feed. Such hospitals now send three quarters of all their babies home at the breast. Some permit the mothers to keep their babies in the same room at all times, rather than have them delivered from the nurseries at regularized intervals. This is in keeping with the theory of breast feeding "on demand"—whenever the baby is inclined.

Babies have always obstinately preferred their own mother to any cow, however contented. But for some years in the 1930s and '40s they had to take a bottle and like it. Busy hospitals preferred to run through a crop of newborns on a routine "house formula" delivered on a four-hour schedule, instead of encouraging the time-consuming art of breast feeding. Doctors have found formulas, routines and charts the easiest way to get an anxious young mother started with a new baby. And mothers often haven't been told the importance to their own well-being of completing the complex reproductive process which sets mammals apart from lower forms of life.

It was big news, about a decade ago, that leading hospitals—from Lying-In in Boston to Franklin in San Francisco—were promoting old-fashioned breast feeding. A high-powered list of doctors, including Benjamin Spock and Milton Senn, have publicized the fact that mothers and babies both profit from the intimacy and warmth that somehow was frozen out of too many streamlined "scientific" nurseries.

Breast-fed babies gain more consistently, have fewer allergies, a longer natural immunity to many diseases, notably fewer skin and digestive disorders. Later on, the breast-fed baby seems less likely to develop into a "feeding problem." Breast-fed babies associate food, from the start, with love and cuddling. They think food is fun.

Are mothers "tied down" by breast feeding? "No," chorus a group of wives of Yale graduate students interviewed· on the subject. Nursing, they say, is so much easier than bottle feeding that there is no comparison. No trotting around on a cold night to get a bottle and warm it for a screaming baby. No fussing with sterilizers and slippery nipples. Nursing babies eat a little oftener than bottle babies—but they are so much more contented in between. "I take my son with me on picnics or to visit Grandma," said one wife, "without having to lug a whole drugstore with me."

The women in recent years who haven't been able to nurse were probably victims of an environment that has been hard on nursing and, in fact, on motherhood in general. Nursing mothers need what mothers have always needed: rest, simple and nourishing food and a joyful sense of their importance as mothers. Hectic headlines and anxieties of all kinds are a bad environment for nursing.

Mothers who have been brought up to believe that a clever girl can toss off a few babies while running the League of Women Voters, redecorating her house and giving the smartest dinners in town are due for a severe inner struggle when they try to slow down to the peaceful rhythm of breast feeding. A woman who can't decide whether she was meant to be a mother, glamour girl or career woman will solve her inner conflict by having no milk or else by finding breast feeding painful and difficult.

Mothers should insist on knowing what is to be done to help them before they enter a hospital; when possible, they should find a hospital that takes a genuine interest in nursing.

Feeding on "demand" is back in full force—the way all babies were brought up until the last fifty years. The mother feeds her baby when he is hungry, instead of letting him "cry it out" until the clock says feeding time. Hunger is actual pain to a tiny baby, and not all babies have the same inner alarm clock. Some get hungry on the usual four-hour shift. Some are hungry every three hours. A few are ravenous the first few weeks, on no apparent schedule at all. Eventually they hit their own rhythm.

There are two advantages in letting a small baby nurse more or less at will. One is that this kind of nursing is very helpful in "bringing in" a mother's milk. Short periods of frequent nursing produce more milk and fewer sore nipples than an ironclad four-hour schedule on which many hungry infants tear at their mothers' breasts like baby tigers.

The other reason is deeply important—and applies to bottle babies as well. Life is a startling and even terrifying adventure to a newborn baby. To make him feel that this new world is a friendly and welcoming place, he needs a great deal of warm and intimate contact with his mother. During his first few weeks, especially, he wants the smell and feel of his mother, the closeness of her arms. Nursed and cuddled when he is hungry or upset, he begins to feel that the world is a pretty fine place after all. Soon he is quite ready to coöperate when family convenience says dinner at six or nap at two.

Like any other career, real motherhood demands a great deal of time at first. But it pays off a thousandfold later on, in happy and responsible children and in mature, confident mothers, enjoying their motherhood.

Pregnant Moments

A NUMBER of magazines and newspapers have had articles on the benefits of breast feeding. When I asked one of my expectant patients if she intended to breast-feed her infant, she replied, "I can't decide—though I know it's the latest thing."   —M.D. in *Medical Economics*

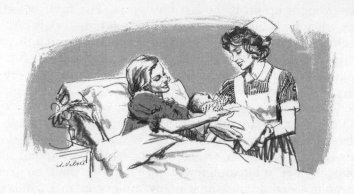

Childbirth without Fear

A CONDENSATION FROM THE ORIGINAL BOOK

by Grantly Dick Read, M.D.

The late Grantly Dick Read, author of this absorbing and controversial book, was an English obstetrician with a Cambridge University degree, a Harley Street practice, and a private clinic in a London industrial suburb. Natural childbirth was a cause that Dr. Grantly Dick Read preached for many years. An earlier volume on the subject almost ruined his practice. "People ran from me like scalded cats," he said.

Dr. Henricus Stander, Professor of Obstetrics and Gynecology at Cornell Medical College, New York, observed: "Dr. Dick Read advocates what is practiced by every first-class obstetrician. His book can do a great deal of good by reminding us that if the expectant mother sees her doctor often, and early, there is no need for fear; and by stressing the fact that every doctor must get his patient's confidence. There can be no harm in doing as Dr. Dick Read suggests, but there is always the possibility of harm, especially to the baby, in the use of anesthetics, no one of which is as yet ideal for all cases of childbirth."

I often wonder if a woman in Whitechapel whose name I have long since forgotten has ever realized the far-reaching influence of a casual remark she made to me.

I had plowed through mud and rain on my bicycle between two and three in the morning, and came to a low hovel by the railway arches. Having groped up a dark staircase, I opened the door of a room about ten feet square. There was a pool of water lying on the floor; the window was broken; rain was pouring in; the bed had no proper covering and was kept up at one end by a sugar box. My patient lay covered only with sacks and an old black skirt. The room was lit by one candle stuck in the top of a beer bottle on the mantel. A neighbor had brought in a jug of water and a basin; I had to provide my own soap and towel. In spite of this setting I soon became conscious of a quiet kindliness in the atmosphere.

In due course, the baby was born. There was no fuss or noise, and only one slight note of dissension: I had tried to persuade my patient to let me give her some chloroform. She refused kindly yet firmly. I asked her why. She did not answer at once, but looked from the old woman who had been assisting to the window through which was bursting the first light of dawn; then shyly she turned to me and said, "It didn't hurt. It wasn't meant to, was it, Doctor?"

For months afterward, as I sat with women who appeared to be in the terror and agony of childbirth, that sentence came drumming back into my ears—"It wasn't meant to, was it, Doctor?"—until finally, even through my conservative mind, I began to realize that in the normal course of health there is no physiological function which gives rise to pain, that childbirth is a primitive function intended by nature to be painless.

Why then should some women suffer and others be apparently free from pain? Was the painfulness of labor responsible for the woman's emotional state, or was her emotional state largely responsible for the pain?

During the last seventeen years I have tried to explain the causes of pain in civilized labor, and also to demonstrate that those evil causes may to some extent be removed. Obviously this explanation applies only to normal and uncomplicated labor, but as over 95 percent of all labors are normal, its influence may be considerable.

The more cultured the races of man have become, the more dogmatic have they been in pronouncing childbirth to be a painful and dangerous ordeal. From a very early age, girls are made aware of this accepted teaching. Their fears and anxious anticipation give rise to protective tensions in the mind, and in the muscles of the body as well.

Various muscles govern the motions of the uterus. One set, the first uncontrollable contractions of which tell a woman that her labor has begun, gradually squeezes the unborn child from the womb. A second set, which guards the exit from the womb, should be relaxed and free from tension during normal, natural labor. If a woman's mind, conditioned since childhood by gossip and mythology, interprets the new sensations caused by the first contractions as "pain," the fancied and expected "pain" results in fear. The fear results in muscular tension, which in turn causes genuine pain, all too often prolonged labor, and unnecessary anesthesia.

Therefore, fear, pain and tension are the three evils which are not normal to the natural design, but which have been introduced in the course of civilization. If pain, fear and tension go hand in hand, then it must be possible to eliminate pain by relieving tension and overcoming fear.

Every clinician knows that suggestion will produce pain. For instance, inquire of a woman in labor where the last pain hurt her; agree that it was a bad pain; put your hand on the uterus and feel it contract, then say, "Now, it's going to hurt. Try and tell me when the pain is at its height. Grip my hand; set your teeth; concentrate on your pain; close your eyes, and suffer!"

"Be brave, darling"—said by the pale, tense mother as she leaves the room—is an excellent pain producer.

"Don't worry, now; plenty of anesthetic when it gets too bad. But you must put up with it as long as you can"—from the cheerful medical man in confirmation of pain.

So let fear creep in to join forces with pain, and by propaganda, deceit and inhumanity, these twin enemies of childbirth destroy the structure and mechanism of labor.

Young women hear about childbirth firsthand from their friends, relations and others who have borne children. It is strange how many women delight in recalling the horrors of their own experiences, and exaggerate by such phrases as, "My doctor said I was one of the worst cases he had ever attended."

I can never forget a stern matron, the tyrannical empress of a family of eight, who exercised her sway over half a county from the baronial mansion of her patient husband's ancestors. Into my consulting room she led, literally by the hand, a fat, red-faced girl of twenty-four, placed her in the chair by my desk, drew herself up to about five feet ten, pulled down her Norfolk jacket with a jerk, shook her neck a little farther out of a stiff collar, and without greeting me opened the conversation in a low, dramatic voice:

"I have brought my daughter to you; I am afraid she has conceived."

I took a hurried glance at the girl's left hand, and was relieved to see a wedding ring. The mother then went on to explain that she had told her daughter all about it, and that she hoped, when her time came, that her daughter would conduct herself with unflinching courage in keeping with the family tradition.

Two months later, the girl had a miscarriage. Two years later she was being treated for alcoholism. I have since heard she is divorced. Can anyone doubt that fear was at the root of all her trouble?

Books, movies, radio, newspapers—all dangle fear-producing presentations before a woman's eyes. Is it not essential, then, that we should create by education the true and natural happiness of motherhood? The mental picture of her anticipated experience should be the image of all that is beautiful in the fulfillment of love. In peacefulness of mind and body she should patiently await the child whose greeting cry imprints such joy that for all time she can return to that sweet music and live again the crowning moment of her life.

And so it is with labor. It is my belief that there is not one feature of normal pregnancy which should in any way mar the health of a woman, or do anything but increase her happiness and her physical stability for all time. If fear can be eliminated, pain will cease. In a long series of cases over the past ten or fifteen years, means have been devised to eliminate fear. In varying degrees, pain has been conspicuous by its absence. I am prepared to state that in the not very far distant future the inevitability of painful childbirth will be a relic of the past.

It is impossible to protect women from fear of childbirth if they are ignorant of the truth. We do not fear facts, but doubts and uncertainties.

Women have never been taught the rudiments of childbearing; when the primitive mind was undisturbed by terrifying associations, such knowledge was unneccessary. No effort has been made to counteract the medieval propaganda. The wonders of reproduction are withheld.

The extent to which some of my patients have been unacquainted with the simplest facts is almost unbelievable. I have known married women who, although well advanced in pregnancy, believed that their baby would arrive by way of the umbilicus. I have made an effort, therefore, to educate women in the facts. I unfold the story of pregnancy and birth gradually as the months go by, giving a general and concise account of the process of development. Before the baby quickens, the mother should be warned that the first faint throbbing is the movement of her child exercising its muscles. I give the mother a stethoscope so that she can listen to the child's heartbeat.

My initial efforts—to make childbirth the natural affair it was intended to be—soon received encouragement, for many women instinctively felt the truth and disbelieved in the necessity for suffering. But that did not appear to be enough. Some method had to be found to overcome this main weapon of the enemy, which was tension. So the practice of physical relaxation was introduced. If the body is completely relaxed, it is impossible to entertain the emotion of fear.

What is meant by relaxation? As an example, as only the first step in a long process, I tell the patient: "Just lie absolutely still and loose on the sofa, and let me have your right arm and let me have it entirely; that is to say, do not take any notice of what I am doing to it and do not try to help me, because any effort you make to help me is going to do more harm than good." I then take hold of the elbow and the wrist and raise the arm just off the sofa. I tell her I want her hand to drop so that there is no life in it at all. It is extraordinary how many people cannot drop their hand; they let their hand slowly fall, and then wiggle a finger or waggle a thumb. This is practiced until complete relaxation of the hand is obtained. The instruction is then extended to other groups of muscles.

Relaxation must be recognized as a necessary part of natural labor, and it should be accompanied by a disassociation of the mind from any active interest in the uterine function. How often have I said to a woman in labor: "You can do nothing to help yet; allow your uterus to get on with its work undisturbed by your inquisitive interest. If you interfere, it will resent it, and hurt you. There is no hurry; the door will open." Almost invariably that advice, when acted upon, results in the relief of pain.

A patient may wish to hold your hand; she may wish to lie with her head on your arm; but most certainly she desires the unwavering strength of the confidence that you share in the success of her trial. And trial indeed it is; for in labor a woman shows her true colors—the patient and the impatient, the courageous and the "gutless." The "I-can-and-I-will" women and the "Oh-please-I-can't-and-what's-more-I-won't" women require different handling, but with one accord they seek comfort in the support of their guide in labor. There is no limit to a woman's courage if you give her faith.

After no more than two years, not only had the results of practicing relaxation established my own belief in it, but—what was far more important—the large majority of the women whose labors had been conducted in accordance with it had an entirely new attitude toward childbirth. They often held the apparatus of anesthesia in their hands with full knowledge of its use, but refused to take it. They were able to differentiate between hard work and pain.

Of course, no woman should be allowed to bear more discomfort than she is willing to bear for her child's sake, and every method discovered by science should be used to prevent such suffering. More women demand anesthesia as an escape from fear than from pain. In the absence of fear, pain indicates abnormality, and should be relieved. But in normal labor, properly conducted, a high percentage of women do not wish for anesthetic.

I emphatically do not subscribe to the "anesthetics-for-all" movement as many obstetricians do. It is a crime to insist upon dulling the consciousness of the natural mother who desires above all things to be aware of the final reward of her efforts—a reward which is happiness and satisfaction too intense for adequate expression. Furthermore, no anesthetics satisfactory for all cases have yet been discovered. Some interfere with the natural forces of labor. Others are not safe for the mother or baby.

Obstetricians have been educated to believe that all labors are painful; they have made a routine of using some analgesic, or anesthetic, whether labor is normal or not; they have made a practice of disbelieving a woman who says that it is not painful.

I picture a crowd of men in white coats and large horn-rimmed glasses, seeking fame and fortune by the searching for a weapon with which to protect all women from an enemy which in 95 percent of cases did not exist. But the more awkward the means of administration or the longer the name, so much more likely was it that fame might be achieved. Simple inhalation of gas, ether or chloroform was soon left behind. Drugs were put under the skin, into the stomach, into veins, deep into muscles, into the rectum, into the spinal cord, into the sacral nerves—in fact, anywhere that things can be put into the human body.

How long, oh, how long will this nonsense go on? Surely it is safer to introduce a mental process than a dangerous drug. The best—and safest—anesthetic is a controlled and educated mind; the next best is the combined use of light-inhalation anesthesia and "suggestion."

I do not hesitate to record that so startling were the results of suggestion when I first employed it in the practice of natural childbirth that I became suspicious of myself, although I have never had any knowledge of mesmerism or hypnotism. Consequently I consulted one of the greatest authorities upon these subjects, and asked him to examine me and my methods. The examination was most carefully made, and I was assured that there was no relation whatever between hypnotism and the application of relaxation in obstetrics.

If their fears are destroyed and they have a calm understanding of the conduct of their own labor, very few women need help either by suggestion or drug.

Again I must stress that I do not wish to encourage anyone to feel that relaxation is the whole secret of natural childbirth. It is not really effective unless a woman understands the phenomena of labor.

I am frequently told by obstetricians, "But, my dear sir, I simply have not time to do all this." My reply is that nothing should be allowed to rob a woman in labor of the undivided attention of the doctor in whom she has placed her confidence. Obstetricians are sometimes busy men, but there is no reason why busy men should not be obstetricians!

Childbirth is a normal and natural function. Its ultimate reward is out of all proportion to the sacrifices incurred. In the natural law it is the perfection of womanhood in the great design for continuity of the species. It is the objective of the strongest emotional experiences of human nature. I have witnessed so often the inexplicable transfiguration of women at the time of their babies' arrival that I have been led, as usual, to ask: Can it be that the Creator intended to draw mothers nearest to Himself at the moment of love's fulfillment? Can it be that it is the natural reward of those who perfect their ultimate purpose in life?

The more I ponder these things, the surer I am of the answer to the question put by that woman in Whitechapel many years ago. *No, it was not meant to hurt.*

Truths and Untruths about Miscarriage

by Edith L. Potter, M.D.

~ ❦ ~

ACH DAY some 2500 American women pregnant for less than six months lose their babies through miscarriage. Indeed, death before birth is the commonest death of all. Now, country-wide research is going forward to curb this tragic wastage of a million unborn babies' lives each year.

I have been concerned with the miscarriage problem, medically called "spontaneous abortion," for a quarter of a century. As a woman, I know the sadness of a hopeful married couple when miscarriage occurs. As a doctor, I know the forebodings concerning future pregnancies. Let me provide a word of reassurance:

Most miscarriages are *not* the result of something seriously wrong with the mother or father; they are the result of bad luck, which is unlikely to strike the same couple more than once. Of the 2500 women a day who lose their babies, at least 4 out of 5 can look forward to an uneventful pregnancy and successful birth the next time.

There are many causes of miscarriage. Sometimes, for example, one occurs because the fertilized egg or ovum has the bad fortune to implant itself in a part of the mother's uterus not properly prepared for a pregnancy. When this happens, the pregnancy may continue for a few weeks or months; then nature erases her mistake, and a miscarriage follows. There is every reason in such cases to be confident that next time everything will be normal.

Sometimes the male sperm reaches the egg at the wrong moment. One egg leaves a woman's ovaries each month, and moves down the tube toward the uterus. To give rise to a pregnancy, the male sperm must reach the egg within approximately twenty-four hours of the egg's departure from the ovary. If sperm and egg meet close to this deadline, a pregnancy may begin—but the likelihood of miscarriage is high. Again, simply bad luck.

Some physicians seek to reassure a woman who has miscarried by telling her that it is all for the best: the egg, they say, probably wasn't a good one and the baby might have been defective had it survived. Far from comforting a woman, this theory often arouses new anxieties. She may say to herself: There is something wrong with my genes; perhaps my next baby will be born with a serious defect.

Having carefully examined more than 1500 embryos from miscarriages, I am quite sure that miscarriages are rarely, if ever, due to "bad genes." Almost all can be attributed to factors which are not inheritable. Studies have established this basic fact: *Even a long series of miscarriages does not significantly increase the chance that a woman's next baby will be born with a defect.*

We have also learned of late that, contrary to an old wives' tale still widely believed, a mother's activities during pregnancy rarely cause damage or miscarriage. An unborn baby is "packaged" in a manner insulating him from the rough-and-tumble of the mother's daily life.

A study which dramatically illustrated the effectiveness of this protective packaging concerned more than 400 wives of men stationed at Robins Air Force Base in Georgia. During their pregnancies these women had traveled an average of 2000 miles each, by car, plane, train and bus. Some had crossed the continent in jouncing trucks; some had driven to Alaska and back. Five had been in serious smashups; one was catapulted out of a car. Twenty had been extricated from houses demolished by a tornado. Yet the miscarriage rate among these much buffeted women was no higher than would be expected among women who spent their entire pregnancies placidly sewing little garments in their own homes.

As a result of such studies, obstetricians increasingly are telling their pregnant patients that they can continue to swim, play tennis, do housework or work at most jobs as long as they feel comfortable and don't get overtired.

What of sexual intercourse during pregnancy? Many a woman, convinced that intercourse during pregnancy was responsible for her miscarriage, is prey to deep feelings of guilt. In the overwhelming majority of cases, such feelings are absolutely groundless. Almost all obstetricians are agreed that intercourse during pregnancy is normal and harmless, and advise against it only during the very last weeks of pregnancy. If a woman has lost two or three babies in succession, however, she may be advised not to have intercourse during pregnancy.

The commonest symptoms of something wrong during pregnancy are bleeding and abdominal cramps. These symptoms, known as "threatened abortion," are perhaps commonest between the tenth and fourteenth weeks, but they may occur earlier. Whenever they occur, a woman should phone her physician immediately and follow his advice precisely.

Threatened abortion is a serious matter. Yet roughly one half of all women with threatened abortion proceed to carry their babies for the full term, and deliver healthy babies. Many physicians prescribe complete bed rest in such cases, and this may be the safest course. However, one recent study of 1797 women with symptoms of threatened abortion showed that the 464 who were permitted to resume moderate activities after the symptoms subsided did about as well as the 1333 who were kept in bed.

All in all, research into the problem of miscarriage shows the wisdom of a promising new policy in medicine: *The time to save an unborn baby's life is before the pregnancy begins.* Just as babies have benefited from the improved prenatal care most mothers now receive, so a good many miscarriages can be prevented by a prepregnancy examination. This examination may reveal some problem in the uterus which surgery can correct. It may reveal that a woman who has miscarried has a previously unsuspected deficiency of some hormone—perhaps that secreted by the thyroid gland. The prescription of a thyroid supplement may help her to carry her next baby for the full nine months.

In the vast majority of cases, a prepregnancy examination turns up no one physical factor responsible for previous miscarriages. Obstetricians therefore concentrate on helping the woman—and her husband—to attain the best possible state of overall physical and emotional health, in anticipation of the next pregnancy. Good nutrition is stressed—a point which should be remembered by all young women.

The method of treatment of a woman who has had several miscarriages may vary widely. Some obstetricians report excellent results with progesterone or other hormones. Some cases respond to a particular combination of vitamins. Obstetricians who use these and other types of treatment may succeed in breaking the miscarriage habit among four patients out of five.

Such diverse treatments have one common factor: the obstetricians' great confidence in them. Confidence is contagious, and patients face their next pregnancy without the fears which formerly plagued them. Can it be that anxiety or fear may cause miscarriage? A number of outstanding obstetricians are beginning to think so.

However, contrary to views once common, sudden emotional shock is rarely responsible for miscarriage. Many women suffer such shocks during pregnancy without ill effect. A husband may desert; their other children may fall ill; death may claim someone they love; they may witness some catastrophic accident—all without any damage to their unborn babies. The kinds of strain which may lead to miscarriage are the chronic, nagging, day-in-day-out problems which breed anxiety, resentment, guilt feelings, lack of confidence.

No obstetrician today believes that we have found all the facts about miscarriage and its prevention. With this as one factor in mind, scientists of sixteen major medical centers from Boston to Los Angeles have launched a collaborative "perinatal research program," financed by a four-million-dollar grant from the National Institutes of Health. This study of the problems of pregnancy and child health is following more than 40,000 women throughout their pregnancies, and their babies for several years thereafter. From this unprecedented long-range research, it is hoped that substantial additional insight into the miscarriage problem will be achieved.

℘

Birth Control

by Albert Q. Maisel

℘

THE U.S. Food and Drug Administration has "approved" the marketing—for birth-control purposes—of a synthetic-hormone drug called by the trade name Enovid.

It was a routine action, for the law requires the FDA to permit the marketing of any drug as soon as adequate clinical tests demonstrate that the new product will be safe to use when properly prescribed and taken as directed. In effect, the FDA merely declared, "This steroid hormone will not harm women who swallow one ten-milligram pill every day."

Yet these pills are not just one more contraceptive. They are the first of a family of birth-control chemicals entirely different from anything ever before available, for they temporarily suppress the reproductive process.

Up to now, all the medically approved birth-control methods

have aimed at preventing male sperm cells from reaching the female ovum, or egg cell. Even the rhythm method of family limitation seeks to prevent sperm from reaching an ovum receptive to fertilization. It does so by restricting sexual relations to those days when a wife is presumed to be infertile because one egg cell has lost its ability to be fertilized and her ovaries have not yet matured another egg cell to replace it.

In the U.S.A., Canada and Europe, the conventional contraceptive methods have been used increasingly during recent decades. But they have proved to be far from completely effective. A 1957 survey of 1165 American couples, for example, showed that even the most reliable of contraceptive devices had proved only 72 to 80 percent efficient.

In crowded, underdeveloped countries such as Ceylon, India and Indonesia, conventional contraceptives have proved almost total failures. Uneducated women find it impossible to perform the mathematical calculation of the menstrual cycle essential for the success of the rhythm method. The proper use of conventional contraceptive devices becomes incredibly difficult where there are no sanitary facilities and where entire families sleep in one room. And countless millions are too poor even to dream of meeting the cost of contraceptive supplies.

Aware of these drawbacks, many physicians and scientists have long sought to develop a birth-control method so safe, simple and inexpensive that it could be used effectively by even the most poverty-stricken and least educated.

Meanwhile, biochemists, endocrinologists and gynecologists were studying a different problem. Far from trying to prevent conception, they were seeking methods of overcoming the infertility which keeps 10 percent of married couples who desperately want children from achieving parenthood. Gradually these studies led to a vast increase in our knowledge of the intricate processes of human reproduction.

And, paradoxically, it was this new knowledge that led to a birth-control breakthrough. By 1950, enough had been learned of the physiology of conception for scientists to be able to spot more than a dozen weak links in the reproductive chain. Some were points at which nature *normally* made conception a temporary impossibility. Others were instances in which some malfunction, in the male or the female, caused either temporary or permanent sterility. But, in theory at least, each of these weak links represents a point at which deliberate control of the reproductive process might be effected.

One of the first to explore these new possibilities was a biologist, Gregory Pincus, codirector of the famed Worcester Foundation for Experimental Biology. Dr. Pincus had won worldwide recognition as a leader in research on the steroid hormones (the chemical messengers which play complex governing roles in the process of reproduction). Early in 1951 he set out to see whether one of these hormones—progesterone—might be the key to a deliberate physiological control of fertility.

It was already known that as soon as a fertilized ovum begins its growth in the womb, nature steps up its output of progesterone. This in turn causes the ovaries to cease releasing additional ova throughout the period of pregnancy. It was also known that progesterone was nontoxic and therefore safe to use as a drug. Physicians, in fact, have been using it for years in massive injections to prevent miscarriages among so-called "habitual aborters."

But injections would never do as a birth-control measure. Dr. Pincus's first experiments, therefore, were designed to see whether orally administered progesterone would retain its ovulation-suppressing power. Female rabbits were fed varying doses of the hormone and, twenty-four hours later, placed with males in mating cages. Whenever the oral dose exceeded 5 milligrams, ovulation was halted and not one of these female rabbits produced a litter.

From rabbits, Pincus and his coworker, Dr. M. C. Chang, turned to laboratory rats because they normally ovulate in cycles similar to those of humans. When the females were fed 5 or more milligrams of progesterone, the single dose was sufficient to suppress ovulation for an entire cyclic period.

But would the same effect occur if women took progesterone

by mouth? To find out, Pincus turned to Dr. John Rock, Clinical Professor of Gynecology at Harvard and director of the fertility clinic at the Free Hospital for Women in the Boston suburb of Brookline. Rock's aim was not birth control, but a means of establishing fertility in his inexplicably infertile patients. For some of these women it seemed that a "make-believe" pregnancy (in that the woman would cease to ovulate), which was established by oral progesterone, might be of help. Of course, ovulation would be suppressed throughout the period of treatments. Thus, the biologist and the physician joined forces.

To twenty-nine barren women Dr. Rock supplied progesterone pills. To avoid an undesired suppression of menstruation, he instructed his patients to interrupt medication after the twenty-fifth day of each treated cycle and not to resume taking the pills until the fifth day after their menstrual periods began. For one month, then two months, then three, tests showed that progesterone, taken orally, halted ovulation in most of these women. Then, with Pincus's theory vindicated, the medication was stopped and Dr. Rock waited to see whether the effect he had hoped for would occur. Soon, he, too, had cause for hurrahs. For among these infertile patients, upon whom all previous therapy had failed, four became pregnant within the next four months.

Now Dr. Pincus paused to review what had been proved. Progesterone pills definitely could suppress ovulation and thus induce temporary sterility. But the drug had to be given in expensive, gigantic doses—up to 300 milligrams a day—to achieve the desired effect. And even then, it worked only 75 to 80 percent of the time. Obviously, this wasn't *the* foolproof birth-control pill that Pincus had been seeking.

So the hunt began again, this time for a steroid that could do what progesterone had done—but do it consistently, at lower dosages. For more than two years the lights burned late in the laboratories at Worcester as Pincus and Chang tested more than 175 hormones. The safest and most powerful, they found, was a synthetic hormone which was later named Enovid—short for 17-alpha-ethinyl-estraenolone. On Dr. Rock's women volunteers, this worked at a dosage only one thirtieth of that required with progesterone. A 10-milligram pill, taken daily from the fifth to the twenty-fifth day of the menstrual cycle, invariably prevented ovulation where progesterone had apparently failed in one case out of five. When treatment was discontinued, all the volunteers promptly resumed their normal pattern of ovulation. And, again, a number found their fertility restored and became pregnant.

But only a mass clinical test among women without the cultural and educational advantages of the Boston volunteers could prove whether the new pills were a practical replacement for conventional contraceptives. The chance for such a test came early in 1956. Dr. Edris Rice-Wray, medical director of Puerto Rico's Family Planning Association, sought out women in a slum-clearance development near San Juan who had already given birth to a number of children and who, for a time at least, wanted no more. As word spread, Dr. Rice-Wray found herself besieged by many times the 100 applicants she had originally planned to treat.

By January 1957, the experimental group had grown to 221. By November 1958, 438 women had used the pills to prevent ovulation through nearly 5000 monthly cycles. Later projects in Puerto Rico and in Port-au-Prince, Haiti, brought the number of participating women to more than 1200. By the end of 1959, the effectiveness of the new pills had been unequivocally established. Prior to the tests, the pregnancy rate had been over 70 per 100 women per year. But among those who took the tablets faithfully, only one became pregnant while under treatment and there was evidence that she had already been pregnant when her treatment began. Even among those who missed taking up to five pills in any single month, the pregnancy rate still remained under 10 per 100 women per year.

When the San Juan tests were first started, a number of endocrinologists feared that prolonged suppression of ovulation might result in permanent sterility. Fortunately 174 women, who dropped out of the project when they decided that they wanted another baby, provided a perfect test. Once they stopped taking

the pills, pregnancy occurred among these women at a phenomenal rate. Many became pregnant within a month.

Some authorities had feared that the prolonged use of powerful
steroids might endanger health and, particularly, might predispose women to cancer. To check these theoretical possibilities,
the women taking part in the Puerto Rican clinical trials received regular and thorough physical examinations and laboratory tests. No rise in the general disease rate occurred and not a
single case of posttreatment cervical, uterine or breast malignancy
was found among the participating women. "Enovid," Dr. Rock
states, "emphatically has not caused cancer."

Other researchers have observed no pathological effects after
administering much larger doses of Enovid than those used in
Puerto Rico. And still larger doses, given for more than a year
to laboratory animals, likewise failed to cause disease. This evidence of safety, together with the favorable reports of researchers
who used the new hormone in the treatment of menstrual difficulties of thousands of women, provided the basis for the FDA's
approval of the drug for general prescription use as a contraceptive.

In all the clinical trials, about one volunteer in five reported
some nausea, headache, weight gain, dizziness or abdominal
pain, especially during the first month of medication. But experiments using inert placebos in place of the hormone showed that,
in many of these women, the side effects had a psychological
rather than a physical basis.

One remaining drawback of the hormone contraceptive has
been its high cost—about 50 cents per single 10-milligram pill, or
$10 for one month's protection from pregnancy. But in Puerto
Rico the full contraceptive effect has been achieved by several
hundred women using only 5 milligrams, and even as little as
2½ milligrams, per day. At the latter dosage, the monthly
retail cost is $2.50. With mass production, according to Dr.
Lee D. Van Antwerp of G. D. Searle & Company, manufacturers
of Enovid, a further substantial drop in cost may be possible.

Meanwhile, other physiological ways of controlling fertility
are currently being explored. In the Population Council Labora-

tory at the Rockefeller Institute, for example, Drs. Warren O. Nelson, Sheldon J. Segal and other researchers have conducted extensive experiments with a nonsteroid compound which, fed to laboratory rats as late as four days after mating, has halted the development of ova and provided 100-percent prevention of pregnancy. Whether it would work as effectively on women—and without causing untoward side effects—is still to be determined.

In Israel and in India, researchers have been studying the use of compounds that prevent the adherence of an ovum to the wall of the womb, thus halting its further development. Elsewhere, research is being directed toward the suppression of sperm development in men. And still other scientists are seeking to develop a vaccine that would temporarily sterilize either men or women.

Whether these or still other lines of research will produce a contraceptive method as good as—or even better than—the present hormone technique, only time will tell.

East Is East . . .

WITH ITS population problem threatening the nation with slow strangulation, the government of India knows it has to make people realize the advantages of smaller families. But this is not easy when so many cannot read. The Bengal government tried the poster approach. One picture showed a dirty hut filled with ragged children and exhausted parents; the other showed a neat cottage with a happy couple and two well-dressed children. The villagers' response to the good example was: "The poor things! Only two children!"   —Taya Zinkin, *India Changes*

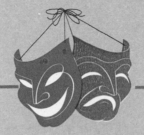

CHAPTER 11

The Body
Battles Stress

WE ALL KNOW about the pace and worry of modern life, but few seem to know what to do about it. Yet the medical world in recent years has turned the spotlight of attention on the effects of stress on the human body, pinpointing it as the crucial element in most of our physical woes. In modern times, we must learn to live—and learn from those who have employed the techniques of modern research to uncover this most elusive truth.

Stress—
the Cause of
All Disease?

by J. D. Ratcliff

The work of a Canadian researcher in a new field of medicine has opened dazzling vistas in medical science. It indicates that there may be common cause for almost all disease, whether it be a heart attack, a mild case of asthma or just the feeling of "being sick." Dr. Hans Selye of Montreal believes the cause is chemical imbalance in the body—*caused by stress.*

"If future events prove this concept correct," says *The Journal of the American Medical Association*, "it will be one of the most significant medical advances of this century." *The Lancet*, a leading British medical journal, agrees.

Reaction to stress, according to Selye's theory, is governed mainly by three tiny glands: the pituitary, which nestles under the brain, and the two adrenals, which sit astride the kidneys. All of them together weigh only about a third of an ounce, yet their unbelievably potent hormones have a huge influence on vital body functions. Selye believes it is the task of the pituitary and adrenal hormones to combat stress and fight off any threat to the body's welfare.

In a hurry-up world, according to Selye, we are subjecting ourselves to too many stresses. We hurry constantly and worry incessantly. The businessman drives himself at his office all day, then worries most of the night. The housewife tries to run her home, maintain a social life and participate in community activities—and at bedtime is so jangled that she needs a sleeping pill.

Glands attempt to adjust to the constant demands of stress. They pour out excess hormones to keep the body going. For a while they succeed. But in the end the defense mechanism itself breaks down. Arteries deteriorate, blood pressure rises, heart disease develops, arthritis strikes. These and other diseases, Selye believes, are all part of the stress picture.

"The *apparent* cause of illness," says Selye, "is often an infection, an intoxication, nervous exhaustion or merely old age. But actually a breakdown of the hormonal-adaptation mechanism appears to be the most common ultimate cause of death." His study of this mechanism, via widespread experiments with animals, set the stage for his far-reaching discoveries.

Austrian-born of a family that has produced doctors for four generations, Hans Selye received his M.D. and Ph.D. from the German University of Prague. Later, when a Rockefeller fellowship brought him to America, he studied at Johns Hopkins University in Baltimore and McGill University in Montreal. Since 1945 he has headed the University of Montreal's Institute of Experimental Medicine and Surgery.

As a medical student he pestered starchy German professors who loved to talk about specific diseases with specific causes, such as pneumonia and the microbe which produces it. "What about *nonspecific* disease?" Selye kept asking. "What about the feeling of just being sick?"

Professors had little patience with such nonsense. But Selye kept at them. Almost all diseases have certain common symptoms: pallor, loss of appetite, loss of weight, for example. "Don't these common symptoms *mean* anything?" he asked. "Don't bother with such things," he was told.

Selye did bother. In 1936, when he was studying at McGill, two female sex hormones were known. Selye thought he was on the point of discovering a third. To test the effects of a new extract he had produced, he shot it into female rats whose ovaries had been removed. He expected autopsy to show changes in the animals' sexual apparatus. Instead, the sight which awaited him was utterly baffling: his rats' adrenal glands were bloated to three times normal size; their lymphatic systems had undergone degeneration; stomachs and intestinal tracts were dotted with ulcers.

Was it toxic material in his chemical juice that was wrecking the insides of the rats? To check, he shot some formaldehyde into a rat. A postmortem showed exactly the same picture: swollen adrenals, ulcers, wrecked lymphatic system. Clearly he was on a false trail in the search for a new hormone.

Then a momentous thought occurred: Would other things besides formaldehyde and his hormone juice wreck rats' insides?

He put caged animals on his windswept laboratory roof. They survived the winter cold for long periods but finally suffered the same kind of internal damage as the others. Next, he wore rats out in motor-driven revolving cages. The same effects occurred again. It seemed that *any* stress to which he subjected the animals produced the same symptoms: bloated adrenals, ulcers, decayed lymphatic system.

Selye thought back to his student days in Prague. What he was now looking at was nonspecific disease—not disease of a single organ, produced by a single factor. Almost any stress seemed to cause the conditions. Stress—could that be the key to everything?

In human beings there were no very good explanations of *why* heart disease strikes millions, *why* hypertension takes such a lethal toll, *why* arthritis and rheumatic fever wreak their devastations. Was it possible that all these things were merely expressions, end results, of stress? Could it be that they resulted from hormonal imbalance within the body? It looked as if this might well be the case. Research would have to be done.

Dr. Frederick G. Banting, the brooding genius who gave the world insulin, was visiting McGill. Selye told him about his experiments and his suspicions that stress might be the cause of many deadly illnesses. Banting listened attentively. "You may have something big," he said. "You will need money to pursue it. I believe I can get you a grant."

The grant came through: $500! It wasn't much, but Selye went ahead with his search, a lone man in a cubbyhole laboratory—one pioneer against traditional medical thinking with its emphasis on specific disease.

The first problem was to find why stress did such dreadful things to rats. Selye thought the pituitary might be responsible. He devised an exquisite technique for removing the gland with a device of his own invention. Then he subjected the pituitary-less animals to cold, heat, fatigue, noise, poisons. With the pituitary gone there was no internal wreckage!

Next he removed adrenals but left the pituitary, and applied similar stresses. This time damage within the animals was small. So the adrenals, too, played a part in what Selye was beginning to call "the stress syndrome."

Gradually the whole picture began to unfold. When an animal was subjected to stress there was an alarm reaction. The pituitary poured out hormones which stimulated the adrenals to pour out others. If stresses continued, the alarm reaction was followed by a period of adaptation during which the animal learned to live with its stress. Eventually, however, the defense mechanisms wore out, the animals sickened and died.

Autopsy showed some striking symptoms. Generally, arteries were thickened and hardened, hearts and kidneys severely damaged. Some had arthritislike diseases; others had diseases similar to rheumatic fever. In sum, they looked exactly like human victims of heart and circulatory disorders. Evidently the wreckage had been caused by the excess hormones produced by the pituitary and adrenal glands as an emergency defense against stresses applied outside the body.

There were, clearly, some remarkable parallels between what Selye had observed in his rats and what all of us have noted in ourselves. Under stress of worry, overwork, fatigue, chronic infections, many of us seem to get along well enough—for a time. Then the thin, quiet type, who keeps his worries bottled up within himself, becomes the victim of high blood pressure. The florid, hard-driving plant manager has his coronary. The always-tired, always-overworked housewife may become diabetic.

Selye wanted to check his belief that the wreckage he observed in his rats was caused by excess hormone. Could similar wreckage be caused by *injecting* excess hormone? Would it throw the body out of chemical balance and bring on disease?

The pituitary gland secretes a number of hormones which have specific purposes. Only one of them seemed likely to play a major role in the stress problem: STH (somatotropic hormone), which is responsible for the body's growth. The adrenals produce about thirty hormones, but here again only one appeared a likely candidate: desoxycorticosterone—DOCA for short.

To rats Selye administered walloping shots of DOCA. In a short time they developed heart and kidney disease and high blood pressure. Their joints became swollen, inflamed, sensitive. With a naturally secreted bodily substance, Selye had produced some of the worst diseases with which man has to contend.

The next step was to see what STH would do. When given in excess it produced much the same diseases: a sickness like rheumatic fever, heart and artery disease, and diabetes. Now he was on the way! Selye reported these results in 1944 to *The Journal of the American Medical Association.*

It was obvious that if STH and DOCA could produce a host of diseases there must be other hormones which would neutralize them and counteract their effects. Otherwise we would all have arthritis, diabetes and heart and kidney disease. Thus Selye's work foreshadowed ACTH and cortisone five years before their actual discovery.

When cortisone and ACTH were announced in 1949 most physicians were astounded by their wide range of activity. How, they asked, could a single medicine such as cortisone be effective on a whole spectrum of apparently unrelated diseases—gout, asthma, skin ailments, arthritis, muscular diseases, eye diseases? To Selye the answer seemed clear enough: the same types of disease had been induced experimentally in his rats by excess DOCA or excess STH. All ACTH and cortisone did was restore chemical balance—and disease magically melted away.

The amount of interest aroused by Selye's stress concept is indicated by the fact that about five thousand research papers are being published each year on the subject. More material evidence of acceptance comes from the financial support being given his research team, by foundations, individuals, pharmaceutical firms and the U.S. and Canadian governments.

What lessons are to be drawn from Selye's discoveries? How can one avoid the stresses that so often lead to disaster?

It is easy enough to advise the hard-driver to take it easy, the worrier to let up—but the advice is difficult to follow. Everyone can be alerted, however, to the fact that stress is a killer—perhaps the greatest of all killers. As this realization grows, the businessman can find relaxing hobbies which will help him slow down, the housewife can learn that it might be more important to take a nap than to launder the guest-room curtains. We can all master any lesson once we know that our lives are at stake.

If Selye's concept proves to be true, it is possible to foresee a day when people may get periodic checks of chemical balance just as they now get checks of metabolism, blood pressure and urine. If imbalance is discovered, perhaps the administration of hormones and other substances will restore the body to normal. When that day arrives Selye sees no reason why our life span shouldn't be upped to a hundred years or more.

THE MAGICAL WAYS TO INNER PEACE

Through the years, The Reader's Digest has published condensations of the most outstanding books and booklets on the subject of living a sane life in a tension-filled world. Here is the carefully selected advice of four famous physicians, the authors of these books.

How to Deal with Your Tensions

CONDENSED FROM THE BOOKLET OF THE SAME TITLE ISSUED BY THE NATIONAL ASSOCIATION FOR MENTAL HEALTH

by George S. Stevenson, M.D.

Dr. George S. Stevenson is international consultant to the National Association for Mental Health, president of the World Federation for Mental Health and former president of the American Psychiatric Association.

E verybody experiences tensions. Anxiety and tension are essential functions of living, just as hunger and thirst are. They are our self-protective reactions when we are confronted by threats to our safety, well-being, happiness or self-esteem.

So, while an occasional bout of anxiety and tension may be unpleasant, it is quite normal, and it need not be a cause for concern. The time to become watchful is when emotional upsets come frequently, shake us severely and fail to wear off after a while. How do you recognize when this is happening? Perhaps your answers to the following questions will give you some indication.

Do minor problems and small disappointments throw you into a dither?

Do you find it difficult to get along with people, and are people having trouble getting along with you?

Do the small pleasures of life fail to satisfy you?

Are you unable to stop thinking of your anxieties?

Do you fear people or situations that never used to bother you?

Are you suspicious of people, mistrustful of your friends?

Do you feel inadequate, suffer the tortures of self-doubt?

If your answer is "yes" to most of these questions, it does not mean disaster. But it does indicate the need to deal with the situation. Here are certain simple, practical, positive actions you can take for yourself.

Talk it out. When something worries you, don't bottle it up. Confide your worry to some level-headed person you can trust— your husband or wife, father or mother, your clergyman, your family doctor, a teacher. Talking things out helps to relieve your strain, helps you to see your worry in a clearer light, often helps you to see what you can do about it.

Escape for a while. Sometimes it helps to escape from a painful problem *for a while:* to lose yourself in a movie or a book or a game, or a brief trip for a change of scene. Making yourself "stand there and suffer" is a form of self-punishment, not a way to solve a problem. But be prepared to *come back and deal with your difficulty* when you are more composed, in better condition emotionally and intellectually.

Work off your anger. If you find yourself using anger as a general pattern of behavior, remember that anger will generally leave you feeling foolish and sorry in the end. If you feel like lashing out at someone, try holding off until tomorrow. Mean-

while, pitch into some physical activity like gardening or car-
pentry, or tennis or a long walk. Working the anger out of your
system will leave you much better prepared to handle your
problem intelligently.

Give in occasionally. If you find yourself getting into frequent
quarrels with people, and feeling obstinate and defiant, remember that that's the way frustrated children behave. Stand your
ground on what you believe is right, but do it calmly and make
allowance for the fact that you *could* turn out to be wrong. And
even if you're dead right, it's easier on your system to give in
once in a while. If you do this, you'll usually find that others will
yield, too. The result will be relief from tension, the achievement
of a practical solution, together with a feeling of satisfaction and
maturity.

Do something for others. If you worry about yourself all the time,
try doing something for *somebody else.* This will take the steam out
of your worries and, even better, give you a warm feeling of having done well.

Take one thing at a time. To people under tension, an ordinary
work load looks so great that it's painful to tackle any part of it.
When that happens, pitch into a few of the most urgent tasks one
at a time, setting aside the rest for the time being. Once you dispose of these first matters, the rest will go much more easily. If
you feel you can't set *anything* aside, reflect; are you sure you
aren't overestimating the importance of the things you do—that
is, your own importance?

Shun the Superman urge. Some people get into a state of anxiety
because they think they are not achieving as much as they should;
they try for perfection in everything. This ideal is an invitation to
failure. Decide which things you do well, and then put your
major effort into these. They are likely to be the things that give
you most satisfaction. Give other things the best of your ability,
but don't take yourself to task if you can't achieve perfection in
them.

Go easy with criticism. Some people expect too much of others,
then feel let down, disappointed, frustrated when another person
does not measure up. The "other person" may be a wife, a hus-

band or a child whom we are trying to fit into a preconceived pattern—perhaps even trying to make over to suit ourselves. Remember, each person has the right to develop as an individual. People who feel let down by the shortcomings (real or imagined) of their relatives are really let down about themselves. Instead of being critical of another person's behavior, search out his good points and help him to develop them. This will give you both satisfaction, and help you gain perspective on yourself.

Give the other fellow a break. People under tension often feel that they have to "get there first," no matter if the goal is as trivial as getting ahead on the highway. Everything becomes a race in which somebody is bound to get injured. Life need not be this way. Competition is contagious, but so is coöperation. When you give the other fellow a break, you often make things easier for yourself. If he no longer feels you are a threat to him, he stops being a threat to you.

Make yourself "available." Many of us have the feeling that we are being "left out," slighted, neglected. Often we just imagine this. Instead of shrinking away and withdrawing, it is healthier and more practical to make overtures yourself. There is a middle ground between withdrawal and pushing. Try it.

Schedule your recreation. Many people find it hard to take time out. For such people a set schedule of hours for recreation will help. It is desirable for almost everyone to have a hobby that absorbs him in off hours—one into which he can throw himself completely and with pleasure, forgetting all about his work.

Often emotional difficulties arise out of practical problems: financial difficulties, trouble on the job, problems of children and parents, marital trouble. But just as often a person's long-standing habits and attitudes may *produce* conflict. These interacting forces outside him and within him tend to build up, each making the other worse—perhaps rapidly so. In such cases we may need more help than we can give ourselves, help of the sort a counseling or guidance service gives.

These services may be found in family welfare agencies, schools, churches, industrial plants, settlement houses, public health departments. They help people clear up practical problems and thus help relieve emotional strains.

However, if an emotional disturbance becomes too distressing, it should be dealt with as an illness requiring professional treatment, just as one deals with a cold when it becomes severe. Go to your family doctor. He may recommend visiting a psychiatrist, or treatment at a clinic or a mental hospital. To find out about counseling and treatment in your community, get in touch with your local or state mental health association.

The quest for peace of mind—or for good mental health, which is another name for it—is universal. Yet few of us are blessed with all the internal qualities and external circumstances that automatically assure it. We have to work to achieve it. This means striving for a better understanding of ourselves and others. It means working out our problems by ourselves when we can, and seeking the assistance of others when we need it.

There is a basic philosophy fundamental to good emotional health. That is the philosophy of faith: faith in the ability of ourselves and others to improve and grow; faith in the desire and capacity of human beings to work out problems coöperatively; faith in spiritual and moral values, in the essential decency of mankind. This faith will carry us through stresses that might otherwise shatter us.

O<small>NCE</small>, as a young man, I undertook to draw up a catalogue of the acknowledged "goods" of life. I set down my inventory of earthly desirables: *health, love, talent, power, riches* and *fame*. Then I proudly showed it to a wise elder.

"An excellent list," said my old friend, "and set down in not unreasonable order. But it appears that you have omitted the one important ingredient lacking which your list becomes an intolerable burden."

He crossed out my entire schedule. Then he wrote down three syllables: *peace of mind.* —Joshua Loth Liebman, in his modern classic, *Peace of Mind*

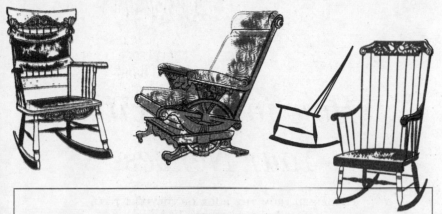

The Gentle Art of Just Sittin' 'n' Rockin'

A FEW YEARS AGO, while rocking contentedly on the veranda of a quiet Florida hotel, I had the happiest inspiration of my life. Lulled in body and soul by the slow, salubrious rocking motion and pleasantly monotonous *squeak-squeak* of the chair, I thought drowsily of the frenetic pace of modern life. "Why can't some of my friends join me in rocking away their fretting and fussing?" I wondered.

From this casual rumination there developed a unique club whose influence today extends from my business headquarters in Stamford, Connecticut, to the jungles of Indonesia. Our membership roster includes a Supreme Court justice, an ex-Cabinet member, housewives, Congressmen, barbers, ambassadors, football coaches, clergymen, judges, policemen, newspapermen.

The Sittin', Starin' 'n' Rockin' Club has no committees, no dues and no *don'ts*. As president I have the honor of presiding over meetings which are never held. Cards are issued to all members "in good sitting," as well as a rocking-chair "operator's license" and a six-month calendar reminding members to rock more, especially on holidays. Thus simply is our membership dedicated to recapture in our daily living one of the lost graces of American life.

I have heard—and firmly believe—that rocking improves circulation and is therefore especially beneficial for the old. Our grandfathers went further, recommending the "to-and-fro" exercise as a palliative for rheumatic pains and a reliable cure for constipation.

Dr. Janet Travell, President Kennedy's doctor, recommends the rocker for any prolonged reading. "The constantly changing position will relax your muscles and rest you," she says.   —Thomas E. Saxe, Jr.

How to Live with Your Nerves

CONDENSED FROM THE BOOK OF THE SAME TITLE

by Walter C. Alvarez, M.D.

ℰℰ

Dr. Walter C. Alvarez is one of the most widely read syndicated columnists in the United States, and author of the best-selling book Live at Peace with Your Nerves.

ℰℰ

To live easily with your nerves, the first thing is to get acquainted with the ways in which they play tricks on you. Often I must say to a worried patient, "There is nothing seriously wrong with you; your symptoms are all produced by your erratic nerves."

Often the most distressing spells follow a trying experience, a sleepless night, a tiring day. For instance, a businessman began to suffer severe heart palpitation the day he had to face the unpleasant task of dismissing an old employe. A woman who woke one night with the feeling that she was strangling had spent the evening arguing angrily with a relative over money. One can easily see why the nerves of these persons were on edge and ready to go on a rampage.

Many times, however, the storm seems to come out of a clear sky. A highly nervous woman tells me that her life is easy—she has a loving husband, a comfortable home, good children, no worries. Why, then, should she have spells in which she is jittery, terribly tired, apprehensive or depressed? Usually in such cases I find marked nervousness in the family. Let us say that you have inherited your father's quick temper or your mother's tendency to worry. You cannot entirely get rid of these tendencies, but you can learn to control them and to live with them better.

When, as a young man, I faced failure and poor health because of my inheritance of my mother's bad nerves, I resolved that I would do the many wise things she did, but would struggle hard never to do the foolish things she did, such as worrying and fretting and living life the hard way. I decided I would hoard my energies. And when I did, I found I had enough for two jobs: one earning a living and the other doing research, writing, teaching and lecturing. I even had enough left over for hobbies. Someone once said our relatives are given us to show us what we shouldn't do and be!

Learn to keep your nervous system as fit as possible with the help of good mental hygiene. By this I mean living sensibly— getting the proper amount of sleep and rest and recreation. People forget that the brain is a delicate and complicated bit of apparatus, and that it should be given care and consideration. Today many of us work too long hours, then stay up much too late. We would be much healthier if we were always in bed by 10 p.m. Our vacations may be so strenuous that we get no real rest or recreation and do not store up energy. Many people, also, abuse their nerves by smoking and drinking too much.

Many nervous persons wear themselves out on nonessential activities. They put too much energy and thought into doing things that another person does almost automatically. That is why some people get so little work done and become so terribly tired doing it. Dr. W. J. Mayo, carrying on a huge surgical and consultant practice, always entertaining visiting surgeons, daily guiding and administering and building up a huge institution, lecturing and writing and serving on many boards, never seemed hurried or impatient. As he once told me, he tried never to waste energy or emotion on things that did not count.

Years ago a woman gave me the key to nervous breakdowns. I asked her why she, who had wealth and little to do, was so worn out. She said, "I wear *myself* out." She wore herself out with petty worries.

Often I find people wasting energy on needless conflicts—especially with themselves. They are full of resentments, animosities, hates, jealousies, envies. Blessed is the man or woman who goes through life easily—not irritable, touchy, impatient, irascible. It is wonderful how helpful this way of life is to the nervous system; and it is wonderful how much energy it leaves free for useful work.

I admire my sensible daughter who is never ruffled by the ceaseless activity of her two little boys. She says, "I would much rather have them active and into everything than sickly or apathetic." One day when she left a can of paint within reach of the baby and he spilled it on the floor, her only comment was that she should have had more sense than to leave it where he could reach it. As a result of such serenity, she always has energy to spare to run a house, play tennis, swim and engage in civic affairs.

If we want calm nerves we must not nurse resentments and jealousies or indulge in envy. In every business one can find envious men who spend more time trying to hold back the leaders among their associates than they spend in studying and working to advance themselves. How much energy they waste and how bad it is for their nerves! I have seen envy of this type wreck a man's health.

One of the greatest curses of life today, and one of the greatest breeders of nervousness, is working under tension. The late Stewart Edward White once built himself a cabin in the California Sierras. An old mountaineer used to come and watch him. One day, as White was sawing violently at a log, the mountaineer remarked that White sawed like all city fellows, going as fast as he could to get the log sawed. "Now," said the old man, "when *I* saw, I just saws."

All of us with tense nerves could almost cure ourselves by learning to "just saw." We must learn to tackle just the job in hand and stay with it quietly. I often have said to my secretary, if she could see in one pile all the letters she is going to write in the next ten years, she might want to jump out the window. But by writing them one at a time, the job is bearable.

When Will Rogers was asked what he'd do if he had only five days to live, he said he'd live each day one at a time. All of us would do well to learn to live each day in a sort of compartment, not weeping over the mistakes of the past or holding constant postmortems over them, and not worrying about the morrow. A man can work efficiently in this way. All he needs then is to do quickly and as well as possible the work that lies right at hand. It is helpful, also, to learn to tackle a difficult job without hesitation and get it done. Don't put it off. Many nervous persons break down after putting off work that must be done.

The same goes for indecision. Nervous persons could save themselves worlds of now-wasted energy if they would only learn to make decisions quickly—and make them stick. Mayor La-Guardia used to call after a man who had just gotten a decision from him about a matter, "And don't bring that back to me!"

A wonderful saver of energy is Sir William Osler's trick that he called "burning one's own smoke." He meant that we should not indulge in the miserable habit of taking out on others our discomforts, griefs and annoyances.

I belong to the Sierra Club of California, which each year takes two hundred members into the high mountains. Their most important but unwritten bylaw goes something like this: "Thou shalt never utter the least word of complaint if it rains all day and all night, or if the pack train is late and thy food does not arrive until 10 p.m." Many a night I have seen the party wet, cold, hungry and without shelter, but always there was fun and good humor and never any grousing. Among those people to "crab" is the unpardonable sin.

There is another hint that we can take from the teachings of Osler, and that is to cultivate equanimity and serenity. As he said, we must learn not to be too upset by the pinpricks—and even the big shocks—of life. We must learn to take them in our stride. As one writer said so wisely and well: "O Lord, grant me the serenity to accept the things I cannot change; the courage to change the things I can; and the wisdom to know the difference."

〜

How to Stand Up under Stress

CONDENSED FROM PSYCHO-CYBERNETICS

by Maxwell Maltz, M.D.

During the last days of World War II, President Harry Truman was asked how he managed to bear up so calmly under the stress and strain of the Presidency. His answer was, "I have a fox-hole in my mind." He explained that, just as a soldier retreats into his foxhole for protection and respite, he periodically retired into his own "mental foxhole" where he allowed nothing to bother him.

He was, in effect, heeding the wisdom of Marcus Aurelius, who wrote: "Nowhere, either with more quiet or more freedom from trouble, does a man retire than into his own soul." And, because he believed this ability to retire within himself was essential for peace of mind, Marcus Aurelius advised: "Constantly then give to thyself this retreat, and renew thyself."

The modern world has conditioned us to respond to so many outside stimuli that we have lost the ability to ignore them. This explains why, in recent years, tranquilizer drugs have become so popular. They erect a "psychic screen" between us and disturbing stimuli. They do not change the environment; all the old annoying elements are still there. They work because they reduce, or eliminate, our own response to these outside stimuli.

All our disturbed feelings—anger, hostility, fear, anxiety, insecurity—are caused by our own responses, not by any external stimuli. If we could learn to control these responses, wouldn't we, in effect, be building our own "psychic screen"? Response means tension: tension in muscles, for example, is a preparation for action. The opposite of tension is relaxation—this is nature's own tranquilizer. Indeed, it has been proved in laboratory experiments that you cannot feel angry, fearful, anxious or insecure so long as your muscles remain perfectly relaxed. And muscle relaxation means mental relaxation as well.

Suppose you are quietly reading at home when the telephone rings. This is a stimulus you have learned from habit and experience to obey, and you leap, without thinking, from your chair to answer it. Why? The phone itself has no power to move you. Let it ring; go on with your reading. By refusing to respond to the phone's signal, you are, in a sense, practicing relaxation.

Later, when confronted by a disturbing stimulus, use this experience as a key thought in overcoming the conditioned response. Picture yourself at home, as before. Let "the telephone ring unheeded," and it will act as a trigger to call up the same relaxed attitude.

If at first you find it impossible to ignore the response, delay it. Delay breaks up the automatic workings of conditioning. "Counting to ten" when you are tempted to become angry is based on this principle. By holding off the emotion of fear or anger, you may be able to extinguish the automatic reflex altogether. I know a woman who used this method to help remove her fear of crowds. Her usual reaction to them was an overpowering desire to flee. Now she would first say to herself: "All right, I'll run, but not right away. I'll wait for a few minutes." And it worked.

Once you have found the secret of relaxation, by learning to ignore the conditioned response, you will have a chance to discover the quiet room within you that each of us needs—and has. It is my belief that each personality is equipped with a center which, like the deep of the ocean, is never disturbed. We need to do what President Truman did—find this quiet center.

One good way to begin is to build for yourself, in imagination, a little mental room. Furnish it simply with whatever is most restful and refreshing to you—beautiful landscapes, perhaps, or a volume of your favorite verse. Choose restful colors. Make the keynotes simplicity, quietness and beauty, with everything neat and in order. Take as much care in planning it as you would in building an actual room. Be thoroughly familiar with every detail.

Then, whenever you have a few spare moments during the day, or whenever you begin to feel tension mounting, retire into this quiet room for a few moments. In your imagination, see all the quiet, restful details; settle down in your favorite easy chair, utterly relaxed and at peace with the world. It will not be time wasted, but time invested.

Mental pictures can be helpful in many ways. On a visit to Yellowstone National Park some years ago, I saw the geyser "Old Faithful" suddenly erupt in a great mass of hissing steam, like a gigantic boiler whose safety plug had blown out. A small boy standing nearby turned to his father and asked, "What makes it do that?"

"Well," said the father, "I guess old Mother Earth is like the rest of us. She builds up a certain amount of pressure, and just has to blow off steam once in a while to stay healthy."

I began using the mental picture of Old Faithful erupting whenever I became wrought up. I would retire into my quiet mental room, then blow my top; I imagined emotional steam bursting from the top of my head, evaporating harmlessly. The picture formed a powerful association in my mind, and at once I relaxed, the tension gone.

I'm often asked, isn't this idea of a quiet mental room merely a form of escapism? Certainly it is; but so is sleep escapism, as are most forms of entertainment. Our nervous systems require a certain amount of escapism, just as we need yearly physical vacations from the old scenes and responsibilities. Why shouldn't you give your soul a small vacation, too, by retiring into your mental quiet room for a few moments each day?

In using a computer, the operator must clear the machine of the previous problem before undertaking a new one. Otherwise, parts of the old problem carry over into the new situation, and the result is a wrong answer. In the same manner, we must clear our own inner mechanisms. Your quiet room is an ideal clearance device for emotions and moods. In my practice of plastic surgery, for example, a high degree of concentration is essential. To make certain I won't carry any personal worries into the operating room, I always clear my mental machinery by spending a few moments beforehand completely relaxed in my quiet room.

Above all, keep in mind that the key to the matter of whether you are disturbed or tranquil, fearful or composed, is not the external stimulus but your own response. In the Ninety-First Psalm there is a vivid word picture of a man who experiences a feeling of security amid the terrors of the night, arrows that fly by day, plagues, intrigues and the snares of enemies—all because he has found the secret place within his soul and is unmoved. This man was, in the words of Marcus Aurelius, "like the promontory against which the waves continually break, but it stands firm and tames the fury of the water around it."

My INVESTIGATION of 600 drivers proves that motor accidents and bruised egos go together. For a car is a most effective salve for emotional hurts. All day long, on the job, perhaps at home, you have been carrying out orders given by others; behind the wheel of your auto you are boss—you step on the gas and great power leaps to your command. You put distance between yourself and your unhappiness—temporarily. Your car never argues; it obeys, and you, like all the rest of us, crave being boss some of the time. All this is fine when things go well for you. But when you're emotionally upset, your car can instantly turn into a lethal weapon.   —Louise Gay Balsam

Your Mind
Can Keep You Well

by John A. Schindler, M.D.

Author of HOW TO LIVE 365 DAYS A YEAR

As a doctor I know that there are a thousand different ailments that this human clay is heir to, and one of them is as common as the other 999 put together. Fifty percent of all the people going to doctors today are victims of this one disease. Many would put the figure higher. At one well-known clinic a report was published reviewing 500 consecutive admissions to that institution; of those, 386—or 77 percent—were sick with this one disease. Persons of any age, in any walk of life, can contract it. Furthermore, as we all know, it is a terrifically expensive disease to diagnose and treat.

I hesitate to give you its name because immediately you will get a lot of misconceptions. The first will be that it is not a real disease. But don't kid yourself. It used to be called psychoneurosis. Now it is known as psychosomatic illness. And it is *not* a disease in which the patient just *thinks* he is sick. The pain you get is often just as severe as the pain you get with a gallbladder colic.

Psychosomatic illness isn't produced by a bacterium, or by a virus, or by a new growth. It is produced by the circumstances of daily living. I have tried to find one word for it, but it takes three, each meaning about the same thing but in different degrees. They are: *cares, difficulties, troubles.* Whenever one has such a thick, impenetrable layer of c.d.t. that he can't get up above it into a realm of joy and pleasure occasionally, he gets a psychosomatic illness.

There are three general groupings of people who suffer from c.d.t. In the first group are the people who are habitually crabby. They get a psychosomatic illness, and get it hard. As a rule they are invalids for the rest of their lives. There is nothing you can do about it.

The second group, where most of us belong, are the people who all day long manage to be concerned, to be anxious, to be worrying about something. If there's nothing around home or the business, they worry about Mrs. Smith down the street.

The third group is made up of those who have an acute case of c.d.t. Maybe they have gotten themselves into some kind of mess, financial or domestic. They are usually easier to treat than those in the second group, who are certainly easier to treat than those in the first group.

Many victims of psychosomatic illness are up and around. Many are in hospitals. Thousands have been in bed at home for years. To avoid psychosomatic illness, we must learn how to make our attitude and thinking as pleasant and cheerful as possible. It would be idiotic for me to tell you that you can be pleasant and cheerful all the time. Of course you can't. But I can offer certain suggestions which will help you to think sensibly about yourself.

First, quit looking for a knock in your motor. Don't be analyzing your feelings all the time, looking for trouble.

Second, learn to like to work. To get anywhere in this world you've got to work. One thing you will escape, if you learn to like it, is work tension, the tension that comes to those who look upon work as something to be gotten over with.

Third, have a hobby. A hobby is an important element in getting your mind off work tension. During the day when you are

hurrying and worrying, just relax for thirty seconds by thinking
briefly about the thing you're making in the basement, that community project you're interested in or that fishing trip you're
taking next weekend.

Fourth, learn to like people. Carrying a grudge or dislike can
have disastrous bodily effects. We had a man in the hospital who
got there because he had to work in an office with a man he
didn't like. He said, "I don't like the way he combs his hair, the
way he whistles through his teeth, the way he always starts a sentence with 'Listen!'" On questioning the patient I found that he
never liked anybody—his mother or his father or any other member of his family. But you've got to live with people, so learn to
like them.

Fifth, learn to be satisfied when the situation is such that you
can't easily change it. A young lady was in a hospital with a psychosomatic illness because she had become dissatisfied with her
life. She had been a secretary, had held a war job in Washington.
There she married an Army captain. After the war she found herself living in a trailer, raising three children. She didn't like to
live in a trailer, didn't like to raise children in a trailer, wasn't
sure that she liked to live with her husband in a trailer. She
wanted to be a secretary, back in Washington. I didn't tell her
what her trouble was. I just advised her to read the four Polly-
anna books. She did, and she returned to live in the trailer and
like it. She had learned that it is just as easy under most conditions to be satisfied as it is to be dissatisfied, and it is much more
pleasurable.

Sixth, learn to accept adversity. In this life you're going to meet
some adversity. You may meet a lot, but don't let it bowl you
over. I had a patient who hadn't worked for a year. Then his
wife died. A month later his son was killed. And he sat around
thinking, "How unfortunate I am—why did this have to happen
to *me!*" He became very sick. A lot of people start a psychosomatic illness after an adversity.

Seventh, learn to say the cheerful, humorous thing. Never say the mean thing, even if you feel like doing so. In the morning, look at your wife or your husband and, even if it isn't so, say, "My dear, you look good this morning." It will make both of you feel better.

Finally, learn to meet your problems with decision. About the worst thing to do is to have a problem and to mull it over and over in your mind. If you have a problem, decide what you are going to do about it and then quit thinking about it.

These are some of the things you have to learn if you want to escape the most common disease of all. The key is: *I'm going to keep my attitude and my thinking as pleasant and as cheerful as possible.* There isn't any better way to happiness.

Few ailments show so clearly as stomach ulcer the close connections between mind and body. At the New York Hospital, Dr. Harold G. Wolff tested 205 patients to see how emotional upsets affected the flow of hydrochloric acid, which aggravates stomach ulcers. While making his tests he led the conversation around to topics he suspected would be painful. The acid count soared when the bankrupt business or the thwarted career was being discussed. It doubled at the mere mention of an estranged wife. —Elsie McCormick

Worry affects the circulation, the heart, the glands, the whole nervous system. I have never known a man who died from overwork, but many who died from doubt. —Dr. Charles Mayo

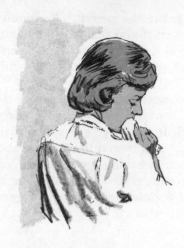

The Case for Crying

by Karl Huber

A college professor told me recently that whenever the pressures and frustrations of life become severe, he puts everything aside and goes to the movies. "I find a particularly sentimental film," he says, "and bawl like a baby."

The young mother of three small sons has a similar practice. When the youngsters have been particularly trying, or the budget simply can't be stretched to pay for another snowsuit, she sends her boys to their grandmother's house for the afternoon, turns on the record player and weeps. "In half an hour," she says, "I'm fit to face the world again."

Maudlin, weak, self-pitying, you may say. Actually, these people have found a harmless and effective way of getting rid of feelings that might otherwise be damaging.

Contrary to what many believe, tears are not necessarily the mark of deep emotion. More often they result from an accumulation of surface feelings—frustration, irritation, fatigue—that need some recurrent release. Crying depressurizes us emotionally, and thus relieves stresses that may affect even our bodies.

There is evidence that certain physical diseases are aggravated by an inability to find release in tears. Some psychoanalysts believe that neurotic asthma for example, has a close relation to the rigid control that prevents crying. An asthmatic attack, characterized by gasping sobs, is very like an attempt to weep in which the relief of tears does not come. Migraine headaches and many common but nameless complaints—the "weight" on one's chest, the "lump" in one's throat, the "band" tightening around one's head—all seem to be connected with excessive control.

Natural as weeping is, Anglo-Saxon society has surrounded it with an extraordinary number of taboos and restrictions. Our men are never supposed to cry except in bereavement. Women are permitted to weep publicly then, and on such sentimental occasions as weddings, and privately at disappointments in love, but it is considered poor taste for them to exceed these limits. Even children are expected to confine their tears to moments of physical pain or fear and are rebuked for crying in rage at the many frustrations of childhood.

Other peoples are more permissive. Italians weep unashamedly on almost any touching occasion. Many Middle Europeans and Latin Americans consider any display of patriotism or heroism ample justification for tears. Even supposedly self-contained Orientals are permitted relief in tears.

Most of us do cry, probably more often than we admit. The most masculine men may be moved to tears after some period of extreme tension or effort. Football players sometimes weep in the locker room after a game, whether they have won or lost. A test pilot told me that on completing a flight he sometimes cannot contain his tears and simply sits weeping in the cockpit of the plane.

Civilized living requires that on many occasions we exercise strong controls on ourselves. We are expected to deal with our children, neighbors and business associates with a show of calm assurance, meet crisis and catastrophe without breaking down.

But constant rigid control is unnecessary. It is important to our happiness and health that we learn to decontrol ourselves within safe limits at appropriate times.

The college professor and the young mother have learned this lesson. Neither of them was crying *about* the situation at hand: the professor was not truly moved by the mawkish scenes on the screen; nor was the woman actually crying over the music. Instead, each had found a device for precipitating tears at a time and a place where the release of their emotions would not be harmful or embarrassing to anyone.

The Bible says there is "a time to weep." If we choose our time carefully—perhaps in church or at concerts, perhaps at the movies, perhaps in the privacy of our bedroom—we can use this natural safety valve to reduce the pressure of our tensions.

If You Need a Drink— Don't Take It !

by Charles Stevenson

Alcoholism is a serious disease for America's 700,000 chronic alcoholics. It is a serious threat to 3,800,000 other excessive drinkers. But the Center of Alcohol Studies (formerly at Yale, now at Rutgers University), which originated the movement for treating alcoholism in public clinics as a disease instead of a sin, has ascertained scientifically that the remaining 73,500,000

Americans who drink moderately can use alcohol with safety and sometimes even with benefit.

Don't order a case of whisky on that! Instead, know the facts about alcohol as Yale discovered them—then govern yourself accordingly, because men and women already on the highroad to alcoholism too often imagine they are moderate drinkers.

There was no shortage of willing martyrs to science at Yale. Both outsiders and staffers have lined up at weird cocktail parties to have whisky poured down their throats while the professors manipulated Rube Goldbergian devices to record reactions and learn that it isn't the amount of alcohol consumed that counts but the percentage showing afterward in the blood; that there are a lot of variables in its effect.

Absorption is slowed and the kick lightened by food in the stomach or cereals in the drink, as with beer. Inversely, carbonated mixtures are absorbed faster. The speed with which the liver burns alcohol depends on the individual and the drink (various distilled spirits show differences); thus the lasting power of the kick varies.

Because a big man's body contains more blood than a small man's, it requires more liquor to put a significant concentration of alcohol in his veins. When the professors fed 4 ounces of whisky each to two men two hours after dinner, the 130-pounder showed a .04 percent alcoholic concentration in his blood while his 213-pound companion was only one half that far along.

Nevertheless, experiments have convinced the experts that, while nearly everyone is sober with less than .05 percent of alcohol in his blood (2⅓ ounces of whisky on the empty stomach of an average 150-pound man) and many may be tipsy at .1, everybody suffers some impairment at .15. The drinker becomes deeply intoxicated at .2 and .3 and passes out at .4, when the alcohol completely depresses that part of his brain governing consciousness. At .5 to .9, when it paralyzes the centers which control breathing, he dies. To achieve such a death means gulping quickly the equivalent of a quart or more of the strongest whisky at one brief sitting and keeping it down. Happily, vomiting would probably halt the attempt before it was successful.

It has been found that most functions take place at lower efficiency even after a small dose of alcohol. For instance, if you feel less tired after drinking, you simply are benumbed. Actually your muscular output drops. On two ounces of whisky, the average subject's errors in reasoning jumped 20 percent; on a half pint, 67 percent. No matter how you may insist liquor stimulates you, it does not.

Alcohol is related chemically to ether. It acts first by deadening the nerves of the brain to relieve physical and mental tension. If some people seem clearer-headed after a drink this is only because they are so tense and self-conscious that, without a sedative, they are inhibited. A lawyer I know does better before the jury if he takes a drink. He could do still better were it possible to get rid of his inhibitions by other means.

Even small amounts of alcohol impair efficiency. Though one motorist can drive safely with enough liquor in him to put another atop a lamp post, the experts caution everyone to avoid the steering wheel for at least an hour after taking two ounces of whisky, two hours after four ounces, then to add an hour for each additional ounce.

However, the experts do not feel that well-motivated, moderate drinking is necessarily a bad habit. They contend that, in relaxing tension, it fulfills a psychological need. Moreover, there is no physiological or psychological ill effect from years of such drinking, whether it involves wine, beer, bonded whisky or fresh blends. The only admonition is: Whatever hard liquor you drink, dilute it.

There is nothing to the old belief that the more you drink the more you must drink to obtain the same degree of relaxation. Unlike the morphine addict, who at first might be killed by one grain and yet in time requires ten to feel like living, the drinker develops no great tolerance for alcohol. He will need no more to relieve his tensions as time goes on, unless his tensions increase.

Moderate amounts of alcohol may aid digestion, although an excess will halt it. "For people past middle age it is one of the safest sedatives," according to a noted physiologist. "Many elderly people get much comfort from a small amount of alcohol;

it relieves the aches, pains and chilliness of age, lessens the tensions and irritations and increases the appetite. It does not greatly affect normal blood pressure but it does prevent pressure from rising in anxiety and mental concentration."

However, any person who has reached the point where he wonders if he should discipline his drinking habits may be in the danger zone of excessive drinking. It is a confusing area. A man may fear he is an addict because his regular 5 p.m. drink has established such a habit pattern that he definitely *wants* a drink at that time. But habit does not necessarily imply addiction. Some genuinely heavy drinkers may be endangering their health, but are not yet addicts. On the other hand, a man may be a problem drinker though he limits himself to an ounce every other day.

What, then, is a problem drinker? What counts is motivation. Let's look at an average sample of 100 alcoholics. About half of them are persons whose drinking is only a symptom of underlying mental disorder; alcohol cannot be blamed for their neurosis, for the fact that they are morons, for their epilepsy, dementia praecox or manic-depressive psychosis. But the other half are those who, starting as apparently well-integrated social drinkers, pamper their frustrations with alcohol until they can't face life except through a whisky haze.

If you rule out the mental misfits who really constitute a problem other than one of alcohol, it still does not suffice for an average drinker to insist it is impossible for him to become a problem drinker. Whether the incipient alcoholic's traits develop or not depends on the pressures to which he is subjected and on the social acceptance of heavy drinking by his circle.

Frustrations offer a fertile field for the alcoholic personality. One man may seek escape from the fact that he lacks energy to achieve his ambitions. Another with the same underlying characteristic will break out in drink only because he can't get a job. Or the reason for drinking may lie in childhood psychological experiences the drinker has forgotten.

There are tests which will help a man analyze his drinking habits. Can you enjoy a party only if there is liquor to release you? Do you long for the time of day when you can drink without hurting your job? Do you turn to alcohol each day to overcome anxiety, disgust, fatigue or frustration? Do you drink to offset difficulties with your wife, your boss, your children or employes? If the answer in any case is yes, you are an alcohol dependent and in peril.

To put it in a nutshell, simply ask yourself: *"Do I need this drink?"* If the answer is yes, don't take it. The problem drinker is the person who drinks not because he enjoys it but because he feels he needs it. He is drinking to escape. He never craves alcohol specifically; but he is developing a genuine craving for anesthesia, which alcohol supplies.

It usually takes ten years to develop chronic alcoholism. Along with it may be liver trouble, or irritation of the throat and digestive system, resulting in alcoholic gastritis and improper assimilation of food. But most of the ills result from dietary deficiency, because alcohol is actually a food which in excessive amounts eliminates hunger. Moreover, it contains no vitamins, only calories—200 to the ounce.

Though persons less than thirty years old rarely can be cured of alcoholism, upwards of 60 out of 100 can be helped in middle age. Nobody, though, ever was cured by nagging. Occasionally successful treatment involves psychological conditioning not of the drunken husband but of his nagging wife.

No remedy is successful unless it seeks out the underlying psychological reasons which prompt the drinking. In a surprising number of cases, their elimination will cure alcoholism. One woman's problem was traced to a mother-in-law allergy and cured by eliminating the latter (by fair means).

There is no recorded instance of an alcoholic without a personal problem which caused him to drink. However, alcohol in sufficient quantities supplies its own problem. If you habitually drink excessively, no matter for what reason, you finally will be drinking to escape the woe caused by your drinking.

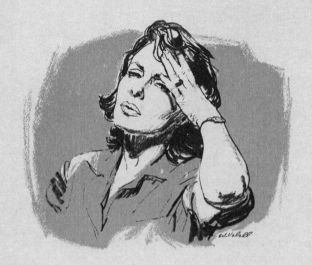

CHAPTER 12

The Big Nuisances

NATURE SEEMS to have arranged a second set of warnings for those who ignore the first: pain or exhaustion. These—fatigue, headaches, insomnia, colds and allergies—are the recurring nuisances that plague us all. Often more puzzling to scientists than the major diseases, they have nonetheless yielded many of their secrets. To a considerable degree they are related to stress, and with proper care and precaution can be handled.

How to Live
without Fatigue

by Marguerite Clark

The patient's voice falters. "Doctor, I'm so tired. What's wrong? What shall I do?"

Every hour, every day, in almost every doctor's consulting room, at least half the visitors voice this complaint. Of all ages, of either sex, rich or poor, they make up the vast throng of fatigued human beings who get little comfort from the pills, shots and examinations they solicit from baffled physicians.

"Fatigue is so common that failure to mention it in an office visit makes me suspect that the patient is holding back," said Dr. Thomas F. Keliher, internal-medicine specialist at Georgetown University Medical School, Washington, D.C.

Dr. David McK. Rioch, neuropsychiatrist of the Walter Reed Army Institute of Research in Washington, reports that "fatigue has become the socially acceptable excuse for not doing things."

It is difficult to measure fatigue or to arrive at its true cause, because no two human beings have the same energy resources, and because the capacities of individuals vary from day to day.

"What different people can do without becoming exhausted is a tremendous variable," said Dr. Robert S. Schwab, of Boston. "And the energy output of a person under one set of circumstances compared with the way he handles exactly the same task under different conditions is a second important variable. On one day an energetic wife and mother may tear through her work with almost superhuman speed. On another, when she is beset by problems—her husband's lost job, her child's illness, a raft of unpaid bills—she may worry herself into exhaustion before midday, with almost none of her housework completed."

Solving the riddle of the tired patients is no easy task. "Theirs is not the pleasant fatigue that follows golf or a rewarding day at the office, from which they emerge after relaxation or sleep feeling like new," says Dr. Schwab. "Often their tiredness is out of proportion to energy spent; and it will not disappear with rest, sleep or a vacation."

People frequently are far more tired than they realize. For a surprisingly long time, a tired man or woman may do as good a job as one who is rested, simply by calling on willpower to keep the energy-controlling thermostat at a high level. But finally, after overexertion of the body or brain, or both, body movements lose dexterity, become automatic. Mental processes are stereotyped; imagination lags; conscious attention wavers; judgment suffers; the whole personality changes. The tired person loses his poise, his social graces and, to a marked degree, his disposition. He may become a victim of *chronic* fatigue, one of the most serious threats to health and happiness.

What Is Fatigue?

To simplify diagnostic procedures, "that tired feeling" has been divided into three spearate categories:

1. *Pathological fatigue:* An early symptom of some serious organic disease.

2. *Physiological fatigue:* From chemical reactions in the blood that leave the muscles of healthy people exhausted.

3. *Psychological fatigue:* From prolonged emotional conflicts, anxiety and boredom.

The tired patient who is sure "there is something terribly wrong with me" may be right. Anyone who is chronically tired should check with his doctor. Most often it is *psychological fatigue* from which patients suffer. In his study of 300 victims of chronic exhaustion, Dr. Frank N. Allan, a Boston internist, found that only 20 percent were tired for purely physical reasons, while 80 percent had emotional difficulties.

Some people seem to be immune to fatigue, even when weighed down by physical exertion or mental frustration. We all know the high-energy man who never complains of being tired. Optimistic, decisive, exuberant, he manages to keep six or seven projects going at the same time—and with vigor to spare. Why do some of us have almost limitless mental and physical drive, while others tire after the least exertion?

Dr. Hans Selye, whose findings on stress are mentioned in an earlier chapter, says that each of us inherits his fatigue pattern. He suggests that everyone should appraise his energy store. Sit down and ask yourself:

1. What are the main stress factors in my life?
2. At what time of the day or night do I have the most energy? The least?
3. When fatigue strikes me, how long does it last?
4. How long can I keep adapting to trying circumstances without growing weary?

Once you have established your fatigue pattern, "try to space out jobs, and reserve energy-demanding tasks for the time when you have the greatest strength," advises Dr. Selye. "Also, it is important to change your pace. If you are too tired to think well, stop and walk around a bit; if you are muscle-tired, sit down and think, or listen to music."

Since high-energy folk are most likely to overcrowd their lives with enticing new projects and responsibilities, Dr. Selye has a word of warning for them, too. "A man may be intoxicated by his own stress-fighting hormones. This kind of drunkenness has caused more harm than alcohol. Even though you love every moment of your work, you may be wearing out your adrenal glands. So watch out for your critical stress quota, just as you would for your cocktail quota. Once in a while, re-examine your fatigue pattern to see if you are exceeding the limit."

The Mechanics of Fatigue

American researchers have spent many years looking for a clue to the mechanics of fatigue. The most intensive studies were those conducted at the Harvard Fatigue Laboratory, backed by the Rockefeller Foundation. Here it was learned that physical fatigue is caused by a complex chain of chemical reactions.

Investigators found that if the human body is to carry a reasonably heavy work load without exhaustion, complete coördination of muscle movements with breathing and circulation is necessary. The muscles rely on glycogen, the energy-producing material, for their power to contract. But, after prolonged muscular effort, the so-called "fatigue materials"—lactic acid, carbon dioxide and other by-products—seep into the bloodstream. (So acute is the chemical change that injections of the blood of a fatigued animal into a rested animal will produce fatigue.)

Metabolism, Weight and Fatigue

Metabolism—regulated by the endocrine glands as their chief function—is the chemical process responsible for the construction of new cells, the destruction of old ones and the rate of release of energy. When a man is excessively tired, his output of adrenalin hormones is greatly decreased, almost to the point of stagnation. However, endocrine studies also explain the system of "the second wind," that unexpected surge of muscular energy under stress. This increase is caused by the action of the nervous system on the adrenal glands. Suddenly there is a release of adrenalin into the tired person's blood.

"What rest will do after an hour or more, adrenalin will do in five minutes or less," commented a gland specialist. "The increased efficiency of the second wind is temporary and the production of adrenalin to take care of a fatigue emergency cannot be substituted *indefinitely* for normal rest and sleep."

At the National Institute of Arthritis and Metabolic Diseases, Bethesda, Maryland, Dr. Elsworth R. Buskirk and his associates have found that people of normal weight can work well for long hours. But in fatigue experiments with obese patients they have learned that obesity is frequently a deterrent to intensive physical work. The overweight patients manage to do one to three hours of "work" on treadmills, or in other walking. But they are "exhausted" for the rest of the day. They lie down, nap or rest heavily in their chairs.

"These obese people just don't take it as well as lean individuals," said Dr. Buskirk. "Lacking the willpower to lose weight, they often have no willpower to exert themselves. Their work capacity is definitely reduced."

Fear and Boredom

Imaginary fatigue, to avoid work, or some other painful activity, is a common ailment, and many a genius has resorted to it. "When faced with work, Samuel Johnson was sometimes so tired, languid and inefficient that he could not distinguish the hour upon the clock," wrote Johnson's faithful biographer, James Boswell.

When he began to compose a new concerto, Robert Schumann, according to his physician, "was seized with fits of trembling, fatigue and coldness of the feet."

These celebrated folk were victims of "motivational fatigue." Gifted though they were, they lacked the incentive to adapt themselves to their callings with courage and patience. A study of chronically tired business executives in their early forties and fifties was made at a Chicago hospital. These men had been full of driving ambition, eager to accept responsibilities, determined to reach the top. But somewhere along the way they had lost their drive, their "incentive to work." All were thoroughly discouraged and fearfully tired. "It seemed that their mainsprings were broken," observed one physician.

Most of them, the doctors found, were more driven by fear of failure than by pride of past accomplishments. What they lacked was a healthy motivation—the stimulus that would help them to fight exhaustion and do their best work in spite of it.

In our modern culture, social and occupational attitudes may have something to do with lack of incentive to work. Dr. Hugh O. Thompson, of Detroit, who has studied "the tired patient" for two decades, believes that these people "represent the transitional period in which we find ourselves, where the exhausted, confused worker sits idly by with the false notion that the world is his without working for it."

Of the forty to fifty patients in Dr. Thompson's office each day, probably 50 percent complain of fatigue. Since careful examinations rules out physical illness in nearly all these cases, the answer must be overwork, worry or both. Dr. Thompson asks each patient, "Is your work too hard for you?" The frequent reply: "No, it's very easy. I don't work three out of eight hours."

"Any economic worries?" asks Dr. Thompson. Far from it. "The patients have cars, TV sets and worksavers in their homes, mostly paid for on the installment plan. When I ask them what might happen in case of a recession, the standard reply is, 'Everybody would be in the same boat.'

"Actually, these people are not tired at all," concluded Dr. Thompson. "They are just bored. They need a revival of true interest in life through purposeful activity—and that means a *full day's work for a full day's pay!*"

Choose Your Goals—and Set Your Pace

In dealing with fatigue it may be helpful to write down on paper the things you want most from life. What is your *goal* for personal happiness? For professional or business success? Estimate the amount of energy necessary for achieving these aims. Some of them will need only a small output; others will demand all the energy you have—and maybe a little more than you think you have.

"Fatigue, actually, is not as bad as some people think," is the consoling conclusion of one neuropsychiatrist. "It does not change our capacities; it just diminishes them temporarily. If the symptoms of exhaustion are recognized and something is done about them, fatigue can be a fine education."

Design for Fatigue

from Newsweek

Some years ago the Mayo Clinic at Rochester, Minnesota, developed a treatment for chronic fatigue. Part of the treatment is a psychological yardstick in the shape of a cross: the four arms show how the patient divides his time in work, play, love and worship. When one of the arms is too long and throws the cross off balance, it indicates that the patient is chronically fatigued because he's living an unbalanced life.

The diagram, adopted by the Clinic's Dr. E. J. Kepler, harked back to a method described in the book *What Men Live By*, written in 1914 by Dr. Richard C. Cabot of Harvard. The arms of the cross symbolize (1) work of a congenial kind, (2) love as typified by happy marriage, (3) wholesome play and (4) worship as devotion to something bigger than self. In the ideal life the four arms are of equal length; when one or more are stubs, the result is unhappiness, a frequent forerunner of fatigue. Thus a businessman's cross may have overlong "work" and "love" arms, and stubby "play" and "worship" arms; a debutante is long on play and short on work; a spinster may be long on work

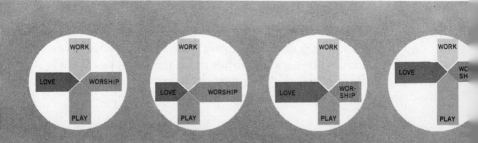

and worship but short on love and play. In the Mayo treatment
the chronic-fatigue patient was asked about his activities, then
shown his cross. Convinced that he had no underlying disease, the
patient found relief in the concept that his main problem was to
strike a finer balance in the allocation of his interests.

Sleep and How to Get More of It

by Robert Coughlan

Insomnia has never killed anyone. But to the people who suffer
from it, insomnia is as debilitating as anemia, as nagging as
an ulcer, as uncomfortable as a leg in a cast. And chronic insomnia has the peculiar distinction of being its own cause. The advanced insomniac approaches his bed in a state of anxiety and
spends the next hours awake because he is fearful that he will do
just that.

No one really knows what sleep is or exactly what causes it or
exactly why it is needed. The process can only be described.

After a normal period of relaxation (up to thirty minutes) the
prospective sleeper reaches a stage of semiconsciousness which is
neither sleeping nor waking. It is a feeling of "floating" or being
"disembodied." If all goes well, sensation ends and the subject
floats over the borderline to unconsciousness. The passage takes
only a few seconds and is marked at the end by an abrupt shift in
the origin of brain waves (minute electrical charges) from the
back part of the head to the front.

With the reversal in the source of brain waves sleep has come, bringing with it mysterious and rather alarming transformations. The sleeper breathes slowly. His eyeballs turn out and up. His fingers grow cold and his toes grow warm. His senses fade. The blood does not leave his brain, contrary to popular belief, but his blood pressure falls rapidly, becoming weakest about three hours after sleep begins. His heart rate also decreases, but often rises again to reach a peak in two or three hours, after which it slackens and becomes slowest about four hours later. His body temperature falls about half a degree Fahrenheit. The sleeper has at first lain quietly, but soon he begins to move—an arm, a leg, now his whole body, shifting from side to side and front to back. In the morning he may declare with perfect honesty that he slept "like a log," but an observer would have recorded that he changed position between twenty and sixty times. It is possible to "sleep like a log" only if one is anesthetized or dead-drunk or feeble-minded.

After a certain time, depending on the sleeper's normal sleep span, the initial process is reversed. Sleep becomes lighter, consciousness flickers, fails, flickers, the brain charge is reversed— the sleeper is awake. Perhaps he yawns, thereby inhaling extra oxygen to lower the proportion of carbon dioxide that has accumulated in his body as a result of his muscular inactivity during sleep.

This, then, is normal sleep, "tired nature's sweet restorer," the insomniac's goal. Why is it so often so difficult to attain? In general, insomnia is a price man pays for having become man. Sleep is not a problem for earthworms, tadpoles, bears or even monkeys, and only rarely for young babies. These lower forms of life lack the intelligence required for insomnia—which means, physiologically, that they lack the highly developed cerebral cortex of the adult human.

Aside from purely physical causes such as disease and organic malfunctionings, it is one word—anxiety—in all its complexities of cause and effect, which explains most sleep aberrations. It usually is anxiety that causes nightmares and "night terrors" in children, and it is the most frequent cause of sleepwalking and sleeptalking. The cure therefore is obvious: Stop worrying, especially at bedtime.

That, however, is easier urged than done. It is not enough, for example, to tell a battle-shocked soldier who relives his war experiences at night to forget them; obviously he would like nothing better. The same is true of the ordinary insomniac. Countless nights have reverberated to his ancient cry, "If I could only stop thinking!" In advanced cases the only cure may be psychotherapy, but for most of humanity there are techniques which can be applied in the privacy of one's own bedroom.

The first and obvious one is to direct the mind by an effort of will away from personal matters. If one must think, let it be about objective rather than subjective things: not about one's own love problems but about the bees and the flowers. Along with this must be a high degree of muscular relaxation. Complete relaxation is, of course, impossible (nor is it necessary; people go to sleep while driving, and exhausted soldiers fall asleep while actually on the march). But the insomniac should aim for as much of it as he can get, with special attention to the muscles of the head, neck and chest. The reason for this is simply that a greater area of the brain is devoted to the incoming and outgoing signals of these muscles than to those of all the others combined. After the eye muscles, the ones to discipline most firmly are the speech muscles. The ability to think is intimately connected with the ability to talk. It is, in fact, almost impossible to maintain coherent thought without activity (minute, to be sure, but present and measurable) in the voice muscles. It follows that if the muscles having to do with speech are relaxed, the mind, in bafflement, will at last give up. The best way to do this is to let the jaw and whole face go slack in an expression of complete stupidity.

Mental vacuity and physical inertness are thus the uncomely handmaidens of sleep. They can be acquired by practice, but not easily: sometimes a year of conscientious application is necessary. They can be helped along by various palliatives, which will be useful to the light and troubled sleepers as well as to the true insomniac.

There are no uniformly effective rules for the best way to sleep. Room temperature, bed coverings, ventilation are all matters of individual preference or habit. Most people sleep better alone. The admonition against lying on one's left, or "heart," side is pure superstition, since the heart is approximately in the middle of the upper body cavity and since, in any case, the normal turnings of the sleeper will inevitably land him on the left side several times during a night. Provided the sleeper enjoys normal digestion, a big meal helps rather than hinders sleep, and for some people the process may be helped along by a cup of good coffee to stimulate the digestive processes. And there is also much to be said for the "nightcap" as a soporific.

Other forms of bedtime nourishment seem to have little effect. Tests at the University of Chicago showed no significant differences whether the subjects did or did not take one or two sandwiches or hot or cold milk before retiring. If a snack, a bath and fifteen minutes of music seem to form a satisfying presleep ritual, then they are useful.

Women, on the average, get more sleep than men, partly because they carry around relatively fewer problems and partly also because of their custom of creaming their faces, brushing their hair and spending a good deal of time in similar pre-bed activities. The ritual itself comes to be associated with sleep and thus helps to bring it. The same associative value applies to the bed itself and speaks against making reading in bed a part of the ritual, especially the reading of mystery novels.

It is helpful to establish a regular time for going to bed and getting up. Dr. Nathaniel Kleitman, University of Chicago physiologist who has spent thirty years probing the mysteries of sleep, has investigated the workings of what he calls "the diurnal sleep cycle." Everyone undergoes a rise and fall of body temperature over a twenty-four-hour period. The drop in temperature brings with it a natural period for sleeping.

Thus the problem sleeper, by going to bed at a regular hour, can establish a temperature cycle which automatically will make him sleepy at that time. He may choose any hour around the clock. Some persons can establish a cycle easily; others may take months and must count on a long period of nightly restlessness before the cycle clicks into place.

Temperature cycles differ. There is the kind that climbs steeply as its owner wakes up, causing him to jump out of bed eagerly. He is a "morning person"; his temperature keeps going up and reaches a peak around noontime, when he is at his most wide-awake. When it begins to fall soon after, he begins to feel less energetic. His temperature continues to fall, reaching the "drowsiness level" fairly early in the evening.

The "evening person's" temperature rises very slowly and does not reach its peak until late afternoon, when he feels at his best. He dislikes getting up, and feels groggy and out-of-sorts in the morning. By the time the "morning person" is looking forward to bed the "evening person" may be wound up and going strong. Dr. Kleitman is fond of the aphorism: "More marriages are broken up by temperature than by temperament."

Dr. Kleitman's tests show that in both mental and physical tasks performance and resistance to fatigue are best when temperature is high, worst when it is low. Consequently it is a good idea to arrange the most important affairs of the day so that they can be handled during the period of maximum temperature.

In the past many experimenters have supposed that fatigue created various "waste products" and "poisons" that numb the brain, and that sleep was needed to eliminate them from the body. There were several drawbacks to this theory. One was that no one could ever find any such poisons in the bloodstream. Another was the evident truth of the familiar expression, "too tired to sleep"; there comes a stage when fatigue is a hindrance rather than a help to slumber. Also, Dr. Kleitman discovered that people of all types usually are least efficient after a night's sleep; it was no longer possible to imagine sleep as a cleanser of poisons. Sleep can take place without fatigue. A completely rested person can fall asleep if he relaxes enough. On the other hand, "healthy fatigue" is an aid to relaxation.

The sleeping pill should be the last resort of an insomniac. The standard barbiturate drugs are not harmful in themselves if taken in medically prescribed doses. But, says Dr. Harris Isbell, director of research at the U.S. Public Health Service Hospital, Lexington, Kentucky, "taken regularly in large doses, they can be habit-forming, and the addiction can be much more painfully difficult to break and more dangerous than morphine addiction."

Suppose that the chronic insomniac has tried all the suggestions given here—in vain. What then? He shouldn't lose any sleep over it. For it is certain that if he keeps at it he will learn the trick, and it is equally true that it will do him no serious harm if he takes a long time to do it. Chronic "undersleeping" is widely supposed to lead to mental and physical breakdown, but almost certainly it can do neither. For tasks requiring short periods of physical or mental coördination, lack of sleep leaves performance as good as ever. In tasks calling for sustained effort, loss of sleep causes performance to fall off drastically. And it does increase sensitiveness to pain.

The common belief that one cannot "pay back" a sleep debt is untrue; the debt, with interest, can be liquidated in one good long sleep.

There is no absolute answer to the question: "How much sleep should people get?" It depends on age, health and activity. Laboratory tests show that sleep needs tend to decline each year from birth to senility. But a fifty-year-old mathematician probably will need more sleep than a twenty-five-year-old ditchdigger, for physical workers usually can get along on about two hours less a night than people who work with their brains. If Jones feels good on three hours' sleep (plus cat naps), he needs no more; if Smith doesn't feel good on eight hours', the chances are that he needs nine or even ten.

Happily for the insomniac, rest can take place without sleep, and so long as he lies down and gets at least a measure of relaxation in mind and body, he can keep going almost indefinitely. He may not feel well; probably he will feel awful; but that will be the worst of it.

❧

What Do You Know about Sleep?

by Gretta Palmer

B etween the ages of twenty-five and seventy the average person spends fifteen years sleeping. Lack of sleep has made generals lose battles, nervous patients lose their minds, wives lose their husbands. Obviously an understanding of sleep is important to us all; but how many of us know the scientifically established facts about it? What's your score on the following statements, some true, some false?

The most refreshing sleep comes early.

True. Studies at Colgate University show that many of the benefits of sleep have been fully obtained by the end of the first few hours.

If you sleep six hours instead of eight, you must expend more energy the next day to accomplish the same work.

True. Laboratory tests show that we use up to 25 percent more calories to compensate for lost sleep.

Men who are able to get along with very little sleep are among the most energetic.

False. Napoleon and Edison went with only a few hours' sleep a night, but they took cat naps during the day. In any twenty-four-hour period they apparently slept a normal length of time.

We fall asleep and also wake up in one split second.

False. When we are half asleep, either at the beginning or the end of the night, we pass through a period when we cannot speak but can clearly hear sounds. Our power to move is then asleep, but our hearing faculties are awake.

It is unhealthy to sleep in summer with an electric fan or an air conditioner in the room.

False. If the fan or air conditioner is adjusted to avoid drafts and operates soundlessly, it will improve your chances of a restful night.

Physical fatigue can make it difficult to get to sleep.

True. A warm bath is probably the best way of reducing the tension that comes from too much unaccustomed exercise before going to bed.

The worst thing about insomnia is worrying about its effects on the next day's work.

True. Dr. Donald A. Laird, who studied sleep habits at Colgate University, suggests that when sleep is difficult you decide to get up later the next day. Knowing that you have plenty of time in which to rest, you will doze off easily.

Mattress and springs should be of medium softness to insure the most restful sleep.

True. A soft bed is the worst enemy of sound sleep, a hard bed almost as bad.

A nap after lunch is sheer self-indulgence and cuts down a person's efficiency.

False. Studies at Stephens College, Missouri, show that when students slept for an hour after lunch their scholastic records were higher than when they used the time for studying.

Mental effort is the worst possible preparation for getting to sleep.

True. A dull evening, ending with a walk to tire your muscles, is the best preparation for sleeping.

I F YOU ARE NOT ALWAYS as bright and energetic as you'd like to be, here's a hint from the famous psychologist, Carl E. Seashore. As an undergraduate at Yale, young Seashore was bothered by daytime loginess. He asked the university's physical director if anything might be done about it, and was told: "A Christian gentleman always takes a nap at noon!" He gave it a trial, and to his delight his energy rose, his efficiency spurted and his spirits sang. Out of his own experience, and from many years of continuing interest, Professor Seashore concludes that fifteen minutes of sleep after the heaviest work and before the main meal count more for efficiency than five times as much late, light sleeping in the morning.   —Ray Giles

I OFTEN THINK this "insomnia" business is about 90 percent nonsense. When I was a young man living in a boardinghouse in Toronto, my brother George came to visit me, and since there was no spare room, we had to share my bed. In the morning, after daylight, I said to George, "Did you get much sleep?"

"Not a damn minute," said he.

"Neither did I," I rejoined, "I could hear every sound all night."

Then we put our heads up from the bedclothes and saw that the bed was covered with plaster. The ceiling had fallen on us in the night. But we hadn't noticed it. We had "insomnia."   —Stephen Leacock

Headaches

WHY YOU HAVE THEM—
WHAT YOU CAN DO ABOUT THEM

by Lin Root

I f you are one of the sixteen million people in the U.S.A. and
Canada who suffer from recurring headaches, you've probably
blamed them on everything from astigmatism to low barometric
pressure. "I should never have read (sewed, watched TV) so
late last night." Or, "Why did I eat that lobster salad?" or,
"Why didn't I take a laxative?"

These usually spurious reasons *seem* to make sense to the sufferers. But experts now believe that practically all chronic headaches are traceable either to dilated blood vessels in the head or to
the effects of muscle tension or to a combination of both. Most
headaches are part of the response to emotional or physiological
stress, which you can do much to control.

A major breakthrough in pinpointing the cause of most recurring headaches has come from the work of the late Dr. Harold G.

Wolff, professor of medicine at Cornell University Medical College. Pioneers in headache research, Dr. Wolff and his associates—not the least of whom were the patients who coöperated—staked out, like surveyors, pain areas in the head and produced or reduced head pains at will. During surgery for intracranial disorders, patients permitted the insertion and inflation of tiny balloons in brain spaces, electrical stimulation and other manipulation of blood vessels and various parts of the brain, then reported the site and nature of the resulting sensations.

Next, Dr. Wolff turned to the chemical front. Drugs called vasodilators, injected into volunteer subjects, produced headaches where none had been before. Nature, Dr. Wolff concluded, makes its headaches the same way—by the vasodilation that you see in bloodshot eyes, swollen nasal passages, distended arteries standing out on the temple.

On the basis of extensive investigations, Dr. Wolff stated that, numerically, "tumors, infections and structural anomalies of the eyes and air spaces in the head constitute a small proportion of the causes of headache. Somewhat less than three out of 100 of the most troublesome headache cases selected at random would fall into this group." All the rest are vascular or muscle-tension headaches.

While arterial hypertension, cerebral arteriosclerosis and other organic troubles are responsible for a small percentage of vascular headaches, more than 90 percent occur in a setting of emotional stress, said Dr. Wolff. He had been able to induce the pain of headache and the clinical picture of measurable vasodilation by introducing to patients distasteful topics that acted as emotional tinder. This means, to put it bluntly, that you yourself probably bring on most of your own headaches.

Worst of the torments in the headache realm is migraine, which the Greeks called *hemikrania*—half-a-head—because the pain rages on one side only, usually radiating from the eye. The pain is continuous, lasting from hours to days.

Research has shown that migraine has a predilection for the educated and intelligent. Dr. Walter C. Alvarez, emeritus consultant in medicine for the Mayo Clinic, refers to it as "something like a Phi Beta Kappa key" in the world of headaches. He also describes migrainous types as "usually perfectionists who want everything done just so and exactly on time." The tendency to migraine is inherited, often reinforced by environment and insistence on inflexibly high standards.

Routine tension headaches usually start in the back of the neck or base of the skull, spreading to localize anywhere—back, front, sides—or even to encircle the head like a vise. Often postural tension sets off this headache. Bookkeepers, stenographers, students bend over books too long; drivers stare intently at the road during too long a trick at the wheel. Although the individual is unaware of it, head and neck muscles become rigid, go into spasm. With sustained contraction comes constriction of the blood vessels and their network of nerves. Decreased circulation adds to the pain of the muscle spasm. The headache begins.

The tension headache seems entirely physical in origin. But why does Betty get it and not Jane—Bill and not John? Because the tense ones hurl themselves with taut nerves and muscles at the columns of figures, the pages of shorthand, the homework, the road ahead.

Thus, whether it is a migraine or tension headache, the villain is the same body-enemy we have met before: *emotional stress*. The so-called "common garden" species of headache may *seem* to be traceable to physical causes—hunger, exhaustion, eyestrain or glare, poor ventilation, hangover, for example. More often than not, however, it results from a combination of physical discomfort and emotional tension. One person reacts to a too bright light by developing a headache—another adjusts to the light. After drinking, one person may acquire a headache through guilt feelings or possibly tension-bearing encounters with his companions—another goes to work next morning clear-eyed and clear-headed. Psychological makeup often spells the difference for, while alcohol causes blood vessels to dilate, hangover appears well after this immediate effect has subsided.

For the physician, modern headache therapy has a short-range and a long-range goal: short-range, to treat the individual attack; long-range, to diminish the frequency and severity of the attacks.

In migraine, the most effective treatment for an individual attack is one or another of the derivatives of ergot, a potent vasoconstrictor which acts on the smooth muscles of the blood vessels, reducing pulsation.

In tension headache, less localized than migraine, treatment of the single attack is aimed at relaxing contracted muscles and lessening sensibility to pain. Heat lamps, hot packs, half-hour soaks in water just above body temperature, massage plus analgesics (from aspirin on up) and even tranquilizers are among the most effective measures.

But the big payoff in the scientific understanding of headaches has come in treatment of the patient himself. While drugs and physical therapy may relieve or control the attack, the basic aim of doctors is to help the patient discover what he is *doing to himself* that brings on his headaches. An important factor here is the relationship between physician and patient. By talking out his problems with his doctor, the patient can gain a greater understanding of the situations that produce his tensions.

Thousands of sufferers have experienced relief once they recognized the headache as a "cease and desist" order for their way of life—and obeyed the order. Does this mean that to exclude pain you must live within boundaries that exclude the fullness of life itself? No, indeed. When you learn the cause and effect of your behavior you stop wasting energy. As one career woman put it: "Once you've charted your boundaries, they, inconsistently enough, begin to expand. You find you can do more because you have yourself under control."

Dr. Wolff and Dr. Robert M. Marcussen, his colleague at Cornell University Medical College, once drew up a few ground rules under the heading, "How Can Headaches Be Cured?" Their principal suggestions are these:

1. Learn to be less fussy about minor details in the day's work.
2. Everyone has days when he feels tired and irritable. Attempting to drive yourself to do as much on these days as on

"energetic, vigorous" days results in much fatigue, tension and headache.

3. Avoid, as much as possible, needless, useless worry.

4. If you feel frequent resentment, anxiety, disappointment, modify your standards. It is essential to get satisfaction out of what you *can* have and *can* do.

In short, all headaches can be useful lessons in sensible living. The more we heed their warnings, the less frequent and less painful they will be.

The Pesky Allergies

Adapted from "They Call It Allergy" *by Lois Mattox Miller and* "Antidotes for Allergy" *by Paul de Kruif*

Mrs. Smith gets asthma every time she goes to the movies. Will Jones has migraine headaches whenever he visits his fiancée. A waitress breaks out with hives regularly on Tuesdays and Fridays. A ship's captain suffers from hay fever at sea and finds relief ashore.

Approximately fifteen million people in the U.S. and Canada, the Allergy Foundation of America reports, are victims of that mysterious backfiring of the body's protective system which we call allergy. In each instance, the "allergen" which caused their

suffering proved to be some commonplace thing—harmless in itself yet having the effect of poison on them.

Mrs. Smith reacted violently to pyrethrum, a disinfectant
sprayed in theaters. Will Jones was sensitive to his fiancée's face
powder and his headaches ceased when she switched to another
face powder. The waitress was allergic to shrimps, served on
Tuesdays and Fridays in the restaurant where she worked, though
she never touched or ate them; their kitchen fumes produced her
skin eruptions. The captain, who slept on feather bedding at
home, was allergic to the kapok in his mattress aboard ship.

The tendency to allergy is inherited in three cases out of four.
Authorities say that over 10 percent of the population are allergic.
Their symptoms vary in persistence and severity.

Only recently have doctors been able to give us a clear picture
of what happens when we are allergic. Essentially it is a drama of
chemical warfare waged amid the cells of the human body.

The body is endowed with a protective mechanism by which
things harmful to the system are excluded or repelled by the skin
and respiratory tract, or chemically changed in the digestive
system. In the allergic individual, some particle in the food he
eats, the air he breathes, the things he touches, slips past these
first lines of defense. Seemingly nothing happens. He experiences
no unpleasant symptoms. But actually, as soon as this foreign
substance enters the body, the microscopic cells and clinical substances go to work, creating antibodies for a single purpose: to
destroy the invader. The initial battle between allergen and antibodies takes place in the bloodstream and the invader is destroyed. But it is a Pyrrhic victory. For the remaining antibodies,
having now no foe to combat, retire to the side lines and attach
themselves to other body cells. There they remain, live and potent
fighters. At that point the allergic individual has become
sensitized.

When he inhales, ingests or absorbs a second dose of the allergen, the veteran antibodies go into action again, not this time in
the bloodstream, but attached to what doctors call *shock tissues:*
the smooth tissues in the nose, the lining of the lungs, the stomach,

intestines, blood vessels. The allergen may be destroyed, but the battle scars are the allergic symptoms, the diseases we call hay fever, some types of asthma, stomach disorders, diarrhea, hives and other allergic skin eruptions.

The doctor, recognizing a disease of allergic origin, is faced with a herculean task of detection. Out of thousands of possible substances, he must find the one or the group to which his patient is allergic. Every type of matter—animal, vegetable, mineral— and such physical agents as heat and cold are suspect.

He begins with a checkup on the patient's family history, environment, living habits, occupational exposures. Any pets in the house may be removed to note the possibility of irritation from animal danders. The patient may have to live away from home for a while so that the effect of changed environment can be observed. A basic diet may be prescribed, to which foods are added or eliminated, with the patient recording his reactions.

The doctor may seek to reproduce the allergen-antibody conflict in miniature, by introducing extracts of foods, tobacco, chemicals, pollens, etc.—one at a time—into a skin test puncture. A hive or wheal developing on the patient's skin indicates the guilty substance, since the antibody reacts only to the allergen for which it was created.

The doctor may be able to *desensitize* a patient by administering small and increasing doses of an extract made from the allergen; or the patient may have to eliminate the offender from his environment or diet. Allergy specialists say it is now possible to desensitize with practically all allergens that are inhaled— pollens, dusts, danders, etc.—with the exception of chemicals. "Contact allergens" such as poison oak or ivy also respond to injections of extract. Seven out of ten hay-fever or asthma cases that persist throughout the year can be given satisfactory relief through injections. And 75 percent of those suffering from food or inhalant allergies that produce hives and eczema can be wholly or partially relieved.

Immunizing by these shots, however, is slow, tedious and expensive. Some persons who are allergic may not be helped by desensitization because their physicians cannot find out to what they are sensitive. Then too, there may be substances against which you cannot be immunized at all.

For years scientists have been groping for a simple chemical answer to the allergic mystery. Lifesaving remedies such as penicillin and sulfa can turn upon allergic patients who have to use them repeatedly. It wasn't until chemists discovered one of the culprits in allergy—histamine, an organic chemical in the body—that an effective antihistamine could be sought. There are numerous such substances now available under different trade names. Two well-known examples of these are benadryl and pyribenzamine—known as PBZ. Both have shown power in relieving a variety of allergies. These antidotes (*not cures*) in some cases allow victims to discard their shots; they also boost the power and lessen the discomfort of these immunizations, and they lessen a great variety of allergic torture where shots are ineffective. Neither PBZ nor benadryl hit at the basic cause of allergy (that's still mysterious), but they do help to combat the poisonous histamine that is released by allergic explosions. While not dangerous in ordinary doses, they should only be used initially under the supervision of a physician.

The effect of either drug is temporary, lasting only a few hours, and of course, as with all drugs, some few people are found to be allergic to PBZ or benadryl itself! Both have definite side effects in certain cases.

For instance, either drug may produce a soporific (drowsy) effect. One patient taking PBZ fell asleep while driving her car and crashed into a bridge. Doctors warn: *Don't drive or engage in any activity that requires concentration or conscious control while taking antihistamines.* Doctors also warn that in some cases of asthma, hives and intestinal allergies the symptoms may increase after taking these drugs.

Experience has shown that PBZ and benadryl will not, as was once hoped, revolutionize the treatment of the nation's most widespread misery, hay fever. The consensus of allergy specialists is that by far the most complete protection against this seasonal plague occurs in people who have been immunized by allergen shots and then—when necessary—also help guard themselves by antihistamines during the hay-fever season or when other allergic symptoms are active.

"One-Shot" Treatment for Hay Fever

by Albert Q. Maisel

In the late 1930s Dr. Jules Freund, of the New York City Health Department, was inoculating horses and other experimental animals to produce antibodies against infectious diseases. Wishing to eliminate the chore of daily injections for each animal, he emulsified his materials in mineral oil so that a single massive shot, deposited in muscular tissue, would gradually leak into the animal's bloodstream. This, he discovered, not only saved him the trouble of administering multiple injections; it also raised the antibody production of his animals far beyond anything he had previously attained.

Would the same technique work on humans afflicted with hay fever? In 1947 the first cautious tests were made on a few pollen-allergic volunteers at New York Hospital. Pollen extract emulsified in mineral oil in doses up to twenty times stronger than ever before were used. And, when the hay-fever season arrived, volunteers found that they benefited as much as they had in earlier years under multi-injection treatment.

One physician in Boston reports that the 4000 most recent injections have produced not a single adverse reaction. Following the first year's shot, 75 to 85 percent of these patients have gone through the pollen season with complete freedom from hay-fever symptoms. A growing number, after two years of successful single-injection treatment, have been able to skip the injection in the third year without suffering a recurrence of hay fever.

Nevertheless, some leading allergists urge caution until more extensive controlled studies can be completed. Dr. Bram Rose, past president of the American Academy of Allergy, points out: "The single-injection method may be associated with certain hazards, such as severe immediate reactions. In addition, nothing is known of the long-term hazard which might arise as a result of the injection of emulsions."

Enthusiasts for the one-shot technique counter with the claim that, in the hands of experienced users, it has brought on reactions no more frequently than has multi-injection therapy. Nor have any adverse long-term effects turned up among patients treated for hay fever by the single-dose method, though some have been under the new therapy for thirteen years. If these reports continue to indicate a consistently low rate of reactions and a consistently high degree of effectiveness, many allergists will undoubtedly adopt the new technique.

೨〜౨

A Word of Difference

THE WEALTHY YOUNG MATRON felt so tired and listless all the time that she wasn't interested in anything. Yet a thorough physical examination revealed nothing wrong. Her doctor—who knew the pampered life she led—advised her to find some kind of work to do. "But, Doctor," she protested indignantly, "how can you ask me to work when I'm so tired?"

"I know you're tired," he answered. "But if you'd only do something you could become tired *from*, there wouldn't be nearly so many things you'd be tired *of*."   —Edward Kardos

The Common Cold

Adapted from "We Can't Cure a Cold" by Herbert A. Reimann, M.D., and "Closing In on the Common Cold" by J. D. Ratcliff

Throughout North America hundreds of millions of dollars are spent on cold "remedies"—everything from aspirin to expensive vaccines—and doctors' fees. Colds account for 32 percent of home visits by physicians and 15 percent of office visits. Yet medicine has no specific treatment that can shorten attacks of colds, grippe, catarrh and influenza. Except in the case of true influenza, there is virtually nothing we can do to prevent attacks.

Colds and their sister diseases are virus infections. Though both the sulfa drugs and penicillin are ineffective against viruses, these expensive products continue to be wasted on colds in huge amounts. Other traditional remedies are equally ineffective. The use of cathartics is unnecessary and exhausting, frequently harmful. Sweating, induced by hot drinks, a hot bath or a drink of good whisky can do little more than give comfort.

Antifever drugs such as acetanilide, phenacetine, quinine and amiopyrine form the chief ingredients of almost every nostrum sold to "break up a cold." They have no possible effect on the infectious process. Medical opinion now holds that a moderate degree of fever is helpful in overcoming infections. Coughing, too, actually serves a useful purpose and should not be checked unless it is unduly harassing. Cough medicines often contain codeine, alcohol or similar narcotics to soothe throat irritation. If such potentially habit-forming drugs are to be used at all, they should be prescribed by a physician. Gargles, sprays or swabs often involve use of irritant antiseptics which remove protective mucus and may actually spread the infection they are supposed to quell, while inhalers, drops and sprays decrease neither the severity nor the duration of colds and related infections. The more we examine the traditional treatments, the clearer it becomes that none of them has any specific effectiveness.

Recent developments in England indicate that a cure for the common cold may be in sight. There researchers have cornered the cold virus in the laboratory and even managed to keep it alive and growing. Their clinical findings using human volunteers indicate that the cold itself is a rather innocuous, three-day affair: slight sore throat, possibly headache and always a watery discharge from the nose. When nasal discharges thicken and become yellowish, this is a sign that bacteria, always present in the nose and throat, have taken over the fertile ground prepared by the virus—the raw, inflamed mucous membranes. The researchers concluded that the virus prepares the way for an attack by bacteria on throat, nasal and other tissues.

Along the way, researchers picked up random facts. It became clear that the cold virus is almost fancifully small, only 1/300 the size of the average bacterium. In the laboratory it could be passed through filter material, the ultramicroscopic pores of which were 50 millimicrons in diameter. And it is remarkably durable. It can be deep-frozen, stored for years and still produce colds.

The British workers checked the generally accepted idea that chilling predisposes to colds. In February weather they asked volunteers to take hot baths, then don bathing suits, allow themselves to be doused with cold water and to stand in drafts until their teeth chattered. Others were asked to wear wet socks all day. Not one of them contracted colds unless the virus material was also dropped in their noses.

Helpful as all this was in building up the most complete picture of the cold ever brought together, the researchers still hadn't managed to trap the cold in a test tube where they could study its wily ways, its points of weakness.

The first real breakthrough came in America when at Harvard

University, Dr. John Ender, Nobel Prize winner, succeeded in growing polio viruses in kidney tissue taken from monkeys.

Following this lead, the British research team developed a virus-growing culture from kidney cells. Researchers now knew exactly what the cold virus liked to eat and at what temperature greatest growth would be achieved. Mankind's tormentor was in the laboratory at long last. Virus was passed from tube to tube twenty or more times with no loss of enthusiasm for growth. Juice from test tubes produced colds in human volunteers after six, seven, eight passages.

The significance of all this? The first step in production of a protective vaccine is to grow virus or bacteria in a laboratory, to grow it readily and in quantity. The virus is then killed (as in the Salk vaccine for polio), or weakened, to make it safe for use.

The time has not quite arrived for this step. More must be known about the varieties of virus that cause colds; nine strains have so far been isolated. The hope is that most colds may be caused by only three or four strains of virus which could be included in a single shot of vaccine.

While we await such new treatments there are a few common-sense procedures which will lessen the discomfort of a cold and minimize the dangers of complications. Best among these is medicine's age-old standby—rest. If fever is present, go to bed.

If we cannot as yet cure a cold, how can we avoid one? Infections of the respiratory tract often occur for no obvious reasons in otherwise robust people. Certain circumstances are thought to lead to colds. These include exposure to wet, to sudden chilling and drafts, volatile irritants and dust, as well as fatigue and other excesses. They should either be guarded against or neutralized by rest, warmth and comfort.

Until a specific treatment for colds is found, we should cease to fool ourselves. If we can't prevent colds and can't cure them, we can at least let nature take its course unimpeded.

A cold is both positive and negative: sometimes the eyes have it and sometimes the nose.   —William Lyon Phelps

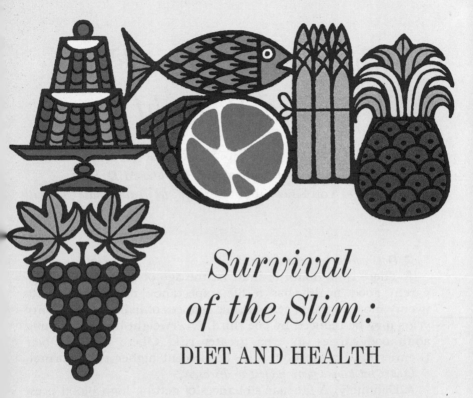

CHAPTER 13

Survival of the Slim:
DIET AND HEALTH

IN AN affluent society such as ours, which produces more food than it can consume, the average person can afford a rich and varied diet. As a result, most of us eat too much.

Unbalanced meals can seriously impair body efficiency and tone, while overweight increases the risk of poor health and serious diseases. We can be just as well fed and satisfied by beneficial foods as by an excess of the wrong ones. What most of us need, perhaps, is to know the modern methods of breaking our old bad eating habits and establishing good ones.

The Facts about Food and Weight

Adapted from "The Facts about Your Weight,"
an interview with Frederick J. Stare, M.D.,
and "What Do You Know about Eating?" *by Judith Chase Churchill*

Q *Does overweight shorten life?*
A There is no doubt of that. At the age of fifty a man in apparent good health has a life expectancy of approximately twenty more years. If he is fat, his chances of living these twenty years may be reduced by one third. Overweight begun in young adulthood carries an even greater risk. Obese men in their twenties have a mortality rate 80 percent higher than normal.

Q *Are fat people more subject to diseases?*
A Definitely. A fat man's chances of getting high blood pressure are three to four times greater than normal. For coronary heart disease, they're two to three times as great. For diabetes, four to five times. His risk in major surgery is two to four times as great.

Q *What is it about overweight that shortens life?*
A If you are carrying around extra weight, whether it's a load of cement or fat, you are putting more work on your heart. Furthermore, a person actively putting on fat may develop atherosclerosis, the condition underlying most heart attacks. In atherosclerosis the walls of the arteries are blocked by deposits of fatty materials.

Q *Is there any easy way to control your weight?*

A No. If you have a tendency to overweight, controlling it will be a lifetime job.

Q *Is the appetite the controlling factor?*

A Yes. An important factor in hunger is the variation in the blood sugar throughout the day. By keeping the blood-sugar level up, you keep the appetite down. For fat persons we advise "scientific nibbles"—a small bite in the morning and afternoon of some food that you ordinarily would have at lunch or at supper. For example, have a glass of milk at eleven o'clock instead of at noontime.

Q *What about drugs?*

A There are several drugs useful in treating obesity, but they are prescription drugs and should be used only on advice of a physician.

Q *What about advertised nonprescription preparations and "liquid diets"?*

A Most "reducing pills" are mixtures of milk powder, sugars and flavoring—a type of expensive candy. You can reduce your appetite just as well with a piece of hard candy or cheese.

As for the 900-calorie "liquid diets," Philip L. White of the American Medical Association says that limited use of such formulas is probably safe for the person whose excess-weight problem is not connected with such ailments as diabetes, heart disease or a gallbladder condition. But when taken without a doctor's supervision, for prolonged periods, or to effect a "crash" weight loss, the liquid diets may be harmful. Most of these commercial diets have enough proteins, carbohydrates, vitamins and minerals to meet minimum dietary needs. However, a liquid diet can never take the place of a well-balanced, conventional diet tailored to the individual's needs. And the only path to permanent weight control is through development of good eating habits, based on a careful selection from the four basic food groups— meats; fruits and vegetables; dairy products; and grains.

Q *Does smoking cut down your appetite?*

A There is no good evidence to support this belief. However, individuals who give up smoking frequently put on some extra weight at first. Food may begin to taste better, so they eat more. If you have a cigarette in your mouth, you get what psychologists call "oral satisfaction" and are perhaps less likely to take so much food.

Q *Is it true that the more you eat the more you want?*

A When you overeat one day you're hungrier the next. Huge meals stretch your stomach and throw your appetite out of proportion. After you become used to smaller intake you may wonder how you could have eaten so much previously.

Q *Would we all be better off if we ate five times daily?*

A Two extra snacks (not large meals), halfway between main meals—the routine of many school children, office workers and Britishers—provide quick-energy pickups, increase efficiency and make us less greedy at main meals.

Q *Should one eat less in hot weather?*

A It's good practice to cut down on indigestibles, but if you exercise a lot in summer and sit by the fireside all winter, you'll actually need more food in the hot months.

Q *Is food a cure for fatigue?*

A Fatigue gives you an abnormal appetite. But never eat heavily when you're overtired. Instead of the quick pickup you're after, the meal is likely to lie undigested and cause some gastric complications.

Q *Is a bedtime snack advisable?*

A A light snack or a cup of soup or milk before bedtime makes for a good rest. It draws blood into the digestive organs and away from the brain. Only if you overeat or choose heavy, greasy foods are you in for trouble.

Q *If most fat people ate what they say they eat would they be thin?*

A Fat people who claim they "eat like birds" aren't deceitful; either they eat little compared with what they'd like to eat or they fool themselves. In recent clinical tests a number of overweight people were put on a diet of what they *said* they ate. They proceeded to shed *five pounds* a day.

What You Should Really Weigh

from U.S. News and World Report

You can throw away those old weight charts. A big U S.-Canadian survey made by the Society of Actuaries has provided a new set of standards to tell you what you ought to weigh for your height and age. Out of the survey has come new evidence that it pays to stay slim—because fat people die sooner than slim ones—and that people with lower-than-average blood pressure live longer-than-average lives.

People are taller than thirty years ago. The report says: "The average heights in the present study suggest that over a period of some 40 years there has been an increase of nearly 1½ inches in height among men, and about ½ inch among women."

Men have grown heavier in relation to height, a trend most evident among short men and young men.

For *young* women the weight trend is just the opposite. At twenty to twenty-four years of age, women 5 feet 4 inches tall now average 121 pounds. In 1929, the average was 126 pounds. For women in their thirties, the comparative averages are 132 and 134. But look what happens in the next age bracket—the forties. Here the average weight jumps to 140—close to the average of 141 in 1929. Women nowadays stay slim longer than men, but put on weight faster once they begin to expand.

The results of the survey are important in assessing the danger of overweight. That danger is calculated by comparing the death rates of slim, average and fat persons. Among men with weights 20 pounds above average, the report shows, the death rate is about 10 percent above average. With added weight, the death rate goes up—to 25 percent above average for men 25 pounds over average weight, and up to 75 percent above average for men weighing 50 pounds above the average. "The lowest mortality ratios among men at ages 30 and over," say the actuaries, "are consistently associated with underweight, often of appreciable degree."

The insurance records confirm that several dangerous diseases are associated with overweight—diabetes, for instance, and certain digestive ailments such as gallbladder disease. And, among those markedly overweight, death rates from heart disease are markedly high. But the survey holds out this hope for the overweight: among those who reduced, the mortality rate went down. In other words, it pays to reduce.

Women, it appears, are better able than men to withstand the effects of high blood pressure. Right now the women's mortality risk is half of the men's. Even so, mortality rates of women, too, go up with their blood pressure.

"Diseases of the heart and circulatory system," the report says, "account for most of the excess deaths among those with elevated blood pressure." The danger is greatest when high blood pressure is combined with overweight; death rates were abnormally high among fat people with high blood pressure. Here, again, heart and circulatory diseases account for most of the excess mortality.

The findings all boil down to this: to live long, stay slim—and keep your blood pressure down.

It's a very odd thing—
As odd as can be,
That whatever Miss T. eats
Turns into Miss T.
　　　　　　　—Walter de la Mare

The New Average Weights

(Height is with shoes on; weight is with ordinary indoor clothing.)

MEN

Height	Age 30-39	Age 40-49	Age 50-59	Age 60-69
5'2"	137	140	142	139
5'4"	145	148	149	146
5'6"	153	156	157	154
5'8"	161	165	166	163
5'10"	170	174	175	173
6'	179	183	185	183
6'2"	188	192	194	193
6'4"	199	203	205	204

WOMEN

Height	Age 30-39	Age 40-49	Age 50-59	Age 60-69
5'	120	127	130	131
5'2"	126	133	136	137
5'4"	132	140	144	145
5'6"	139	147	152	153
5'8"	146	155	160	161
5'10"	154	164	169	*

*Average omitted because of lack of sufficient cases.

Food for Thought

A DOCTOR in Berkeley, California, is making a name for himself by his success in reducing overweight women. Asked his secret, he replied, "I get a head start on a case, that's all. On the patient's first call I spend only a few minutes with her, just long enough to weigh her and instruct her to keep a complete written record of every bite she eats during the two weeks until her second appointment. And," he smiled, "by the end of those two weeks most patients have already lost about ten pounds!"

—John C. Sergeant

How to Reduce– the Question of Eating

by Robert P. Goldman

When I was eighteen years old I weighed 185 pounds, obviously too much for my 5-foot 11-inch frame. In 1957, when I was thirty-two, I weighed 206. Had I continued at that rate, I'd be grossing 212 today. But, starting in 1957, I shed 41 pounds and, even more difficult (as anyone who has lost weight fast knows), I've kept it off. I used no crash diets, no vibrating tables, no appetite depressants. While losing weight, I ate (and drank) just about everything—meat, butter, potatoes, dessert, even beer and whisky.

Fortunately, as a science writer, I had the latest findings in weight control to draw on when I formulated my reducing plan. Even so, it took some jolting experiences to propel me into action. Now I know that the person who would reduce (and stay reduced) must be motivated strongly enough to embark on a lifetime plan involving new habits.

In my case, the motivation was fear. My father had several heart attacks, which led to his death. When my mother developed cardiac symptoms, I realized that my chances of escaping some form of heart disease were greatly reduced.

Then a close friend, a man of forty, collapsed with a suspected coronary thrombosis. He was 30 pounds overweight. As I sat at his bedside in the hospital, we discussed our families; and the rather terrifying prospect crossed my mind of what my young son's future would be like without a father. I knew that the death rates for overweights were higher than for those of normal weight. I remember walking out of that hospital room saying to myself, "This is it. I'm going to start losing weight *now*." And I did it. My decision was literally a matter of life and death.

I believe that you can do what I did, no matter how much you weigh. Furthermore, what I learned can prevent overweight from becoming a source of misery in the first place.

Since overeating is the basic cause of overweight in most cases, the first step in any program is to determine *why* you overeat. Emotional needs, feelings of inadequacy, disappointment, anger can send people scurrying for food and its physical solace. In my case the trigger was tension. When deadlines loomed, when I had a tiff with my wife or my boss, I relied on food as a cushion for my wounded feelings. But I found that once you face the reasons for your overeating, they lose much of their hold on you.

Because boredom and frustration can lead to overeating, try coördinating the launching of your weight-loss program with a change in your way of life. A new job or a switch of tasks in your present one, almost any new pursuit—gardening, golf, even preoccupation with minor home-repair jobs—can provide satisfactions formerly assuaged by food.

Seek help with your plan, from your spouse or, if you are younger, your parents (though mothers tend to overstuff their children). A good family doctor is an invaluable asset—one who is willing to help you explore your emotional as well as physical needs over a long period.

Then, if your motivation is strong and you've come to grips with your emotional needs, the changing of your food patterns shouldn't be difficult.

I'm opposed to rigid, printed diets, one-food diets (the steak diet, egg diet, fat diet), calorie-counting devices, weight-reducing preparations and gimmicks of all kinds.

What you weigh now is most likely the result of your long-term eating patterns. It follows that weight control must be a lifelong activity, of which you are constantly aware. This is the key to the failure of short-term crash diets. They do nothing to change basic eating patterns of years' standing.

With the help of your physician, learn *something* about caloric values—how much to cut your own eating and which foods provide necessary vitamins and minerals. The high-calorie foods are easy to remember (you know them already)—fat meats, pork, ham, bacon, lamb, butter, fried foods, gravies, anything creamed, the macaroni family, potatoes, some salad dressings, alcoholic beverages and most sweets.

Armed with this information, you can revise your eating habits. But to make the new habits stick, don't change too drastically. Think about the change first and it will come more easily. Reorienting my own eating patterns, I devised four basic rules:

Decrease the size of all portions. Have a smaller slice of roast beef, a smaller piece of pie. I used to eat two large lamb chops; now I eat one and a half. I switched from three teaspoons of sugar in my coffee to one. Instead of two predinner highballs, I have one. I cut portions of peas and string beans, too, but because such foods are less caloric I decreased them less sharply.

A corollary to the habit of eating less is the habit of eating *slowly.* When you take your time, savoring each morsel, the appetite is more readily appeased than it is when you bolt your food.

Leave a little of everything on your plate. This is an easy method of cutting down, especially if you are dining out and don't have control of the size of portions. No one minds. Your hostess will be more likely to notice that you ate everything she served than that you left a few mouthfuls.

Eliminate some foods—at some meals. For instance, when I was heavy, I ate potatoes every day. I cut that to two or three times a week. I eliminated one pat of butter a day. I switched to open-face sandwiches—one slice of bread instead of two. From fried foods five times a week, I cut down to fried foods twice a week (the same foods can usually be sautéed, broiled or boiled).

Notice that I gave up no single food entirely; yet this cutting down reduced my daily intake by some 425 calories.

Try using substitutes for high-calorie foods some of the time. Try, for instance, poultry and seafood for the meats; skim milk for whole milk and cream; cottage cheese for the richer cheeses; broccoli, beets, carrots, green beans and spinach for the potatoes and lima beans; fresh fruits for the sweets. If you simply cannot do without certain specific foods—say, ham or sweet potatoes— eat them, but cut the portions and compensate by using substitutes for some other foods you can give up more easily.

The total reduction I achieved with these four steps was about 800 calories a day. (Your doctor will help determine the right number for you.) Then, in addition, I supplemented my food regulation with one other important weight-control measure— greater physical activity.

Weight is determined by the number of calories you put into the body machine balanced against the number you expend. Thus, new eating habits can only reduce the intake. Greater body activity can increase the output. Your best bet is to combine the two. The important thing to remember is that energy expenditure *every* day, *every* week, *every* year *will* make a difference in the long run. To make physical activity pay, *stay with it—for life.*

In any weight-losing program, expect some backsliding. In my case, after a regular loss of one and a half pounds a week for five months, I was suddenly unable to lose more. This, explained the doctor, is common; the body may be adjusting to its new weight before letting go of more. I stuck to my guns for ten discouraging weeks before I started to lose again. From then on the weight loss was steady. When I reached the desired weight for my frame, I tapered off. But I was constantly vigilant.

"Bobbing and weaving" is a matter of going after the two or three pounds as *soon* as they creep back, then relaxing a bit. The real backslider is the man who tells you that he lost twenty or more pounds, then, to his infinite disgust, regained them. This means that after dieting he relapsed into his old habits; that he had no plan for steady, permanent caloric reduction.

Are the results worth all the effort? The answer is a resounding yes. You'll like yourself better. In addition to improved appearance and a new buoyancy, you'll have an immeasurable sense of accomplishment, a feeling that you've overcome forces that threatened your peace of mind and physical well-being—and a gratifying sense that you've contributed to the preservation of your life.

Does Exercise Help or Hinder?

by Blake Clark

Should we try to combat weight exclusively by diet? Forgoing exercise, millions of us in our sit-down civilization expend so little energy that we cannot eat enough to satisfy our appetites without putting on weight. We condemn ourselves to a choice between accumulating fat or going hungry.

But results of experiments by Dr. Jean Mayer at the Department of Nutrition of the Harvard School of Public Health now show that combating overweight by diet alone is fighting with one hand behind our back. Exercise, he declares, is the other fist that would enable us to deal the knockout blow.

The National Research Council of the U.S.A. has recommended dietary allowances that range from 2400 calories daily for sedentary men to 6000 or more for laborers and athletes. This admittedly wide variation, Dr. Mayer says, proves the unquestioned value of physical activity in maintaining normal weight.

Dr. Mayer's former colleague, Dr. George Mann, dramatically underlined this point at Harvard. Four medical students agreed to eat twice as much as they needed, and then to exercise enough to keep themselves from gaining weight. The students normally ate 3000 calories daily. Dr. Mann saw to it that they had three big meals every day, and enough candy in between to swell their total to 6000 calories.

Then they swam vigorously, repeatedly ran sprints, played basketball and raced on bicycles. Even gorging themselves with twice as much as they normally ate, they scarcely gained an ounce. Their complexions became ruddy, their tolerance to cold increased and, unanimously, they claimed to feel relaxed and rugged. Moreover, they slept better and studied more efficiently.

"Exercise is self-defeating," say the lazy dieters. "It makes you eat more than usual and immediately gain back what you lost."

Scoffers continually repeat that to take off a pound of fat by exercise you must perform some prodigious feat, such as walking thirty-six miles or splitting wood for seven hours. Knowing that we could not possibly go through such an ordeal, we despair of getting any help from exercise. But, Dr. Mayer points out, we do not have to hike the thirty-six miles in one forced march. If we walk a mile a day, we burn up a pound of fat in thirty-six days.

Dr. Mayer selected a sample of 213 men representing all ranges of activity, from sedentary to overworked. The light-activity engineers, foremen and drivers of small electric trucks *ate less* and *weighed less* than the sedentary supervisors, clerks and salespeople. Trash collectors, who hoisted heavy loads head-high all day, ate almost twice as much as men of their same weight doing less strenuous work. Finally, a group of extremely hard-pressed laborers, shoveling ton after ton of coal all day and over-time, steadily lost weight despite a high intake. In all the 213, the only ones noticeably fat were in the inactive group.

If you are a city dweller, you can walk your way to normal weight. Fat creeps up on most of us by just a few calories a day. A dietary excess of only 80 calories—the amount in a slice of bread—will cause a 165-pound, chair-borne man to gain at least 13 pounds in five years. But he would expend about 80 calories during a one-mile stroll. He could keep himself at a trim 165 by walking fifteen minutes to the office in the morning and back in the afternoon instead of taking the car. Swimming dissolves away 150 to 350 calories in a half hour; cycling, as many as 300.

Anyone, anywhere, can do calisthenics—still the most convenient way to keep fit. Though boring to some, calisthenics bring rewards in weight control (as much as 200 calories a quarter hour), and in limberness and the good feeling that comes with stimulated circulation.

I Never Saw a Fat Woman in Bali

How do the women of Bali keep their lovely, graceful figures? An important factor is the custom of frequent nibbling rather than eating three meals a day. Breakfast is a cup of coffee with a good deal of sugar at six or so in the morning. An hour later the Balinese will take a *mouthful* of cold boiled rice packaged in a banana leaf. In another hour they will eat a piece of fruit. Throughout the day they nibble on fermented soybean cake, beans, a piece of fish, coconut meat, cassava, more rice, or sweetened colored water. The quantities are very small—any solid food is only a tablespoon or two wrapped in a banana leaf.

This custom of keeping lean by eating several small meals a day supports Dr. Jean Mayer's theory, developed in our laboratory, that the level of sugar in the blood is important in regulating those cells in the brain that regulate appetite. When the sugar in the blood is below a certain level, the "appestat"—as Dr. Norman Jolliffe terms those cells—is turned on and you are hungry. As soon as the blood sugar rises above this level, your appestat shuts off and you are not hungry. By their frequent nibbling, the Balinese keep their blood sugar at a level that minimizes the desire for eating and thus reduces food intake.

Eat three moderate meals a day, with emphasis on breakfast. Save part of what you would normally eat at lunch or dinner for snacks. Then you can nibble without adding more calories.　　—Frederick J. Stare, M.D.

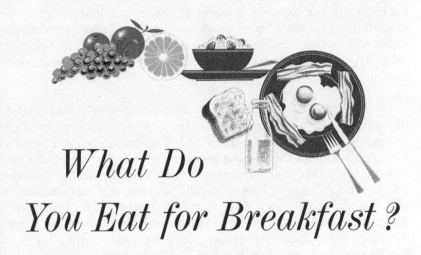

What Do You Eat for Breakfast?

by Frederic Sondern, Jr.

Two out of three of us eat too little for breakfast. Medical surveys indicate that this bad habit of skimping on what nutrition experts consider the most important meal of the day is causing a noticeable loss of efficiency at work and of fun at play, much ill health, many industrial accidents and a lot of bad manners.

A canvass of 50,000 students from first grade through college revealed the startling fact that approximately 65 percent habitually ate a breakfast entirely inadequate for their physical needs; 8000 of them were eating none at all. Believing that much of their trouble with inattentive and fractious pupils can be traced to that cause, educators in increasing numbers are teaching youngsters the importance of proper breakfasting.

Industrial concerns searching for the causes of decreasing production found that half their employes arrived in the morning with no food in their stomachs. For men and women who do manual work, particularly heavy labor, this is not only detrimental to health but actually dangerous. Army efficiency engineers, investigating almost 1000 accident cases in ordnance depots, found that a large majority of the injured workers had come to their jobs without breakfast; resulting fatigue and carelessness had struck them down.

Hidden hunger—which is no advertising catchword but a phrase that many doctors use—is a pernicious malady, according to such authorities as Dr. E. V. McCollum of Johns Hopkins University, one of the leading investigators of food effects on the human body. My own experience with it was typical. Formerly a heavy breakfaster, I had gradually reduced my morning meal to a slice of toast and a cup of coffee. Normally energetic and pleasant enough at 9 a.m., I began to feel myself running down mentally and physically as the morning passed. By 11 I was grouchy and no longer on my toes. By noon I was irritable, scatterbrained—and hungry. But anything more than a light lunch would almost knock me out with sleepiness for an hour. Obviously something was wrong. I went to my doctor.

After a thorough examination which revealed nothing organically out of order, he asked me what I ate for breakfast. "That's your trouble," he said. "You're suffering from hidden hunger."

I glanced at my ample midriff.

"Oh, you're fat enough," he added ungraciously. "But you're undernourished because you don't eat correctly. Most people don't. They expect a hasty, meager breakfast and then a quick, equally careless lunch to carry them through the eleven hours during which mind and body are working at top speed. Then they stoke up at their big meal in the evening with the food elements they should have had during the day. Experiments at the University of Chicago have established that at night, mostly spent in sleep, the body transforms the food not into useful energy but mainly into fat."

For the trial week that the doctor ordered, my wife and I got up half an hour earlier than usual. We set an attractive table, prepared a stout breakfast of fruit, cereal, eggs, toast and coffee—and ate it slowly, without watching the clock. A relaxed and cheerful mood set in, and my morning's work went along with no sign of the old weariness, no more barking at people. After a sensible lunch the afternoon passed as satisfactorily. Breakfast has remained my most important meal ever since.

To determine the effects of breakfast habits, University of Iowa scientists tested a group of volunteers of various ages with special devices which measure exactly an individual's work output, mental alertness and inclination to fatigue. For the first two weeks the volunteers were given a heavy breakfast. For the next two, none at all. Then only a cup of coffee. And finally a light breakfast.

The results were startling. The unsatisfactory effect of the light meal in comparison with the heavy one was apparent enough: work output and mental alertness decreased, and muscle tremor—a measure of the fatigue responsible for so many industrial accidents—increased sharply. And with no breakfast or only coffee, output and alertness fell away to less than half of what they should be, and the dangerous tremor became violent in almost every case.

From the results of these and many other studies, leading nutrition experts are pretty well agreed that breakfast should provide between a quarter and a third of the day's food requirements, and that the minimum breakfast essential for the average sedentary worker should consist of fruit or fruit juice, hot or cold vitamin-enriched cereal with sugar and milk or cream, whole-grain or enriched white bread with butter, and a beverage, preferably milk or cocoa. (Coffee is an enjoyable waker-upper, but its only nutritional contribution comes from the sugar and milk put into it.) Boys between thirteen and twenty—in a class by themselves for expenditure of energy and chemical needs for their growing bodies—and physically active men and women need meat or eggs in addition.

Each one of the recommended breakfast staples does an essential job. Fruits and fruit juices contain the vitally important Vitamin C, which among other things starts our metabolism— our whole chemical process—working again after the night's slowdown. This vitamin is also essential for the proper growth of children, and helps keep our joints flexible in later years. Cereal contains a variety of essentials. One is the Vitamin B complex—thiamine, riboflavin and niacin. Lack of the Vitamin B family may produce irritability, fatigue and decrease of efficiency, as well as loss of appetite and sleeplessness. Whole-grain cereal is also rich in the proteins, which build energy; in phosphorus and iron, which build and repair human tissue; and in Vitamin A, which helps to keep the skin healthy, pliable and attractive. Insufficient intake of any of these at breakfast cannot be made up at other meals without overeating.

Many women today seem to have the idea that skimping breakfast or omitting it is an easy way to reduce weight and generally improve their appearance. Nothing could be further from the truth, according to the consensus of modern medical thinking. Insufficient intake of the vitamins and minerals in cereal and bread, for example, is likely to cause anemia, in which the blood thins, the skin may become sallow and rough, the complexion suffers from pimples and sores, circles develop under the eyes.

Milk, another must, contains calcium for the building and repair of bone structure. Without it, bones may become malformed and brittle. The U.S. Department of Agriculture's Bureau of Human Nutrition and Home Economics, after exhaustive research, came to the conclusion that a pint of milk a day for adults, whole or skim, and a quart for children is the necessary minimum. Bread and butter or their variations—buttered rolls, toast, pancakes, muffins, waffles—supply additional proteins, fats and carbohydrates that make up the calories we expend in energy. So do eggs and meat.

There is no excuse for a skimpy breakfast. With automatic cooking apparatus, conveniently packaged and scientifically enriched breakfast foods, frozen fruits and fruit juices, the housewife who allows her family to suffer from hidden hunger is not doing her job. And that job is one of considerable importance to the health and welfare of the nation.

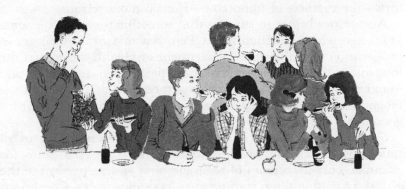

Starving Teen-Agers

by Myril Axelrod

For a number of years nutrition experts have been quietly checking on an alarming condition that still seems incredible despite mounting evidence. In the United States, land of abundance, *far too many boys and girls between the ages of thirteen and nineteen are undernourished.*

Investigators are now convinced that teen-age malnutrition is nationwide. Their studies show that the average American child is properly nourished only up to the age of two; thereafter his diet declines steadily until it hits an alarming low in the teens. Teen-agers, with plenty of pocket money and allowed to eat anything they like away from home, become meal-skippers and food faddists. They do not get enough protein to build sound tissues, enough calcium for strong bones and good teeth, enough vitamins and minerals for steady nerves, normal blood and efficient vision.

Result: The boys make a sad showing in physical examinations, as physical fitness tests indicate, but the nutritional status of the girls—the mothers of tomorrow—is even more serious.

Authorities began to suspect that something was wrong some years ago when nutritionists at Pennsylvania State College, in coöperation with the state Department of Health, examined the food intake of 2536 teen-agers over a typical seven-day period and found that only about one quarter of them had diets that met the recommended allowances of the National Research Council for good nutrition.

Subsequent studies of more than 59,000 boys and girls in 38 states revealed the nationwide situation. In New York State, for example, only 21 percent of teen-age boys and 12 percent of the girls were getting the recommended food allowances. Conditions are no better in the rural areas than in the big cities, and bear no relation to poverty. There is even evidence that children from poor families are often better nourished than their more affluent classmates—who can fill themselves up on candy and soft drinks.

Most nutritionists, doctors and teachers agree that, basically, two factors are to blame: dietary ignorance and a lack of parental direction or discipline, which enables adolescents to indulge their own dietary whims. The youngsters, when left to their own devices, often go haywire.

For example, the luncheon generally favored by the high-school set consists of a hot dog, a bag of potato chips and a bottle of pop. After school the youngsters consume candy bars and soft drinks. They get so full of "empty calories" that they have neither appetite nor capacity for the evening meal.

I made a tour of high schools, ate in school cafeterias and visited the adjacent snack bars and soda fountains that are youth's favorite hangouts. In one school lunchroom I found a well-balanced meal being offered for less than the price of a hot dog and a soft drink. But of 1500 students *only 90 ate in the cafeteria!* The crowds flocked to the nearby snack bars, juke joints and hot-dog wagons.

I stood on the balcony of a large cafeteria opposite a boys' high school and watched the trays go by. While the counters displayed soups, meats, salads, vegetables and fruits, the students' trays bore, instead, macaroni, baked beans, bread, cake, pies, ice cream, coffee. Out of fifty students at one sitting I saw only two drinking milk.

Everybody today knows that nutrition is the basis of health, and that nourishing food is never more important than in the formative years when the bones and tissues that must serve us through a lifetime are being manufactured. Still, as one physician stated, "We are allowing our adolescents to cultivate deficiencies that can plague them with illnesses the rest of their lives."

There is nothing tricky or difficult about the balanced diet. Girls need about half a pound of meat, fish or poultry a day, boys a couple of ounces more. Both need an additional three-ounce serving of liver once a week. Both need, every day, a quart of milk, one egg, an eight-ounce glass of orange, grapefruit or tomato juice, and two servings of leafy green or yellow vegetables, plus at least a pound of other fruits and vegetables.

Most doctors feel that the real consequences of teen-age malnutrition may not become fully apparent for years. One immediate effect, however, is poor resistance to infectious disease. Tuberculosis has been decreasing steadily in other age groups, but it is still a serious problem among teen-agers, particularly girls.

The food habits of girls are a major cause for alarm. One third of today's brides, and one quarter of mothers bearing a first child, are under twenty years old. Many of the doctors I consulted mentioned childbirth complications as a consequence of teen-age malnutrition. The cases they offered all had a tragic sameness—indulgence in empty calories followed by attempts to reduce.

Two hospitals in Washington, D.C., which have made special studies of teen-age mothers report that *one out of five* girls developed toxemia, a serious complication of pregnancy. An authority on maternal diets speaks bluntly: "A girl whose nutrition is not adequate for her own body cannot expect to develop a good baby."

What can be done to make American teen-agers see the light? At the Children's Bureau in Washington I was convinced that much is being done, although not yet on a wide enough scale.

Some schools are now successfully teaching children the facts about the food they need. At a high school in Newton, Massachusetts, the boys' eating habits improved markedly after the captain of the Harvard football team talked to the assembly about his training diet. In New York the kids are being taught that even their hot-dog snack can be made nutritionally sound simply by substituting a milk shake for the soda pop, coleslaw for the potato chips, and adding an apple!

The Children's Bureau urges PTA and civic groups to put pressure on the local snack bars to serve more milk, fruit juices and meat sandwiches. The schools themselves should put milk and fruit juices in their vending machines.

Wherever the problem has been tackled with imagination, the youngsters have responded. Texas State College for Women put on a dramatic demonstration with 122 teen-age girls as guinea pigs. They were chosen because their malnutrition was apparent in poor teeth, sallow complexions and lack of stamina. A year on optimum diets—which included, to the girls' surprise, desserts and even Southern fried chicken—produced spectacular results. The girls not only felt and looked much better but, said one, "We even think better! This is *fun!*"

Parents are urged to plan the evening meal carefully, featuring more desserts made with milk and eggs, and appetizing casseroles with lots of vegetables. There should be more fruit juices and less soda in the refrigerator, and more fresh fruit and carrot and celery sticks available for between-meal snacks.

These vitally needed changes in teen-age diets are a matter of proper food selection and proper cooking rather than the addition of expensive foods. The balanced diet is often less costly than the poor diet.

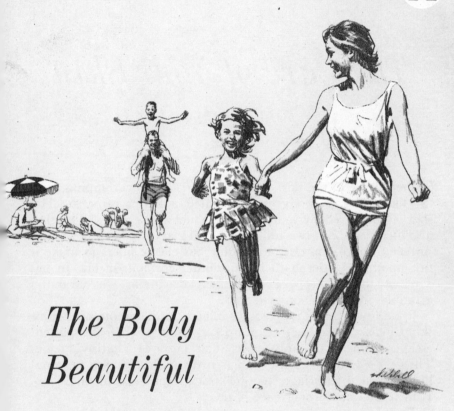

CHAPTER 14

The Body Beautiful

T HAT OLD ADAGE "Handsome is as handsome does" is a scientific fact as well. Skin, eyes, teeth, hair, feet and muscles —each of these has a remarkable nature that we should understand. When we do, it is far easier for us to give the little time and effort needed for good care. If the speed of modern living results in neglect, we pay for it. If we are victims of old wives' tales or of the fictions of modern quacks, we pay for it.

And fiction and fancy are not nearly so fascinating as the scientific discoveries about the care of our human body.

The Care of Your Skin

by Elsie McCormick

The surface of the skin is an armor made of overlapping, fish-like scales. Nobody ever invented a better raincoat. The skin is punctured by millions of tiny holes, the pores. The skin also includes about two million tiny oil glands to keep the horny surface from drying out, and numerous elastic fibers to make it fit smoothly. Underneath lie insulating cushions of fat. In old age these tend to disappear, which explains in part why Grandpa grumbles so much about the cold.

In addition the skin is closely related to the emotions. Minor skin diseases sometimes clear up surprisingly when the patient escapes from an unhappy love affair or finds a satisfying job. Thus the condition of the skin is tied up closely with personal happiness—in marriage, in one's social contacts, in one's job. How, then, take proper care of it?

There's not much anyone can do about a wrinkled skin, according to the experts. Late in life the fat disappears from under the skin, and those elastic fibers become as unresponsive as a worn-out girdle. And no cream, massage or washing with May dew can save the face from falling into folds.

Fortunately there are methods of preventing oneself from looking old before one's time. Do you know the quickest way to age your face? Just bake it in the summer sun. This dries out natural oil, encourages wrinkles and speeds up the life cycle of the cells, so that skin hastens to grow old. Grandma might have looked odd with her parasol, but she was doing a scientific job of cheating the years. If you can't resist sitting bareheaded on a broiling beach, you should save your face by using a chemical parasol—a preparation to absorb the damaging rays.

You can also acquire unnecessary wrinkles by spending the winter in an overheated, dried-out house, by removing the natural oil through excessive use of soap and skin tonics and by habitually wearing a sour or anxious expression. If you're on the far side of forty you can fight encroaching lines by cutting down on the use of salt. When people reach middle age, excreting salt becomes more difficult. The residue in the system stretches the skin, eventually causing wrinkles.

Cold cream protects the skin from dirt, and prevents it from drying out. But creams won't "nourish" your exterior; the only adequate way to do that is through the digestive system. And there isn't a cream on earth that can really reduce large pores on the face. These pores are exits for the oil glands, and become larger as a person grows older.

Any organ as complicated as the skin is bound to develop diseases. Of the dangerous ones, skin cancer comes first. Each year it kills about 4200 of us. Yet dermatologists say that practically every one of these deaths could have been prevented. Skin cancers develop out in plain sight. They can be recognized at an early stage, and removed by surgery, radium or X rays.

The most important avoidable cause of skin cancer is probably excessive exposure to the sun. The disease occurs most frequently among persons who work outdoors and sunbathers who try to bake themselves into a soufflé. It affects about nine times as many blonds as brunets. Moderate sun exposure can be beneficial, but don't be a contestant for the most ferocious burn on the beach.

Another bit of advice: Keep a careful watch on moles and warts. The average person possesses about forty moles. The vast majority of these small pigmented spots are never dangerous, but the gray or slate-blue mole, occurring most frequently on the head or feet, sometimes turns darker or rougher or begins to enlarge. If this occurs, rush to the doctor.

You needn't worry about the warts that occur in early youth, for they are never a prelude to cancer. They can be routed by various kinds of medical treatment. Dermatologists have evidence that they can also be removed by suggestion— something that children, with their mumbo-jumbo treatment, have known for centuries. Doctors have caused large numbers of warts to disappear by painting them with colored water. Other warts have vanished after supposed X-ray treatments, in which the machine did no more than make a noise. Why? Nobody really knows.

Emotional upsets rank high among the causes of both eczema and hives. If you are not in a position to express what you think, your skin sometimes does it for you. Children unhappy at school sometimes develop Monday-to-Friday eczema, which improves miraculously over the weekend. Hives and eczema are also often caused by allergies.

If you want to keep your exterior in first-class condition, just follow a few simple principles. Get plenty of vitamins, especially Vitamin A, give attention to physical cleanliness, worship the sun with moderated enthusiasm, cultivate a good disposition and refrain from painting the town red. Maybe you won't have as much fun, but you'll have a better skin.

Of ALL THE THINGS you wear, your expression is the most important. The next time you catch a glimpse of yourself in a store window or a counter mirror, skip the glance at your hat angle and check up on the expression just below. Then decide if it isn't worth a little time and effort to exchange that look of grim determination for something a little more appealing.   —Janet Lane

Facts about Eye Care

Adapted from "Facts and Non-Facts about Eye Care"
by John Kord Lagemann
and "What You Should Know about Your Eyes" *by Carle Hodge*

D o you believe that reading in dim light will ruin your eyes?
That television can harm a child's eyesight? That cheap sunglasses injure the eye? That excessive reading causes nearsightedness? That you would not need glasses today if you had worn
them as a child? That parents need not worry about a child's
cross-eyes because he'll soon outgrow them?

All these statements have this in common: They are untrue.

Since the eye can be examined more precisely than any other
organ of the body, it may seem strange that so much misinforma-
tion about it should still exist. Even eye specialists are occasionally
responsible for perpetuating some of the fallacies. But this becomes less surprising when the nature of sight is understood.

We do not see with our eyes alone. We see with our minds
and, indeed, with our entire personalities. What we think of as
eye ailments, therefore, can be the result of emotional difficulties
or physical malfunctioning, or both. Emotional factors actually
predominate in some eye ailments.

"Eyestrain," for instance, sends more patients to eye practitioners than any other complaint. Called asthenopia, it is blamed
for a bewildering variety of aches and pains, including nausea,
insomnia, headaches and loss of appetite. Yet medical authorities

have discovered in recent years that eyestrain is almost never responsible for these ailments attributed to it.

"The patient with asthenopia," said the late Dr. Edward Weiss, of Temple University, an authority on psychosomatic medicine, "needs a change in his outlook on life and not in his lenses."

This does not mean that eyestrain is simply a product of the imagination. Eye muscles may ache when you use them excessively and they get tired, especially if you need glasses or are using improper lenses, or if you do close work under inadequate light. But straining to see under these adverse conditions affects only the muscles, and can no more damage your eyes than listening to a whisper can damage your ears.

Instead of resting the eyes to relieve strain, many ophthalmologists encourage patients to use their eyes all the more—provided no inflammation or disease is present—in a kind of disciplined training. The theory is that with greater use the muscles of the eyes will become stronger and will tire—and ache—less frequently.

What, then, is the explanation when people complain of headaches after reading under improper light? Most specialists today are convinced that there is no physical basis for such claims. "I recall a young girl who developed terrible headaches while studying," says Dr. John McLean, professor of ophthalmological surgery at New York Hospital-Cornell Medical Center. "But on close questioning it turned out that the headaches occurred only when she studied Latin, and no other subject."

Headaches attributed to eyestrain often disappear after the patient has been fitted with glasses—even though it is later discovered that the lenses are not well fitted and fail to aid the person's vision. While properly fitted glasses make reading less tiring, it is often not the glasses but the patient's feeling of relief at having been helped that "cures" the headaches.

While the eye is extremely responsive to emotional influences, it is astonishingly tough and resilient in adjusting to external factors. Television and movies both have been blamed for harm-

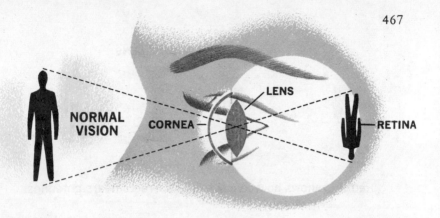

ful eyestrain, but ophthalmologists deny that either medium inflicts any damage. Neither, under most circumstances, will sunlight (unless, of course, one stares directly at the sun). Nor will cheap sunglasses. Tinted or smoked lenses—the color is irrelevant—cut down glare at a beach or in the snow, but in ordinary sunlight they are unnecessary for healthy eyes.

Light enters your eye through the lens, which focuses it on a light-sensitive surface called the retina. In an imperfect eye the images are defective because the lens is warped (astigmatism); or the retina is too close to the lens (farsightedness); or too far away (nearsightedness); or the image from one eye is so blurred or off-beam that it cannot be fused with the image from the other eye (strabismus, or cross-eye). Apart from injury or disease, care of the eye itself boils down mainly to the correction of these four kinds of defects.

Since none of us has a perfectly formed lens or cornea (the transparent "skin" which covers the colored part of the eye), all of us have a certain degree of astigmatism. If the flaws aren't too bad, the brain can unscramble the distortions in the image. If the distortions are handicapping, specially ground lenses can compensate for the flaws and provide clearer pictures.

The other focusing defects—near- and farsightedness—are largely a matter of eyeball dimension. The eyeball normally measures exactly 24 millimeters from lens to retina. If the eyeball

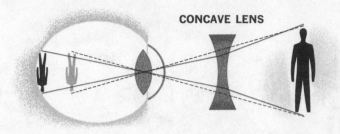

Red line shows how concave lens corrects nearsightedness

is large, the light focuses at a point slightly in front of the retina, causing nearsightedness, or myopia. If the eyeball is small, the light hits the retina before it comes into focus, causing farsightedness, or hyperopia.

Few of us have eyeballs with perfect dimensions. But as long as the eyes are only slightly farsighted or nearsighted, they can still focus on objects at varying distances. Ciliary muscles squeeze the lens in each eye to thicken it and adjust for increasing nearness. This ability to thicken the lens is called "accommodation." For reading and other close work the farsighted person has to use it constantly. Thus when the lens becomes less elastic in middle age the farsighted person must often wear glasses to see things that are nearby.

We inherit the size of our eyeballs. At birth they are small;

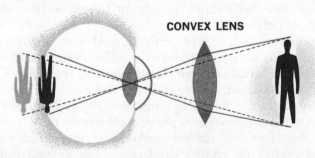

Red line shows how convex lens corrects farsightedness

thus almost all of us start out life farsighted. Then, as growth proceeds, children who inherit large eyeballs develop myopia. Since the growth period coincides with schooling, parents often blame the myopia on too much study. Actually, reading can neither cause it nor make it worse. But myopia does seem to predispose a child to read a great deal. Severe myopia shrinks the clearly visible world to an area no more than a foot or two from the tip of the child's nose. Unless he wears glasses constantly he is disqualified from activities that require distance vision. Reading, then, is often his major link with the world beyond the blur.

A leading sight killer is glaucoma, which usually attacks people approaching middle life. Normally, the eye's lens and cornea are fed with a fluid called aqueous humor, which forms behind the colored iris, flows forward into the front part of the eye and then drains back into the blood system. In glaucoma the eye's drainage system clogs up. The aqueous humor causes pressure against the retina, a membrane at the back of the ball which picks up light rays and helps transmit them along the optic nerve to the brain. As the pressure pushes the retina and nerve, light is slowly squeezed out.

Among the symptoms of glaucoma are blurring of vision and the appearance of colored rainbows like halos around bright lights. But because the onset of glaucoma first affects side vision, and is often without pain, it is a stealthy villain. The National Society for the Prevention of Blindness says that one out of every fifty persons over forty has glaucoma, quite frequently without knowing it. The society suggests that the middle-aged have a thorough eye examination every other year. Vision once blotted out by glaucoma cannot be restored, but physicians can check the disease with medicinal drops or with surgery.

Cataract, more prevalent but less damaging than glaucoma, is a clouding of the eye's lens which may affect a person at any period of his life—even before birth. The most common form, however, afflicts the old. Cataract can develop because of shock, an injury to the eye as the result of disease or because of atomic radiation. (Ten percent of the survivors who had been within a few meters of the Hiroshima blast developed cataract.) Whatever the cause, the patient's sight can be restored by an operation which now is almost always successful. The clouded lens is removed. Extra-thick glasses compensate for its loss.

Blindness among children has been gradually decreasing, thanks mainly to the power of new drugs over infectious maladies. Silver nitrate, prescribed by law for the eyes of newborn infants, has all but stamped out "babies' sore eyes"—a scourge which, passed on by mothers infected with venereal or other germs, once blinded babies by the thousands.

Another blight on young lives, cross-eyes, is no longer the problem it once was. Orthoptic exercises, corrective glasses or simple surgery usually can help if treatment begins early enough.

But antiblindness organizations are not happy with the eye care our children are getting. At least a fourth of the country's school-agers need glasses or eye treatment. All children need regular testing by a qualified eye physician.

There are millions of people (about one man in 15, one woman in 100) who are "color-blind"—which means that they confuse some shades of reds, greens and yellows with other shades. The condition cannot be cured or treated.

Most of us pay little attention to our eyes. This is a mistake, as eye defects and diseases can become gradually worse. Here are some tips from the ophthalmologists: Never rub your eyes with your hands, nor touch them with a towel that is not clean. A cinder or other particle in the eye calls for the skilled hand of an eye physician. If sun glare annoys you, get sunglasses. You can read in bed as long as you keep a comfortable posture and proper lighting. Don't read or work under a patch of light; the whole room should be evenly lighted. Keep your whole body healthy—and happy. Excitement and anxiety can cripple your eyes. And remember—much bad vision is caused by worry.

People are willing to pay almost anything to save sight when they know it is in danger. But timely checkups against disease and simple precautions against accidents are worth more than the finest medical skill after the accident or disease has occurred.

What You Should Know about Your Hair

by J. D. Ratcliff

Pluck a hair from your head and examine it carefully. You are looking at something quite extraordinary—something which has inspired poets and painters for centuries and is the daily concern of more ordinary mortals. We probably devote more time, thought and money to hair than to any other constituent of the human anatomy. We cut, curl, tint and shave it, and industries worth hundreds of millions of dollars result. In the past decade medical research has learned more about hair than in all previous time.

Hair has some remarkable attributes. It is as strong as aluminum. If the hairs of your head were woven into a slender rope it could support a suspended weight of 2000 pounds—more than that of a small car. Head hair grows three eighths to three fourths of an inch a month—faster in summer than winter, faster during day than night.

Scattered over your body are some half-million hairs—the only major hairless areas are palms of hands and soles of feet. Under the microscope a cross section of a hair looks something like the cross section of a tree. The outer cells overlap like shingles. The next layer consists of long, filamentlike cells which give hair its strength and elasticity. This layer also contains the pigments which give hair its color. In the center is a marrow canal.

Hair is formed in follicles—little tubes folded into the skin. At the bottom of each follicle is a bulb-shaped tissue connected with blood vessels, so cells can form and grow. The new cells push the old ones up the follicle, and these old cells then undergo a process called keratinization which turns them into hair. (Keratin is a chemical found in such places as fingernails and the horns of a cow.) Because hair is no longer composed of living cells, it may be said to be "dead." That's why cutting it does not hurt us. And while hair tonics serve a purpose in grooming the hair and lubricating the scalp, there is nothing in a tonic that will stimulate the hair root to grow new hair.

Tiny muscles run out from hair follicles; when you're frightened or cold these muscles contract, giving a prickly sensation. Thus the expression: "My hair stood on end."

The shape of the follicle determines what kind of hair you will have. If the follicle is round, your hair will be straight. If it's oval or flattened, curly hair results. Many Negroes have elliptical follicles, which give their hair its characteristic appearance.

Look at some further facts about hair:

Dandruff: Dandruff is by far the most common hair complaint. Dead cells are continually being shed from the body. When this shedding becomes excessive on the scalp we have dandruff. Several medications are effective in stopping burning, itching, flaking. Among the most widely used are selenium sulphide, sulphur, resorcin and salicylic acid. If simple shampooing does not control the dandruff, your doctor will prescribe a remedy.

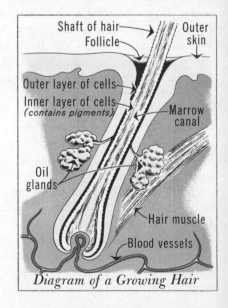

Diagram of a Growing Hair

Graying Hair: The old saying that in times of great stress hair will turn white overnight is probably untrue. Pigment is built into hair deep in the scalp. After the hair emerges at the surface pigment cannot be altered. However, as we grow older, pigment production slows and finally stops. Then hair grays and eventually whitens. From present evidence, a tendency to premature graying is an inherited characteristic and nothing can be done about it.

Falling Hair: Individual hairs in the head live two to five years. Then the follicle that produced them shrinks and goes into a resting phase and the hair drops out. Thus, a certain amount of loss is normal—in the neighborhood of eighty hairs a day. When the follicle returns to action, a new hair grows. At all times something like 10 percent of the follicles in the scalp are resting, and 90 percent are active. On other parts of the body the reverse is true—the greater number resting most of the time. But for this fact we would all be shaggy as sheep dogs.

What about excessive hair loss? Almost everything has been blamed for the balding process: wearing hats, not wearing hats; too much sexual activity, too little; too much exposure to the sun, too little; too frequent washing, too little. Dandruff has been charged with hastening the balding process. Yet countless people have dandruff all their lives and go to their graves with full heads of hair.

Today it is believed that we inherit a tendency to baldness. A man can look at pictures of his grandfather and get a clue as to what the future holds for him. Estimates indicate that baldness affects 43 percent of men, 8 percent of women. Can anything be done to restore hair to bald pates?

Several years ago the American Medical Association's Committee on Cosmetics made the flat assertion: "If the general health of a man is satisfactory and loss of hair is progressive . . . medical science does not know of any device, substance or method which will regenerate hair." There is still no practical way of treating common male baldness, although some amazing results have been achieved in treating a rather rare patchy type of baldness called *alopecia areata*.

Physicians have long noted the effect of hormones on hair growth. They observed, for example, that during pregnancy balding women often had a luxuriant growth of hair, only to lose it at the termination of pregnancy. In these cases hair growth was apparently the result of abundant female hormone secreted during pregnancy. Male hormone appeared to have an opposite effect. In recent years women have been given male hormone as a treatment for breast cancer. Many of them developed male hair patterns—facial and body hair increasing and head hair decreasing.

It appeared that nearly all the glands had some degree of influence on hair growth. A tumor of the adrenal had a powerful effect, increasing hair growth in some areas, decreasing it in others. A lagging thyroid often led to hair loss.

Then it was discovered that the corticosteroid hormones, such as cortisone, were powerful agents for hair growth, probably by counteracting *alopecia areata*. In one experiment 68 people suffering from the disease were treated with these hormones. Some of the patients had been bald for twenty-five years. About 60 percent grew complete heads of hair! And the other 40 percent had some regrowth. However, as soon as hormone doses were stopped, hair follicles became dormant again, and hair dropped out. In addition, hormones sometimes had undesirable side effects, ranging from psychosis to a swelling of the face called "moon face."

Injecting hormones directly into the scalp is currently under trial at the world's only hair clinic—at University Hospital, a division of New York University-Bellevue Medical Center. Dr. Norman Orentreich, in charge of the hair clinic, has found that growth of hair is profuse around the injection spot and there are few if any side effects. The difficulty is that several hundred such shots would be needed to grow a full head of hair, and the injections would have to be repeated every few months. This method is more practical when used in special circumstances:

to grow eyebrows, or hair in some cases of patchy baldness.

Superfluous Hair: Almost as much time and money are spent to get rid of hair where it is not wanted as are spent in attempts to grow it. Women apply waxes, chemicals that are often hazardous, and even resort to risky hair-destroying X rays. Actually there is only one way of removing hair permanently with reasonable safety—electrolysis. A tiny needle is inserted in the hair follicle and a spark of electricity brings destruction. But the process is tedious—about 100 hairs in a half-hour session—and expensive. Also, in inexpert hands it can be dangerous.

Hair Dyes: Most dyes are reasonably safe. The greatest danger is that the scalp may be sensitive to a particular dye—which can lead to severe irritation and even temporary loss of hair. A simple test can determine sensitivity: a bit of the dye is placed on the skin behind the ear. If within forty-eight hours no redness or soreness develops, the dye is probably safe.

Hair Care: Many people think too frequent washing "dries" the hair. Actually, it stimulates secretions from the oil glands opening into the follicles. In the main, good hair care consists of washing in soft water with a good shampoo at least once a week. If hair is too oily, a diluted alcohol preparation will remove excess grease; if it's too dry, a few drops of oil should be rubbed in. Scalp massage—brushing for ten minutes a day— is excellent.

Good hair care does not promise to eliminate the theater's bald-headed row. But it will improve the condition and the appearance of our hair while we have it.

THE BEST cosmetic in the world is an active mind that is always finding something new.   —Mary Meek Atkeson

If You Really Want Healthy Teeth

by J. D. Ratcliff

The dentist's chief aim today is to preserve your teeth through preventive care, and there are things you can do to help. The first task is to reduce the decay rate.

There is conflicting evidence as to the cause of tooth decay. It is attributed to poor diet, yet some of the earth's poorest people have only a fraction of the decay that strikes the best-fed. Decay is rampant in New Zealand and the United States, rare in Mexico and India.

Tooth decay has been attributed to soft diet. Yet Polynesians subsist on soft foods—fish and fruit, mainly—and aren't bothered with tooth troubles. Sugar is widely blamed, but West Indian natives chew sugar cane without courting decay. Oral hygiene? Samoans and Eskimos, who never saw a toothbrush or a bottle of mouthwash, have some of the world's best teeth.

Heredity? Heredity does appear to play a part. People of English stock are unduly susceptible to tooth decay. American dental ills possibly arrived on the *Mayflower*.

There are two major theories. The most widely accepted is that a mouth bacterium attacks carbohydrate foods (starches, sugars) to produce an acid which gradually eats away tooth enamel. A second theory is that bacteria slip through microscopic fissures and attack the dentine under the enamel.

Wherever we place blame for decay, the fact remains that 9 out of 10 American children have decay by the age of six. By the age of sixteen, the average American has 14 decay spots.

A great deal can be done about *preventing* decay. Latest evidence indicates that decay is highly active immediately after meals, then tapers off. This suggests two methods of control.

Excellent results have been obtained by reducing or eliminating sugary and starchy foods. With less for decay bacteria to eat, their numbers dwindle. A second approach is to brush the teeth, or rinse the mouth, immediately after each meal instead of night and morning. The American Dental Association recommends a medium-sized brush with a small head and flat brushing surface. Bristles should be firm, but not hard enough to injure gums. Always brush your teeth the way they grow—*from* the gums.

Although decay is the chief enemy of teeth in early life, most teeth lost after the age of thirty-five go because of gum disease.

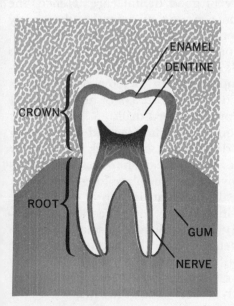

This condition, also known as periodontal disease, may be acute and painful (gingivitis) or chronic (pyorrhea).

In a few cases, the disease may be traced to a diet poor in vitamins. One study showed gingivitis seven times as common among smokers as among nonsmokers. Food particles lodged between teeth irritate gums and open the way for invasion of bacteria. Teeth that mesh improperly, high teeth that work excessively, or low teeth that do no work may result in breakdown of tissue.

The causes of periodontal disease suggest the cures. If teeth mesh poorly, high spots should be ground down—a painless procedure. If gums protrude so that they trap food, excess tissue may have to be trimmed. Extreme care should be taken to keep teeth as clean as possible. In cases of severe infection the dentist, of course, always has penicillin or other antibiotics to bring bacteria under control.

Wisdom teeth are another source of trouble. They usually appear between the ages of seventeen and twenty-one. They are seldom perfect. They impact—become imbedded in bone and fail to come through—jam other teeth and often decay rapidly. It is usually best to have them out if they cause trouble.

To forestall the host of difficulties resulting from crooked teeth, the modern orthodontist can accomplish wonders. Extensive straightening takes time—maybe two or more years—and often costs a lot of money. But most dentists are willing to adjust fees to fit your purse.

For years dentists have recognized fear of the dental chair as a major obstacle in the way of good dental care. Hence, the enormous effort expended on conquest of pain. Until recently most dentists depended on one pain-killing standby: novocain. But many people feared the needle as much as the drill. Today's progressive dentist has a wide assortment of methods of combating pain. High-speed drills operating up to 300,000 revolutions per minute and equipped with cooling sprays of air and water have replaced the painful, slow low-speed drills.

At such speeds, tiny diamond-faced burs, instead of requiring two pounds of pressure as old types did, can whisk away decay with a half ounce of pressure. Dentists can shape cavities so accurately that fillings and inlays remain in place longer.

Dentists have long known that a great portion of dental pain is psychic—imagined. More important, they have found a number of ways to combat it. My dentist plugged a small switch in his dental machine and handed it to me. "*You* are now in control of the drill," he said. "Push the button and the drill stops." Knowing I could turn pain off at any time, I let work proceed rapidly. Everyone, apparently, reacts about the same way.

Many dentists, realizing the value of distracting a patient while drilling, have wired music programs or automatic phonographs in their offices. Others have added television, and a few, whose main practice is with children, have movies.

For several years now, dentists have used acrylic resin plastics for dentures, crowns and bridgework. Older dentures of porcelain teeth imbedded in hard rubber were heavy, awkward and so porous as to absorb unpleasant odors. With artificial teeth made entirely of resin, or porcelain teeth inserted into a resin bed, the denture is light and almost completely nonabsorbent—a quick brushing banishes odor.

Plastics as tooth-filling materials have been developed. They "set" at mouth temperature. Tooth color can be matched almost exactly. From present evidence, they appear to be far more permanent than either porcelain or cement. They do, however, have drawbacks: Chewing gum may stick to them and they may stain. Further research is being done on these materials.

The American Dental Association suggests that perhaps the most important dental advice of all is urging parents to give children a good start. "Baby" teeth, which may be highly subject to decay, should not be neglected, or pulled unless absolutely necessary. They guide permanent teeth into proper place. Fluoridation of the public water supply has proved a great boon in the preservation of teeth throughout life. Countless communities have now adopted this measure.

If the child's teeth are not in perfect alignment they should be straightened. Sweets and starches should be limited, particularly between meals. The habit of brushing teeth *after each meal* should be established early in life.

Adults should follow much the same set of dental rules. The dentist should be visited twice a year. A recent Gallup Poll showed that over half of all people over twenty-one had not been in a dentist's office for two or more years!

None of the rules proposed is excessively hard to follow. If we would all observe them carefully we should have an excellent chance of keeping our teeth where they belong—in our mouths instead of in a bowl on the bathroom shelf.

∗

Fluorides:
YOUR FAMILY'S PROTECTION
AGAINST TOOTH DECAY

by Merle E. Dowd

∗

In more than two thousand American communities a fluoride which helps protect the growing teeth of children against decay is added to the public water supply. But in many communities, as in the Seattle area where I live, public fluoridation has been repeatedly voted down even though the nation's leading dental, medical and public-health groups affirm that it provides more protection at less cost than any other known dental-health measure.

Concerned about preserving my young sons' teeth, I have been heartened recently to find that children can be given protection even if public fluoridation is not available, or if the family is dependent—as are nearly 40 percent of the people in the United States—on private wells or water systems.

While fluoridation of public water supplies, which ensures the daily ingestion of fluorides by children wherever they are—at home or in school—provides the *best* protection, one's dentist or pediatrician can prescribe sodium fluoride drops to be added to milk or fruit juice every day. When mixed by a pharmacist, a year's supply can be obtained at relatively modest cost. Or the dentist or pediatrician may suggest one of several commercial products now available on a prescription basis.

Distribution is controlled by prescription because fluorides in large doses are poisonous. But with ordinary care—keeping them out of children's reach—there is little hazard. As an extra precaution, the druggist may be instructed to package the compound in quantities so small that no ill effects could result even if an entire prescription were swallowed at once.

These prescribed dietary fluorides work well *provided* they are begun when children are very young and continued faithfully over long periods. A U.S. Public Health Service doctor who has given his children fluorides since birth told me that in thirteen years his five children developed only one cavity among them.

In the Washington, D.C., area, tablets of sodium fluoride were given daily to children over a five- to eight-year period. At the end of the period their dental records, compared with those of children drinking fluoridated water from birth, revealed that individual prescription of fluorides cuts cavities just as well as fluoridated water. Health-agency officials point out, however, that a prescription program is *generally* less satisfactory, since carelessness may interrupt the intake. (In this study, for example, the parents of half the original group did not persevere in the program. This despite the fact that the group was chosen from a scientifically trained, highly educated segment of the population.)

In coöperation with the U.S. Public Health Service, devices that will fluoridate individual home water systems are being tested. As in public fluoridation plans, these devices can be adjusted so as to add enough fluoride to the naturally occurring fluoride in the water to raise the concentration to one part per million. (Fluoride is found in varying amounts in all drinking water. In only a few areas, however, does it occur in concentrations capable of protecting the teeth.) If the child gets all his drinking water at home, this concentration provides about one milligram of fluorine per person daily, the amount that has been proved to give maximum protection without undesirable side effects. Once installed, the fluoridators can be serviced and reloaded periodically, at a cost of about $2 to $3 a month. One drawback, however, is that children don't get all their water at home.

Another way to build decay resistance, especially during the years from six to twelve, when teeth are erupting, is to paint the teeth with a fluoride solution. This "topical application," done by a dentist generally at intervals of six months to a year, makes tooth enamel more resistant to the acids formed in the mouth by fermentation of food. Such applications have been found to reduce cavities by 30 to 75 percent—variations in technique and frequency of application accounting for the wide spread in effectiveness.

Applied to newly erupted teeth at six-month intervals, both sodium fluoride and stannous fluoride provide substantial protection. The cost: about $4 to $6 per treatment.

Even in areas where public water supplies have been fluoridated, topical applications can be helpful. In one study, in an area where drinking water had been fluoridated for six years, the cavity rate in children's teeth was reduced about 60 percent. Then teeth were painted with stannous fluoride. A follow-up after thirty months showed an additional 15 percent reduction in the cavity rate in the group, in comparison with that of the children drinking fluoridated water but not receiving topical applications.

Proper care of teeth still means regular brushing. Until recently, brushing teeth served mainly to remove food particles from between the teeth. For this, all kinds of dentifrices—or none at all—were equally effective. Now the American Dental Association has recognized one *stannous* fluoride toothpaste as an added benefit in prevention of decay.

Once teeth are fully developed, fluoridated water has only a meager effect. But the long-range benefits from drinking fluoridated water as children extend to at least age forty-four, as demonstrated in a study of persons living in Colorado Springs, where water contains natural fluorides, and persons living in Boulder, Colorado, where water contains no fluorides. Colorado Springs adults in the forty-to-forty-four age group averaged only about 3 teeth missing, compared with almost 15 teeth missing for a similar age group in Boulder.

Topical application of stannous fluoride to adults' teeth reduced cavities by 24 percent in one Indiana test. Topical application of fluoride to another group, at three-month intervals, reduced cavities 56 percent after fourteen months, compared with a group that did not receive the applications.

In a test of young adults brushing with a stannous fluoride toothpaste, cavities were reduced by 42 percent. But no toothpaste is a cure-all. Maximum protection results from using a combination of all the various methods of decay prevention.

Mind Your Own Two Feet

by Lin Root

Take your hat off to your feet. If you're a 165-pound male with an average job, your feet carry you some 7½ miles a day and take a sledge-hammer pounding of more than 1000 tons. If you're the little woman around the house, credit your feet with roughly 10 miles and 1500 tons of jolts.

No wonder your poor feet sometimes rebel. And when they

do, foot pains often cause the sufferer to alter his posture. If the new stance becomes habitual, other parts of the body may be thrown out of plumb, leading to backache, headache and other symptoms. Authorities agree that these miseries can largely be prevented or cured—by better knowledge of the foot and by following sensible rules for its health.

The foot is constructed of an astonishing number of parts, a fact which accounts for its resiliency. One fourth of all the body's bones are in the feet. Each foot contains 26, cunningly linked through 33 joints and lashed together with ligaments. The biggest bone, one of the 7 tarsals, is the heel. It sits solidly on the ground with 6 chunky dovetailed tarsals arching in front of it. These bones meet the 5 long metatarsals whose heads form the ball of the foot.

Heel bone and metatarsal heads are the weight bearers. The five toes serve as a launching pad. When you walk, the body weight strikes the ground through the heel and travels swiftly along the outside of the foot to the ball, across the metatarsal heads to the first metatarsal, where it is transferred to the big toe, which sets you in motion.

At birth, 99 percent of all feet are perfect. Yet, according to a ten-year study by the Podiatry Society of the State of New York, 8 percent have developed troubles at one year, 41 percent at age five, and 80 percent at twenty. We limp into adulthood on corns, calluses, bunions, ingrown toenails, hammer toes, plantar warts and dozens more groan-getters.

Many authorities believe that the main trouble with feet is shoes. (The incidence of foot defects among barefoot peoples is only 7 percent.) Because it takes ten years to grow the foot bones and twenty years before the heel is fully finished, preschool children need larger-size shoes every two months or oftener. Six- to ten-year-olds need larger shoes every two to three months; 10- to 12-year-olds every three to four months; 12- to 15-year-olds every four to five months; 15- to 20-year-olds every six months. Yet how often do growing feet get the larger size that they demand?

Feet, at rest and in motion, were studied for some thirty years by the late Dr. Dudley J. Morton, of the College of Physicians and Surgeons, Columbia University, and by Dr. R. Plato Schwartz, emeritus professor of orthopedics, University of Rochester School of Medicine.

Dr. Morton blamed most foot ailments on a too-short first metatarsal, found in 40 percent of a long series of X rays of foot patients. Normally the first bears twice as much weight as each of the others. When it is too short, the weight falls on its weaker neighbors, causing strain and pain. Dr. Morton devised a special leather insole as a corrective.

Dr. Schwartz looks to the foot-leg relationship. The weight-bearing axis of the heel is about five eighths of an inch to the outside of the weight-bearing axis of the leg bone. Thus the body weight, coming down the leg bone to the inside of the heel axis, makes the heel bone roll inward. This effect, called pronation, does not necessarily cause pain, but, if neglected in children, it can lead to trouble. As a specific aid to combat pronation, Dr. Schwartz and his colleague, Arthur L. Heath, have devised principles for the design of better shoes.

Though millions of people groan, "My feet are killing me!" only 2 percent of the footsore multitude seek professional care. The rest pay out some $350,000,000 a year for arch supports, lifts, plasters, pads and "corrective" shoes. ("There is no such thing as a ready-made corrective shoe, or an appliance that suits all feet," one authority says.) Otherwise sensible people consult shoe salesmen about nonexistent ailments: "flat feet" (the true flat foot functions well, gives no pain, as many athletes can testify); "dropped metatarsal arches" (there are no metatarsal arches to drop); "fallen arches" (the longitudinal arch can break but rarely falls).

Dr. John Martin Hiss, director of the Hiss Clinic in Los Angeles, says, after more than half a million examinations of feet, "There is no such thing as a fallen arch, and 'arch supports' are not corrective."

Public confusion reflects professional controversy and lack of intercommunication between interested groups—shoe dealers, podiatrists or chiropodists (the two terms are synonymous, both referring to the foot specialist who is not a physician or surgeon), and orthopedists (M.D.s). "The big job facing the medical profession and the shoe industry," says one observer, "is to erase all the current mythology about foot health and to replace it with research-based fact from which *real* help—preventive and curative—can come."

Meanwhile, there is general agreement on the proper treatment of some common complaints.

Corns and calluses are nature's angry defense against continued pressure. A thin doughnut-shaped pad for the hard corn, a bit of lamb's wool changed daily for the soft corn between the toes, afford some relief. If pain persists, consult your physician or a qualified podiatrist. Never be a bathroom surgeon; infection often follows. Never apply corn salves, drops or medicated pads: the caustic acid which burns away the horny top may consume the surrounding flesh. Always cut toenails straight across since curved cutting encourages ingrown toenails, which need professional care.

A bunion is a chronic inflammation of the protective fluid sac over the joint, caused by rubbing against the shoe. Bunions are aggravated by short, pointed shoes, and by high heels, which allow the feet to slide forward. Soft all-leather shoes help, and specially designed shoes provide "bunion pockets." Surgery is a last resort.

It's good practice to bathe your feet at least once daily (using a soft brush to remove dead skin), dry thoroughly and dust on foot powder. Never wear the same shoes, socks or stockings two days in a row. Always change promptly if your feet get wet from rain or perspiration. Such hygiene, incidentally, will often clear up minor attacks of athlete's foot, a fungus infection which usually begins between the toes.

Properly fitted shoes are essential. Here are a few points to keep in mind: Shoes should allow about half an inch of space beyond the longest toe, and the widest part of the shoe should correspond to the widest part of the foot. Buy your shoes late in the day; your feet will be bigger then. Don't regard your feet as shoe-stretchers; properly fitted shoes never need "breaking in." Keep the heels of your shoes, which in normal gait wear out along their outer edge, in repair.

To the ladies: Let your best shoes be your work shoes, which you wear long hours. Economize if you must on dress shoes whose main function is eye catching. Even here, avoid the extremely high heel—anything over two inches—which wrecks the shock-absorbing function of the foot's arch.

There is evidence that women are getting wiser and buying roomier, more comfortable shoes. And as custodians of the foot health of the younger generation, women are urged by the experts to apply the same wisdom to their children's feet.

To BEAT TENSION and fatigue, some doctors are currently prescribing the easiest treatment a patient was ever asked to take: "Take off your shoes whenever and wherever you have the chance."

The medical head of a large sanitarium says, "I'm forever telling people to take off their shoes. A woman, manager of a big store, complained of tenseness in her legs, said she couldn't sleep. I told her to take off her shoes every opportunity she got. Now she sleeps fine. Thing to remember is, there never was a shoe to fit the step unless it had moving parts."

An orthopedist says, "There's a very true saying that when your feet hurt, you hurt all over. It's no joke to say that shoes are at the base of a lot of trouble."

So if you feel the urge to take off your shoes, obey it. It's nature politely making a request, and nature's often got more common sense than you have.   —Howard Van Smith

IF YOU WISH to add to your charm, bear in mind that you appear more youthful standing than sitting down. When seated—especially in modern, low-slung chairs, not only are you tempted by love of comfort to assume an incorrect posture, but you are in a passive state and less alert mentally. More than this, you are in a position of physiological disadvantage. When standing up, you are likely to be positive, alert, ready to act. The clever woman will let her younger rival sit down while she remains standing.
                                                            —Gelett Burgess

Are Americans Physically Fit?

by Max Eastman

The Soft American. The Flabby American. Are We Becoming a Nation of Weaklings? Are We Raising a Generation of Marshmallows? Such headlines are becoming more and more common. The problem needs a thorough going-over.

Ever since the invention of the wheel, men have been contriving to substitute machines for their own labor. They have succeeded so well in highly industrialized countries that strenuous physical exertion has become largely unnecessary. The effect of this upon the muscles and general health of the body is reaching the point of disaster.

In the United States this process has gone farther than anywhere else in the world. We don't walk any more, we ride; we don't climb stairs, we take the elevator; we don't sweep the floor, we use a vacuum cleaner; we don't shovel coal into the furnace, we shift a thermostat; and so on. The word "chores" has almost gone out of use. We forget that daily physical chores were an essential part of a healthy life.

The resulting inferiority of our muscular development was first demonstrated statistically in 1956, when physical-fitness tests devised by Drs. Hans Kraus and Sonja Weber were applied to American and European children. Of the American children, 58 percent failed one or more of the tests, while less than 9 percent of the European children failed.

Call for Vigorous Action

Now President Kennedy is demanding that physical fitness be given urgent attention. He has called for vigorous action to arrest "the physical degeneration of American youth." "The relation between soundness of the body and the activities of the mind," he has said, "is subtle and complex. Intelligence and skill can function at their peak only when the body is healthy and strong."

How healthy and strong are we? There has been shocking confirmation of the Kraus-Weber findings. Physical educators devised a more elaborate series of tests: pull-up; sit-up; shuttle run (running back and forth); 50-yard dash; 600-yard run-walk; standing broad jump; softball throw. These tests were given to 8500 American and 10,000 British young people. We beat the British youth only in ball throwing; with that exception, their all-around fitness was 24 percent better than ours. British boys were far superior to American boys; British girls were far superior to American girls; and in some instances British girls were superior to American boys!

The Unlimber American

The urgency of this problem is pointed up in a recent book by Drs. Hans Kraus and Wilhelm Raab entitled *Hypokinetic Disease*. The doctors show that other debilitating conditions besides "softness" or "flabbiness" result from the lack of sufficient muscular action. Rigidity, or "tightness," and actual shortening of the muscles also result. These cause some of the most painful and crippling of human ailments.

If you watch a cat when she is alarmed, you will see her tense practically all her muscles. Then she will either spring upon the thing that alarms her, or scoot away. When we are worried or alarmed, we also tense our muscles for the flight-or-fight reaction. But in our civilized life the reaction does not occur. The tension persists, and it is that sustained tension that tightens and shortens the muscles. Only by exercise can we limber up and lengthen them. In short, it is not only the "soft" or "flabby" American that presents a national problem, but the *unlimber* American.

A survey was conducted by physicians in a clinic visited by thousands of people suffering from "lower-back pain"—one of the commonest of human ills. It was found that 80 percent of them had no disease or injury whatever, just weakness and/or stiffness of the muscles due to a lack of activity. These patients found relief in exercise.

Muscles Need Movement

The same condition with the same cause may arise in other parts of the body. Wherever there is a muscle, there is need of movement. The heart beats all the time but, in our modern sedentary life, hearts are not beating vigorously often enough. It seems significant that in West Germany, where the economic recovery has permitted an exceptionally rapid "Americanization" of living habits, the number of cardiovascular deaths mounted within two years (1950 to 1952) from 80,000 to 183,000.

It is an easy guess that the young people of the Soviet Union, which is still far behind mechanically, are ahead of even the West Europeans in muscular fitness. If we were to have an Olympic contest of average people, not only would we be beaten out by England and the West European nations but the Soviet Union would win out against the whole Western world. In Russia, people still "do the chores."

There is another reason for this alarming difference, however—a reason very much less to our credit. In some countries the danger in this by-product of industrialization is fully recognized, and measures are being taken to guard against it.

In Germany, for example, such measures have been taken not only by governmental and philanthropic enterprises but by insurance companies—telling evidence that exercise is essential to health and life. A reconditioning center for 200 sedentary persons was founded in Upper Bavaria in 1953 by Dr. Peter Beckmann. A year later the regional insurance organization took over financial responsibility for this venture. Today fifteen such institutions are operated in West Germany by insurance or industrial organizations. Approximately 15,000 employes are taking courses in these centers, lasting four to six weeks—systematic calisthenics and breathing exercises, running, swimming, hiking and climbing. A person goes upon the recommendation of his insurance physician and at the expense of his insurance group. Similar institutions are being developed in Austria, Switzerland and other European countries.

Less Than One Percent

We, on the contrary, have delayed almost fatally long in taking action against industrialization's menace to the body. Look at a frightening fact: a U.S. Government study reveals that our high-school students average less than an hour a *month* in physical education classes! Grade-school students fare no better. Lack of facilities and understanding have weakened many gym classes to "folk dancing" and "social games."

According to Charles B. Wilkinson, special consultant to the President on youth fitness, less than one percent of the average American youth's time is spent on physical education, and only a fraction of that time is spent in vigorous activities that produce fitness.

One thing we must do—now, before it's too late—is to make physical education a part of the regular curriculum of our schools, on the same terms as mental education. We must provide adequate space and equipment for both. A similar testing and grading of pupils according to their gifts and their progress should become standard procedure.

First Steps

In a special report to the nation President Kennedy outlined the first steps:

- Identify the physically underdeveloped pupil and work with him to improve his physical capacity.
- Provide a *minimum* of fifteen minutes of vigorous activity every day for all students, boys and girls alike.
- Use valid fitness tests to determine pupil physical ability and to evaluate progress.

The adoption of these three measures, the President said, "will ensure the beginning of a sound basic program of physical development."

That is true, but it is only the beginning. Some states already require their schools to allow fifteen minutes a day for "physical activity." But those fifteen minutes are largely spent talking, standing around, playing some game or making preparations to play it. They differ little from turning the children out for "recess" as a relaxation from their studies. What our bodies need in this "push-button civilization" is not relaxation but *vigorous muscular effort*, like running and calisthenics. Where schools don't have adequate gym facilities, children can take a short but hard workout in the school yard; in bad weather, the classroom itself can be adequate for modified calisthenics.

Let's start a crusade in pursuit of muscular health and attendant well-being, a crusade toward more enjoyment of living, and also toward our adequate leadership in the defense of the free world. For the indubitable muscle gap between us and those who would bury us may well in the long run prove more disastrous than any alleged missile gap ever will be.

....

To measure your child's physical fitness,
see tests on following pages.

....

How Do Your Children Measure Up ?

Reprinted from "Youth Physical Fitness"
by the President's Council on Youth Fitness

·· SIT-UPS ··

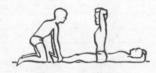

NUMBER OF SIT-UPS—BOYS								
Age:	10	11	12	13	14	15	16	17
Excellent	60	67	78	73	99	99	99	99
Good	47	50	51	54	60	60	73	63
Satisfactory	30	31	37	40	44	45	50	50
Poor	22	23	28	30	33	35	40	38

NUMBER OF SIT-UPS—GIRLS								
Age:	10	11	12	13	14	15	16	17
Excellent	50	50	50	50	49	37	40	42
Good	33	34	30	30	28	26	27	25
Satisfactory	22	25	22	21	20	20	21	20
Poor	15	18	17	17	15	15	16	15

START: Pupil lies on back, hands behind neck, while another pupil holds his ankles. ACTION: Sit up, turn trunk to left, touch right elbow to left knee, return to starting position. Sit up again, turn trunk to right, touch left elbow to right knee, return to starting point. Repeat, not to exceed number of times shown as "excellent" for pupil's age and skill.

··············· STANDING BROAD JUMP ·················

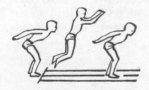

SPAN OF JUMP—BOYS								
Age:	10	11	12	13	14	15	16	17
Excellent	5'-6"	5'-10"	6'-2"	6'-8"	7'-2"	7'-8"	8'-0"	8'-4"
Good	5'-0"	5'-4"	5'-8"	6'-0"	6'-7"	7'-0"	7'-3"	7'-8"
Satisfactory	4'-8"	5'-0"	5'-4"	5'-8"	6'-1"	6'-5"	6'-11"	7'-2"
Poor	4'-4"	4'-7"	4'-11"	5'-2"	5'-7"	5'-11"	6'-4"	6'-8"

SPAN OF JUMP—GIRLS								
Age:	10	11	12	13	14	15	16	17
Excellent	5'-4"	5'-7"	5'-8"	5'-9"	6'-0"	6'-2"	6'-5"	6'-6"
Good	4'-10"	5'-0"	5'-2"	5'-4"	5'-6"	5'-6"	5'-8"	5'-10"
Satisfactory	4'-5"	4'-8"	4'-9"	4'-11"	5'-0"	5'-0"	5'-2"	5'-3"
Poor	4'-1"	4'-3"	4'-5"	4'-6"	4'-7"	4'-8"	4'-10"	4'-10"

START: Pupil stands with feet comfortably apart, toes just behind take-off line. Before jumping, flex knees and swing arms back and forth in rhythmical motion. ACTION: Jump, swinging arms forcefully forward and upward, taking off from balls of the feet. Allow three trials, record the best mark.

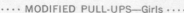

·········· PULL-UPS—Boys ··········   ···· MODIFIED PULL-UPS—Girls ·····

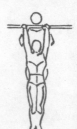

START: Grasp a bar, of sufficient height, with palms facing forward. Hang with arms and legs extended, feet free of floor.

ACTION: Pull body up with arms until chin is placed over the bar; lower body until elbows are fully extended. Repeat as many times as possible. Knees must not be raised; kicking or swinging the body not permitted.

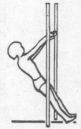

START: Adjust height of bar to chest level. Grasp bar with palms facing out. Extend legs under bar, keeping body and knees straight, heels on floor, arms extended to form 90-degree angle with body line.

ACTION: Pull body up until chest touches bar, lower body until elbows are fully extended. Repeat, attempting to reach "excellent" score for age, but not exceeding that number.

NUMBER OF PULL-UPS

Age:	10	11	12	13	14	15	16	17
Excellent	6	6	7	8	10	10	12	13
Good	3	4	4	5	6	7	9	10
Satisfactory	2	2	2	3	4	5	6	7
Poor	1	1	1	2	2	2	3	4

NUMBER OF MODIFIED PULL-UPS

Age:	10	11	12	13	14	15	16	17
Excellent	45	45	45	45	45	45	45	45
Good	40	40	40	40	40	40	40	40
Satisfactory	30	30	29	30	29	22	25	25
Poor	17	20	20	20	19	12	14	15

⌔

Today my heart beat 103,389 times, my blood traveled 168,000,000 miles, I breathed 23,040 times, I inhaled 438 cubic feet of air, I spoke 4800 words, moved 750 major muscles, and I exercised 7,000,000 brain cells. I'm tired.   —Bob Hope

⌔

A teacher who regularly makes a practice of hunting up the most unattractive child and whispering in her ear, "You're getting prettier every day," says it always works; almost at once the child begins to blossom into something close to beauty.   —Marcelene Cox

Don't Just Sit There— Exercise !

by Curtis Mitchell

I n response to President Kennedy's charge that young Americans were getting soft, and that lack of physical fitness is a national problem, citizens by the thousands began to study their unpatriotic paunches with a view to reducing either sag or surplus. Unfortunately, the President did not tell them how to do it.

Medical men are of varied opinion about exercise. Dr. Theodore Klumpp, New York City specialist in aging, says, "The activity should be something a person likes, such as golf, swimming, hiking, gardening or tennis." Dr. Howard Sprague, Boston heart specialist, specifies regular exercise and "lots of it." Dr. Howard Ross, of the Michigan State Medical Society, says, "Every muscle and joint that has the power to wiggle must be made to wiggle more." Whatever form the prescription takes, it emphasizes *body movement and regularity*.

As for the right sports, doctors are reluctant to be specific because so much depends on individual physical makeup. But the medical consensus affords some guide to the average man or woman.

From 20 to 30 years. Tennis, squash, golf, swimming, skiing and badminton are ideal. Any of them played hard will dissipate surplus energy and damp down tensions. Estimates made at the Harvard Fatigue Laboratory say that tennis uses energy at a rate of 4000 calories per hour when you are jockeying for a smash at the net, and 9000 per hour when sprinting to make a "save." Slow skiing, moderate swimming and brisk walking up a slight grade use 500 to 600 per hour.

31 to 40. Add handball, horseback riding or ice skating to your skills. These are excellent "two-sided" sports—exercising both sides of the body, as opposed to tennis. During these years, added pressures are inescapable for most men. Golf, though it does have opponents, is widely recommended because it has two prime benefits: First, it performs that most useful of functions—sending the blood circulating throughout the entire system. Second, it is helpful in taking the mind off tensions built up in the workaday world.

41 to 50. Authorities advise keeping up whatever sports you enjoyed in early life: swimming, skiing, tennis, golf. They stress the danger during these years of becoming a weekend athlete. Midweek play should be maintained if you expect to be active on Saturdays.

Tapering off usually is recommended in this decade; play fewer sets of tennis, more doubles, and play with partners your own age. You might install a rowing or pedaling machine in the garage for midweek use. It helps if one night each week is devoted to bowling or to swimming at the "Y."

More than ever, physicians who have studied the subject recommend a brief exercise period every day. Dr. Paul Dudley White prescribes stair climbing as a tranquilizer and rarely misses a chance to use his legs. Arriving at the National Press Club in Washington D.C., to make a speech a few years ago, he was greeted in the lobby by a press delegation assigned to escort him to the auditorium. "Where is it?" he asked. "Thirteenth floor," they replied, ringing for the elevator. "Let's walk," he said, and led his panting hosts up twelve flights of stairs without drawing a deep breath.

51 to 65. Dangerous years, these. Fatty food plus inactivity has sealed off thousands of miles of blood-distributing capillaries in the average person. Doctors urge the average man to avoid strenuous or prolonged sport. Nor should he try to clear his driveway of snow.

By all means, they say, keep swimming, keep walking. Do it daily. Dr. White recommends bicycle riding. Supreme Court Justice William O. Douglas spends twenty minutes daily with weights and dumbbells. Sundays, he walks 10 to 20 miles, rain or shine. He is over 60. George Romney, president of American Motors, insists on daily golf. At Bloomfield Hills, near his home, he tees up two balls each sunrise, winter and summer, and drives them over hill and dale. Between holes, he lopes.

William H. Danforth, a St. Louis manufacturer, was once the sickliest boy in his class. Calisthenics, he claimed, built up the strength that enabled him to establish industrial plants in twenty-five cities.

"Bend over until the tips of your fingers touch the floor. Do it 50 times," he commanded. "Do the liver squeezer, twisting around back and forth, 50 times. Do you like it? I don't. I hate exercise. But exercise is good for me, and I'm going to do it religiously every morning and night."

When he died at the ripe age of 85, he had outlived every classmate. The hundred-million-dollar Danforth Foundation of St. Louis, dedicated to human betterment, is his monument.

Over 65. For fun, try croquet. Composer Richard Rodgers, just out of his 50s, recommends it for any age and practices what he preaches at his Connecticut estate. Gardening lifts the spirit and supples the body. Add to it one hour of walking per day, and any grandfather will be conditioned to knock the tar out of his grandchildren.

Is any single exercise best for all the decades of life? Most authorities will say it is swimming. The virtue of swimming is that it exercises all the muscles, but the weight of the body is buoyed up by the water. Walking is a close second, and as free as air. But walk as if you were going somewhere, authorities say;

ambling along a country lane may please your soul but it strengthens your sinews not one whit.

If the experts are agreed on anything, it is that the human body can be salvaged as long as disease is not present. Any noon at the West 63rd Street YMCA in New York you will see a band of businessmen—average age 50 years—dogtrotting around an indoor track. After running a mile or so, they will zip through a calisthenic drill followed by a twenty-lap stint in the pool. They are typical of groups in three hundred other Ys, where thousands of businessmen are learning that a life of vigor can be beneficial.

Experts say any exercise that makes a person move enough to push his blood into every nook and cranny is good. They say you can take strenuous exercise without fear *if you work up to it*. Dr. Thomas Cureton, of the University of Illinois, who worked out the regimen used at the Ys, states, "If hard exertion of this type could precipitate a coronary attack, we would have had a good many, but we have never had one. In testing over 50,000 men of all ages since 1941 we know of not a single case."

The drive for physical fitness should do much for our nation. Fortitude, courage and daring are by-products and a national resource to be guarded as carefully as a stockpile of plutonium. But perhaps the greatest benefit will accrue to the men and women who rediscover the pleasure of a conditioned, alert body.

～

SATCHEL PAIGE, the St. Louis Browns' pitcher of indeterminate age, once gave his six rules for staying young:

1. Avoid fried meats which angry up the blood.
2. If your stomach disputes you, lie down and pacify it with cool thoughts.
3. Keep the juices flowing by jangling around gently as you move.
4. Go very light on the vices, such as carrying on in society. The social ramble ain't restful.
5. Avoid running at all times.
6. Don't look back. Something might be gaining on you.

—Collier's

Even Six Seconds Will Help

by Keith Monroe

Without workouts at a gym or a "daily dozen" every morning, we can still get all the exercise we need and keep ourselves in top trim by using odd moments during the day—those few seconds spent waiting for a traffic light, telephoning, standing in line.

"What *kind* of exercise is more important than *how much*," says Dr. Arthur H. Steinhaus, dean and professor of physiology at George Williams College. "In a German laboratory where I worked, it was discovered that a very small amount of the right exercise will start a muscle growing. If you contract any one of your muscles to about two thirds of its maximum power and hold that for six seconds once a day, the muscle will grow just as fast as it can grow.

"Every day there are bound to be intervals when you have six seconds to relax. They can make a tremendous difference. Pull in your stomach. Pull up your chin. Wriggle. Yawn. Stretch. Do these exercises on company time. Do them while going from one place to another. Weave them into the day's routine."

Gene Tunney says what so many experts say: "Take regular exercise—not violent weekends of too much golf, or sporadic bursts of squash, but a daily drill that becomes as much a part of your life as brushing your teeth."

Many show-business stars make idle seconds count to help their health and appearance. Hugh O'Brian, the TV Western hero, has an unobtrusive habit of pressing the clenched fist of one hand forcibly into the open palm of the other, at waist level, whenever he stands talking with someone. It keeps his forearms and biceps powerful. Jane Powell, Frankie Laine and other singers have an exercise for the moments when, sitting in their cars, they wait for traffic lights to change. Borrowing an idea from Indian yoga, they slowly pull in the stomach, sucking the diaphragm up and up until the whole abdomen is flat from groin to chest—then little by little release it. When you first try this, it can make you lightheaded if you tighten too hard, Miss Powell warns. "Begin gently. But keep at it. It's the simplest trick I know for building good posture and a flat tummy."

For muscle tone, Dr. Steinhaus advocates a few seconds of planned exercise while toweling yourself after a bath. "Loop the towel behind your neck," he suggests. "Then pull your chin in, pull forward on both ends of the towel and resist the towel with your neck, as hard as you can, for just six seconds. Do it only once. No more is necessary with this sort of workout if you keep it up daily. Now slide the towel down to the small of your back. While pulling forward on the towel, resist by contracting the muscles in your buttocks and your belly. Push back hard against the towel and count six. Now that's done. Loop the towel under your toes and pull up with both hands while your toes push down. Hold it for six seconds, then let go. Once on each foot and you're done for the day."

U.S. Navy submariners, cramped into small space, have learned to keep fit without moving more than a few inches. Lying flat on their bunks, they put hands under head, lift the head while resisting with the neck, and keep lifting until chin touches chest. Then they let the head down slowly. Or, in rising to a sitting position, they arrest the motion partway up, hold it a few seconds and sink back again. These brief drills are good for anyone.

You may want to try a few moments of similar exercise yourself. At night in bed, stretch all over slowly and luxuriously, like a cat. Then start at your toes and work up to eyelids and scalp, tensing each muscle for a moment, then relaxing it. You'll probably be almost asleep when you finish.

In the morning, a simple breathing exercise can help rouse you and clear out cobwebs. As you lie half awake take the deepest breath you can; fill your lungs with air. Then close your mouth, pinch your nose and lie still. Time it, and you'll be amazed to find that you can hold your breath without discomfort for twice as long as usual. And when you finally let your breath out you'll be wide awake.

Now you can limber up before getting out of bed. Lie on your back, stretch your arms overhead till you feel the pull all the way down to your waist. Hold them there a moment; then drop them limply. Next kick the covers off and raise your legs. Then lower them—but don't let your heels quite touch the bed. Repeat this several times. At first you'll feel a strain on your stomach muscles, but after a few days your midsection will begin to firm up.

While dressing, stand on one foot as you put on your shoe and tie the shoelaces. You may have to start by putting your foot in the shoe on the floor, and leaning against a wall while tying the laces. However you do it, daily repetitions will tighten your stomach and give you stronger, suppler legs and feet.

When you think about it, you'll be surprised to notice how many brief periods of idleness there are in your day: riding to work, waiting at a counter for a clerk's attention, sitting at your desk or standing by your workbench between chores. Put some life into those intervals! Use them for a "seventh-inning stretch."

If you want to firm a flabby chin, you can. Push your chin out, pull it back, drop it, lift it. Then give yourself a five-second massage under the jaw. To tone the muscles around your midriff, draw your abdomen up and in whenever you think of it, whether sitting or standing. At the phone, instead of doodling, use your free hand to knead your belly or give it a gentle pummeling. Dave Garroway holds an umbrella or golf club out in front of him with the heavy end away, flipping it up and down. You'd be surprised how this, or similar action, tightens the torso muscles.

Perhaps you bulge and wobble at the seat. Ever notice that truck drivers nearly always have firm hindquarters? So do cowboys. That's because they constantly bounce up and down. Try it yourself. Pick out a hard chair in home or office. Bounce on it a few times whenever you're alone. Vary the routine by extending your legs and shifting your weight from side to side.

For spine straightening, stand with your back to a wall and try to push firmly up against it so you're touching from head to heels—buttocks, shoulder blades, if possible every vertebra. You'll feel a strong pull along your backbone and neck. This stretching is recommended by physical culturists to improve posture, get rid of aches in back or neck and make you feel alive all over.

The "heel stretch" is a favorite of health experts for use while sitting at a desk or table. You needn't get out of your chair to do it. Just lift your feet and push the heels forward as if trying to push a wall away. Bring your toes up—so you feel the muscles in back of your knee pulling like a rope—count six, and slowly relax. This also relieves general tension.

Dr. Jay A. Bender, director of the physical-fitness program of Peoria, Illinois, says, "All you need do is *use your muscles correctly* as you go through a routine day at home or office." If you pick up something from the floor, for example, don't spraddle your legs and bend. Put one foot forward and kneel erectly. Or, when it's a light object, keep your knees stiff and reach straight down. For variety, squat and rise like a jack-in-the-box; it tightens flabby legs.

When you must wait in line, teeter on your toes a few times to uncramp foot and leg muscles. Put your hands in your pockets and clench and unclench the fingers to get the blood speeded up. Take a whopper of a breath and see how far you can expand your belt. Deep-breathing exercises should be employed every day. When you go up stairs, climb slowly with head and chest high and stomach muscles tight. If you can, walk up two steps at a time, or even three.

Basically, there are nine essential exercises which authorities advise you to take every day, in doses of a few seconds at a time:

1. *Stretch*—while sitting, lying or standing.

2. *Straighten your spine*—while standing with your back against something straight.

3. *Roll your neck*—up, down and around.

4. *Suck in your stomach*—while sitting or bending over.

5. *Expand your chest.*

6. *Flex your arms*—by pushing, pulling and reaching.

7. *Bend your legs*—by squatting, climbing and walking.

8. *Limber your toes and feet.*

9. *Firm your muscles*—by bouncing, pinching, kneading, pummeling.

A little of each of these every day, and you'll be slimmer, stronger and peppier. Try them and see!

WHEN WE ENCOUNTER the rare individual whose conduct is inspired by a moral ideal, we cannot help noticing his aspect. Moral beauty is an exceptional and striking phenomenon—one never forgets it. This form of beauty is far more impressive than the beauty of nature. It gives to those who possess its divine gifts a strange and inexplicable power. It increases the strength of the intellect. Much more than science, art and religious rites, moral beauty is the basis of civilization.   —Alexis Carrel

· · · · *Index* · · · ·

Picture Credits

Page 11, engraving: The Bettmann Archive. Page 83, Pain chart: adapted from data gathered by John Lear. Page 157, engravings: Culver Pictures. Page 189, photo: Dr. Harold E. Edgerton, from *Flash!*, Charles T. Branford Co., publisher. Page 289, Changes in Form and Proportion chart: adapted from *Today's Health,* published by the American Medical Association.

RD